Qìgōng Grand Circulation

Don't be afraid!

不用害怕!

Dare to challenge.....

敢於挑戰...

Dare to accept.....

敢於接受...

Dare to dream.....

敢於夢想...

Qìgōng
Grand Circulation

大周天氣功與神通

FOR SPIRITUAL ENLIGHTENMENT

Dr. Yáng, Jwìng-Mǐng

YMAA Publication Center
Wolfeboro, NH USA

SUSTAINABLE FORESTRY INITIATIVE Certified Sourcing
www.sfiprogram.org
SFI-00756

YMAA Publication Center, Inc.
PO Box 480
Wolfeboro, NH 03894
800 669-8892 • www.ymaa.com • info@ymaa.com

ISBN: 9781594398452 (print) • ISBN: 9781594398469 (ebook)

This book set in EB Garamond and Avenir.

Copyright © 2022 by Yáng, Jwìng-Mǐng
Content editing by David Silver
Copyedit by Leslie Takao and Doran Hunter
Cover design by Axie Breen
Photos by YMAA Publication Center unless otherwise noted.
Illustration enhancements by Quentin Lopes and Axie Breen

20210301

Publisher's Cataloging in Publication

Names: Yang, Jwing-Ming, 1946- author.

Title: Qìgōng grand circulation for spiritual enlightenment / by Dr. Yang, Jwing-Ming.

Description: Wolfeboro, NH USA : YMAA Publication Center, [2021] | Text in English, with some Chinese characters included. | Includes bibliographical references, translation and glossary of Chinese terms, and index.

Identifiers: ISBN: 9781594398452 (print) | 9781594398469 (ebook) | LCCN: 2021945494

Subjects: LCSH: Qi gong--Therapeutic use. | Qi (Chinese philosophy) | Mind and body. | Well-being. | Meditation. | Taoist philosophy. | Buddhist philosophy. | Breathing exercises--Therapeutic use. | Pulmonary circulation--Alternative treatment. | Cardiovascular system--Alternative treatment. | Spiritual care (Medical care) | Spirituality. | Medicine, Chinese. | Holistic medicine. | BISAC: BODY, MIND & SPIRIT / Healing / Energy (Qigong, Reiki, Polarity) | BODY, MIND & SPIRIT / Spiritualism. | PHILOSOPHY / Mind & Body. | PHILOSOPHY / Taoist. | PHILOSOPHY / Buddhist. | SPORTS & RECREATION / Martial Arts / General.

Classification: LCC: RA781.8 .Y3636 2021 | DDC: 613.7/1489--dc23

Printed in USA.

Dedication

To those who are searching for spiritual freedom and enlightenment.

観音菩薩六字大明心咒

Guānyīn Púsà Liùzì Dàmíng Xīnzhòu

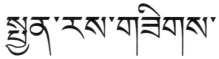

Guānyīn Bodhisattva Six-Character Great Bright Heart Mantra

嗡姆麻扲帕的美哈姆（吽）

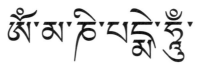

oṃ maṇi padme hūṃ
Connect self-being to lotus flower, I pray
(I pray that my inner self-being may be as pure as a lotus flower.)

My Mottos

心靜如水 (Xīnjìng Rúshuǐ)
My heart (emotional mind) is as calm as water.
(心平氣和) (Xīnpíng Qìhé)—The heart is peaceful and the Qì is harmonious.

性純如蓮 (Xìngchún Rúlián)
My temperament is as pure as a lotus flower.
(一塵不染) (Yìchén Bùrǎn)—There is not even a single speck of dust of contamination.

神定如松 (Shéndìng Rúsōng)
My spirit (Shén) is as steady as a pine tree.
(守中抱一) (Shǒuzhōng Bàoyī)—Keep centered and embrace singularity.

意明如鏡 (Yìmíng Rújìng)
My Yì (wisdom mind) is as clear as a mirror.
(毫不疑惑) (Háobù Yíhuò)—There is not even the slightest doubt.

氣和如旭 (Qìhé Rúxù)
My Qì is harmonious like the rising sun.
(氣調和順) (Qìtiáo Héshùn)—Qì is regulated harmoniously.

息深如淵 (Xíshēn Rúyuān)
My breathing is as deep as an abyss.
(息如抽絲) (Xīrú Chōusī)—The breathing is slender as if drawing silk.

志高如泰 (Zhìgāo Rútài)
My will is as high as the Tài Mountain.
(鵬程萬里) (Péngchéng Wànlǐ)—The roc flies myriad miles.

情誼如流 (Qìngyí Rúliù)
My relations with others flow like the current.
(順其自然) (Shùnqí Zìrán)—Follow the Nature.

楊俊敏博士 (Dr. Yáng, Jwìng-Mǐng)
YMAA CA Retreat Center

Contents

Editor's Note

David Silver

The term enlightenment is often used in casual conversation, or as an adjective to describe an eye-opening experience. Traditionally, however, enlightenment specifically refers to a rare and difficult transformative mental and physiological process resulting in nothing short of omniscience and escape from the cycle of rebirth.

Practitioners for thousands of years have recognized that the powerful energy aroused by our desire is an indispensable resource for enlightenment. Because human life is inseparably linked with desire, we must transform and repurpose this tremendous energy.

Recent decades of gradual opening of Buddhist culture to the world has resulted in more details of the practices becoming available to the public. "Subtle body" energy work had been known long before the word Qìgōng was used and is a common component—though this is usually kept quiet—of major religions, including the Daoist, Buddhist, and Hindu philosophies. In the Buddhist sutras, or sacred texts, the winds (Qì/energy), channels (meridians/pathways), and drops (essence/chemistry) are referred to and can sometimes be mistranslated metaphorically by those unfamiliar with Qìgōng Grand Circulation.

Along the journey of inner cultivation, whether in yoga, meditation, or Qìgōng, over time one may experience deeper levels of meditative absorption that can fundamentally transform the mind and body. This may sometimes result in supernatural abilities or spiritual powers, alternately considered a gift and an obstacle along the path. These Siddhis (translated from Sanskrit as "fulfillment" or "accomplishments") are a natural manifestation of our innate mind-body potential, resulting in clairvoyance, psychic powers, mind over matter, and ultimately reopening the Third Eye. Dr. Yáng has spent his lifetime developing and revealing a modern scientific understanding of this complex mental and physiological process that we undertake in tantric practice.

The topic of partner Qìgōng dual cultivation, or partner meditation, is sometimes popularized as tantric sex and has been visualized most prominently as the "Yab-yum" image. Vajrayāna Buddhists and the Nyingma School of Tibet specialize in this esoteric or "secret" technique. This sometimes confuses people, as the general understanding is to subdue desire and attachment to end our lifetime of suffering, as expressed in the Buddha's first teaching of the Four Noble Truths.

Logically, this desire-based practice is trained only after years of fundamental discipline. It is considered very difficult and kept only for the most skillful practitioners and is therefore often practiced only as a visualization by most students. This intimate technique utilizes the heightened energy and chemistry of arousal while teaching you to conserve the accumulated Qì and has been described as the "highest yoga":

When the completion stage practices have been mastered and we have gained control over our subtle energy winds and so forth, there will come a time when the dakas and dakinis will come . . . physically embracing such a consort is necessary to bring all the pervading energy winds into the central channel, a prerequisite for opening the heart center and experiencing the profoundest level of clear light." —*Thubten Yeshe (1935–1984)*

If one is capable of calmly abiding within this pinnacle of energy, while unifying the mind and body into a single point of awareness free of all concepts, remaining present in an infinite moment, this practice can powerfully transform the body and spirit. Whether solo or with a partner, the practice of Qìgōng Grand Circulation will benefit all aspects of your life.

David Silver
Cape Cod, MA 2021

Foreword

Thomas G. Gutheil, MD

"...to marry the past and present, and give birth to the future." p. 19

"Qìgōng practitioners in scholar and medical Qìgōng societies are aiming for a calm, peaceful, and harmonious mind..." p. 69

In the late 70s, I was watching the first *Star Wars* movie with a friend and encountered the first explanation of "the Force" that plays such an important role in the story. When Obi-Wan Kenobi revealed how the Force permeated and flowed through everything, I leaned over to my friend in the adjoining seat and whispered (we were, after all in a theater), "Sounds like Qì." "I thought so too," he replied.

The force, though fictional, conveys a number of instructive images. A flow of energy, able to affect the material world (as when Luke Skywalker summons his light saber to his hand); a self-development process, as when Luke exercises under Yoda's guidance; and the description of the Jedi concept as an "old religion." Recurrent mention is made of the need for "balance in the Force"; these ideas and images from a totally different realm provide a mental framework on which to build an understanding of energy flow, physical strengthening, balance of forces, and spiritual development. This framework helps to convey the essence of the topics in this book, exploring the theoretical roots of Qì and its related applied practice, Qìgōng.

The reader of this work is entering into a subject that—although clearly ancient—involves new concepts, new language, and new terminology – a daunting prospect. Fortunately, there is at hand one of the foremost interpreters of this ancient material in Dr. Yáng, Jwìng-Mǐng, whose extensive experience and wide research have pulled together many separate elements of the field to make them accessible to any reader, Western or Eastern; through many related publications he has shared his understanding with a wide audience. Step by step, leading the reader by the hand as it were, he takes you from the basics to a more complex and deeper understanding.

The complexity of this subject, indeed, defies summary, but there are certain points and trends discussed in this introduction that may serve for the beginning reader as an orientation to the topics covered. First, the book attempts to link the ancient and the modern, connecting traditional Chinese theories such as Qì and Qìgōng with modern concepts of bioelectricity. Adjusting Qì flow is at the heart of Chinese medical science and principles of health, as well as regulating the disturbed "emotional mind." Just as the more familiar term, Gōngfū (sometimes Kūng Fū) means energy (effort) over time, Qìgōng involves energy, time—and patience.

Like those of blood and lymph, Qì is understood to have its own circulation, described in appropriate detail in this book and clarified by helpful analogies and metaphors as usual. Qì circulation is best understood by a dominant analogy in this text: an electric circuit. Electric circuit imagery is one of several analogies that aid in the understanding of Qì principles. Another is the notion of the factory, where things are produced. But these concrete images are not the whole picture: fire and water imagery also illustrate, respectively, excitement/inflammation versus cooling, calming, and centering. Water imagery may also clarify: as water may have reservoirs and pipes, Qì has storage locations in the body and channels through which to flow.

In this book Master Yáng crafts a didactic braid from a multitude of strands. These include Buddhism and Daoism and their respective differences; connection to acupuncture theory, meridians, Qì channels, cavity theory, and martial arts (Grand Circulation has special application to this last practice). The various forms of spirit and their relationship to breathing are also described.

The book itself benefits from copious photos and diagrams that aid in picturing the processes being described. For each Chinese term employed, an English transliteration and the corresponding Chinese ideograms are supplied; in addition, in many cases, the original metaphoric translation is provided, offering insight into the roots of the terminology. Useful supplementary references appear throughout.

In sum, it is unlikely that a deeper exploration of Qì and Qìgōng theory can be found anywhere. The reader in search of deep understanding has found the perfect guide.

Thomas G. Gutheil, MD
Harvard Medical School

Foreword

Roshi Teja Fudo Myoo Bell

When asked, "Who are you? A god, a saint, an enlightened master?" Siddhartha Gautama—the historical Buddha—did not answer with personal information; instead, he simply said, "I am Awake!" This was not an arrogant statement but one of lucid recognition and humble self-realization. In this declaration is an embodied understanding that liberation from delusion and "waking up" is not about a system of belief but a direct experience that is based on the real spiritual insight that arises from practice. In their radical engagement with the path of liberation, earnest seekers of truth continue to evolve both their level of insight and the quality of their practice. This liberation is, in part, breaking free of habitual personal and cultural patterns that keep us from the direct recognition of our true interconnected nature with the universe itself—the Dào. Dr. Yáng has referred to this process as "letting go of your mask." Letting go, indeed!

From the time Buddhism first arrived in China, Buddhist philosophy, along with its insight meditation techniques and mindfulness awakening practices, has had a most auspicious connection to the existing Daoist culture. Each system and tradition of practice positively impacted the other without either losing its fundamental identity. This was not about competition but rather a mutual appreciation—not so much a marriage but learning and enhancing each other.

The Axial Age (between the 8th and 3rd centuries BCE) saw the appearance of great teachers like Lǎozi, Zhuāngzi, Confucius, and the historical Buddha—Siddhartha Gautama. Their teachings were radically new and transformative for humanity, having had a profound impact on world culture and spiritual understanding right up to the present day. Within certain of these Daoist and Buddhist traditions, and intimately connected with the teaching and the methodologies of meditation and mindfulness, are the profoundly integrating, coherency-creating, and well-being promoting work that we have come to know as Qìgōng. This process of transformation is the fulcrum point that potentially integrates cognitive understanding with embodied direct knowing and in its finer expression is called Internal Alchemy. Qìgōng meditation helps to establish a first-person knowing and trust in the universe that is beyond doubt. Together, the cognitive and scholarly engagement, along with the direct personal and transpersonal experience of the Dào—by any name the Dào may be known—is the foundation and the expression of what we might call enlightenment. Understood in this way, enlightenment is not a single momentary experience but an unfolding process that may include stages of personal psychological and moral development as well as dimensions of transcendent state experiences that arise from contemplative training, including the finer stages of Qìgōng practices like the principles of *Yìjīnjīng* and the spiritual endeavor of the *Xǐsuǐjīng*. Experienced practitioners know this to include the transmutation of the three treasures, the Sān Bǎo—Jīng to Qì to Shén.

As a Buddhist priest and a Daoist practitioner, as well as a teacher of these traditions and practices, I have found Dr. Yáng's teaching and in-depth research to be invaluable to my experiential understanding of Qìgōng and my dharma heritage.

Dr. Yáng's research and translations are extraordinary in themselves, yet he has also brought something else equally relevant and necessary to a grounded actualization of Qìgōng meditation: a clear and legitimate voice of modern science and the scientific method. Dr. Yáng has been able to explain Qì in terms of bioelectrical energy, has clearly distinguished the differences between internal and external martial arts, and has recognized important modern discoveries like the second brain in the field of the Lower Dāntián, to name just a few contributions. Through his work, Dr. Yáng has been able to successfully create a bridge to ancient Eastern wisdom for those of us with empirical-leaning Western minds.

The pathway that Dr. Yáng has opened up for us in *Qìgōng Grand Circulation for Spiritual Enlightenment* (大周天氣功與神通) is a rare and incomparably valuable map for the process and the methodology of authentic awakening to our true nature—by any name.

It is a confluence of the rivers of intellectual understanding and direct nondual experience through the meditation practice portal. The scope of the three books in the Qìgōng Meditation series ranges from the essential foundations of Qìgōng and the clarification of guiding principles to the very advanced aspects of physical, mental, and spiritual transformation in Internal Alchemy. The richness of the themes and practices in *Qìgōng Grand Circulation for Spiritual Enlightenment* sets this book apart as a well-spring of coherent material for study and practice that one may engage in for a lifetime.

This text is a culmination of a lifetime of practice, research, and teaching. Building on the previous two texts, *Qìgōng Meditation: Embryonic Breathing* and *Qìgōng Meditation: Small Circulation*, Dr. Yáng delivers a consummation of practical and spiritual insight from his endless hours of comparative research and translation of ancient texts and, most importantly, his own direct experience. The outcome is *Qìgōng Grand Circulation for Spiritual Enlightenment*.

I would call this book a treasure, as it reveals a depth and scope of material that is vast, detailed, and trustworthy. Relevant to any sincere seeker and explorer of human potential, it is presented in a way that is systematic, inspirational, accessible, and non-dogmatic.

As humanity now appears to have arrived at a point where the choice between the two paths of evolution and extinction is presented before us, what is more important than giving priority and our heart's attention to genuine transformation? If we are to make this evolutionary change to a sustainable and inhabitable planet, it must be in harmony with nature and not through more manipulation and self-centered greed. By synthesizing the ancient and the modern, the compassionate and the wise, and the true and the liberating,

Dr. Yáng reveals for us this evolutionary pathway that is a treasure of well-being and internal harmony.

Qìgōng Grand Circulation for Spiritual Enlightenment is ultimately about wholeness and the actualization of our potential as individual human beings on the path of an evolving awakening realization of our inextirpable connection to the heart/mind of the universe—the Dào.

Roshi Teja Fudo Myoo Bell
Rinzai Zen Lineage—84th Ancestor
QigongDharma.com
Fairfax, CA July 2021

Preface

I have been interested in Qìgōng since I was in my teens. Like many others, I was confused about the spiritual world and wondered about the meaning of life. I have inquired into existing religions, hoping to find answers. From my understanding at that time, it seemed that since all religions were created to study and understand the spiritual world, I should have been able to find answers. Unfortunately, the information I found was disappointing and led me into more confusion. I felt there was too much bondage connected to the dogma or doctrine, and if I followed the path they guided me toward, my spirit would be in that bondage and my spirit would not evolve. I began to meditate and search my own feeling. I also collected available information and ancient documents from Qìgōng masters and Buddhist and Daoist monks, and studied them hoping to find a correct path for my spiritual cultivation.

After more than fifty-five years of studying, pondering, and seeking understanding, I found that in order to understand the meaning of life, I could not just use the concepts of the material world to define the meaning of life. If I did so, I would miss one half of my life, the spiritual life.

In the last twenty years, I began to pay more attention to developing my spiritual feeling and understanding. Amazingly, through meditation and the available ancient documents, I was able to find this path. Now, I am walking on this path and hopefully I will achieve the final goal before the end of my life.

As we know, due to the lack of material satisfaction in the early twentieth century, peoples' minds and science were focused on developing and pursuing material satisfaction. Now, our material satisfaction has reached unprecedented levels. Most of the world has access to plenty of food and luxury items such as cars, airplanes, refrigerators, televisions, cell phones, computers, and so on. These were the dreams of people in the last century. Unfortunately, even though we have all of these material enjoyments, we still feel that life is not fulfilling. In addition, in the course of the development of material science, we have also created and stockpiled so many powerful and destructive weapons that we are able to exterminate the entire human race a hundred times over. This dissatisfaction and dangerous condition exists because we have not balanced material advancement with advancement in the spiritual world.

Since the beginning of this century, more and more people have felt this dissatisfaction and joined in the search for the other half of the meaning of life, the spiritual life. I know the mission of my life is to share what I have understood from studying ancient documents written by these ancient Qìgōng masters or Buddhist and Daoist monks. These documents have provided guidelines to approach the final goal of spiritual understanding.

Before you study this book, I highly recommend you first study two books: *Qìgōng Meditation—Embryonic Breathing* and also *Qìgōng Meditation—Small Circulation*. These two books will help you build a firm foundation of understanding for this book,

Qìgōng Grand Circulation for Spiritual Enlightenment. In the first part of this book, I will begin by reviewing some basic Qìgōng concepts. If you have already studied the two books recommended, then you may skip this first part.

Dr. Yáng, Jwìng-Mǐng
YMAA CA Retreat Center
January 16th, 2019

PART I

Foundations

CHAPTER 1

General Qìgōng Concepts

1.1 INTRODUCTION (JIÈSHÀO, 介紹)

Qìgōng has been studied and practiced for more than four thousand years in China. It has always been a part of Chinese culture. After such a long time of development, Qìgōng has been popularly practiced in medical, scholar, religious, and martial arts societies. Though the theoretical foundation remains the same, the development, especially in applications and goals, is different. For example, medical Qìgōng pays more attention to health maintenance and healing, scholar Qìgōng is looking for a peaceful and calm mind, religious Qìgōng aims for spiritual enlightenment and Buddhahood, and martial arts Qìgōng focuses on the cultivation of both physical strength and mental concentration for power manifestation, alertness, and awareness.

All Qìgōng studies have one thing in common: they cannot be separated from their roots in the philosophies expressed in classic documents such as *The Book of Changes* (*Yìjīng*, 易經), *Lǎozi Dàodéjīng* (老子道德經), Confucius' *Analects* (*Lúnyǔ*, 論語), and Dharma's Muscle/Tendon Changing and Marrow/Brain Washing (*Dámó Yìjīnjīng/Xǐsuǐjīng*, 達磨易筋經/洗髓經). If you wish to understand Qìgōng at a profound level, you must also study these classics; otherwise, you will have missed the roots of the theory of Qìgōng. For example, if you don't study *The Book of Changes*, you may miss the important concept of Yīn and Yáng theory. If you don't have an idea of scholar classics, you will not understand how the scholars cultivated their temperament and tried to comprehend humanity through mediation. If you don't understand Muscle/Tendon Changing and Marrow/Brain Washing classics, you will not have a clue or guideline in achieving the final goal of spiritual cultivation.

Unlike medical and scholar Qìgōng, spiritual and martial Qìgōng were usually kept secret in monasteries. It was not till the 1980s that most of the secrets were revealed to the lay society. Now, we have all these ancient practices in our hands. The question is how do we absorb this ancient knowledge and experience and apply them into today's society. This is especially true in spiritual cultivation.

As we know, even though we have reached a high level of understanding in material science, it is undeniable that we are still ignorant about the spiritual world. Through our material sciences, our weapons have been developed to a stage that we are able to destroy the entire human race a hundred times over, yet we still don't pay much attention to spiritual development. Without spiritual development, we have lost the balance of Yīn and Yáng.

I believe that while the twentieth century was the material century, this twenty-first century should be the spiritual century. If we don't catch up in our spiritual development, it will possibly be the end of our world. Borrowing and learning from ancient study and experience in spiritual cultivation is more important than ever.

We cannot deny that in order to reach to a high level of spiritual cultivation, we have to isolate ourselves from all emotional bondage and dogmas that we have created in our lay society or matrix. However, if all of us can recognize the cause and the truth of these emotions and dogmas, we will be able to create a society that is fertile for spiritual cultivation without entering the mountains to live a secluded life.

In this chapter, I would like to help you build a foundation of Qìgōng practice. From this foundation, you will be able to understand the subsequent chapters. If you have already read my other books, *Qigōng Meditation—Embryonic Breathing* or *Qigōng Meditation—Small Circulation*, you may skip this chapter since it is a review of the Qìgōng concepts discussed in those books. However, if you have never read the two books, it will be hard to understand the rest of this book, and I highly recommend you comprehend this first chapter before moving on.

In Section 1.2, we will go over the most basic concepts of Qì and Qìgōng from both the traditional and the scientific understanding. After you have a clear idea of Qì and Qìgōng, move on to the important concepts of general Qìgōng practice in Section 1.3. In order to comprehend how Qìgōng works, we review the body's Qì network in Section 1.4. The main crucial keys to practicing Qìgōng is how to build abundant Qì and also how to manifest Qì efficiently. We will summarize these two key practices in Section 1.5. Then, we will introduce the traditional procedures of Qìgōng practice, five regulatings, in Section 1.6. To avoid confusion between Buddhist and Daoist Qìgōng practices, we will review the concepts of both Buddhist and Daoist Qìgōng practice in Sections 1.7 and 1.8.

1.2 WHAT IS QÌ? WHAT IS QÌGŌNG? (HÉWÈI QÌ? HÉWÈI QÌGŌNG? 何謂氣？何謂氣功？)

To define Qì and Qìgōng clearly, we must include both the traditional definition and modern definition. As known, traditional knowledge and practices were accumulated from countless experiments and experiences which led to defining the correct path. We are now living in a modern scientific society and human science has developed to a stage that enables us to interpret and verify many of these ancient practices with logic, commonsense, and scientific understanding. Theoretically, if those ancient Qìgōng practices are accurate, they should be able to accept the challenge of modernity and submit to modern scientific verification.

However, we should recognize an important fact. As mentioned earlier, though we have understood material science to a high level, we still don't know much about the spiritual world. We are still confused about what is the spirit and the spiritual world. Therefore, we should keep our mind open and at the same time continue to use science to uncover the mysteries of the spiritual world.

In this section, we will first review the traditional general definition and narrow definition of Qì and Qìgōng. After that, we will discuss the modern definition of Qì and Qìgōng.

Definition of Qì

In this subsection, we will first give the traditional general definition of Qì, followed with the narrow definition of Qì.

> *Qì is the energy or natural force that fills the universe. The Chinese have traditionally believed that there are three major powers in the universe. These Three Powers (Sāncái, 三才) are Heaven (Tiān, 天), Earth (Dì, 地), and Man (Rén, 人). Heaven (the sky or universe) has Heaven Qì (Tiānqì, 天氣), the most important of the three, which is made up of the forces that the heavenly bodies exert on the earth, such as sunshine, moonlight, the moon's gravity, and the energy from the stars. In ancient times, the Chinese believed that weather, climate, and natural disasters were governed by Heaven Qì. Chinese people still refer to the weather as Heaven Qì (Tiānqì, 天氣). Every energy field strives to stay in balance, so whenever the Heaven Qì loses its balance, it tries to rebalance itself. Then the wind must blow, rain must fall, even tornadoes or hurricanes become necessary in order for the Heaven Qì to reach a new energy balance.*

Under Heaven Qì is Earth Qì (Dìqì, 地氣). It is influenced and controlled by Heaven Qì. For example, too much rain will force a river to flood or change its path. Without rain, the plants will die. The Chinese believe that Earth Qì is made up of lines and patterns of energy, as well as the earth's magnetic field and the heat concealed underground. These energies must also balance; otherwise disasters such as earthquakes or hurricanes will occur. When the Qì of the earth is balanced and harmonized, plants will grow and animals thrive.

Finally, within the Earth Qì, each individual person, animal, and plant has its own Qì field, which always seeks to be balanced. When any individual living thing loses its Qì balance, it will sicken, die, and decompose. All natural things, including mankind and our Human Qì (Rénqì, 人氣), grow within and are influenced by the natural cycles of Heaven Qì and Earth Qì. Throughout the history of Qìgōng, people have been most interested in Human Qì and its relationship with Heaven Qì and Earth Qì.

In the Chinese tradition, Qì can also be defined as any type of energy that is able to demonstrate power and strength. This energy can be electricity, magnetism, heat, or light. For example, electric power is called "Electric Qì" (Diànqì, 電氣), and heat is called "Heat Qì" (Rèqì, 熱氣). When a person is alive, his body's energy is called "Human Qì" (Rénqì, 人氣).

Qì is also commonly used to express the energy state of something, especially living things. As mentioned before, the weather is called "Heaven Qì" (Tiānqì, 天氣) because it indicates the energy state of the heavens. When something is alive it has "Vital Qì" (Huóqì, 活氣), and when it is dead it has "Dead Qì" (Sǐqì, 死氣) or "Ghost Qì" (Guǐqì, 鬼氣). When a person is righteous and has the spiritual strength to do good, he is said to have "Normal Qì or Righteous Qì" (Zhèngqì, 正氣). The spiritual state or morale of an army is called "energy state" (Qìshì, 氣勢).

You can see that the word "Qì" has a wider and more general definition than most people think. It does not refer only to the energy circulating in the human body. Furthermore, the word "Qì" can represent the energy itself, but it can even be used to express the manner or state of the energy. It is important to understand this when you practice Qìgōng so that your mind is not channeled into a narrow understanding of Qì, which would limit your future understanding and development.

A Narrow Traditional Definition of Qì

Now that you understand the general definition of Qì, let us look at how Qì is defined in Qìgōng society today. As mentioned before, among the Three Powers, the Chinese have been most concerned with the Qì that affects our health and longevity. Therefore, after four thousand years of emphasizing Human Qì, when people mention Qì they usually mean the Qì circulating in our bodies.

If we look at the Chinese medical and Qìgōng documents that were written in ancient times, the word "Qì" was written "炁." This character is constructed of two words, "旡" on the top, which means "nothing," and ",,," on the bottom, which means "fire." This means that the word Qì was actually written as "no fire" in ancient times. If we go back through Chinese medical and Qìgōng history, it is not hard to understand this expression.

In ancient times, the Chinese physicians or Qìgōng practitioners were actually looking for the Yīn-Yáng balance of the Qì that was circulating in the body. When this goal was reached, there was "no fire" in the internal organs. This concept is very simple. According to Chinese medicine, each of our internal organs needs to receive a specific amount of Qì to function properly. If an organ receives an improper amount of Qì (usually too much— too yang, or on fire), it will start to malfunction, and, in time, physical damage will occur. Therefore, the goal of the medical or Qìgōng practitioner was to attain a state of "no fire," which eventually became the word Qì.

However, in more recent publications, the Qì of "no fire" has been replaced by the word "氣," which is again constructed of two words, "气" which means "air" and "米" which means "rice." This shows that later practitioners realized that, after each of us is born, the Qì circulating in our bodies is produced mainly by the inhalation of air (oxygen) and the consumption of food (rice). Air is called kōngqì (空氣), which means literally "space energy."

For a long time, people were confused about just what type of energy was circulating in our bodies. Many people believed that it was heat, others considered it to be electricity, and many others assumed that it was a mixture of heat, electricity, and light.

This confusion lasted until the early 1980s when it gradually became clear that the Qì circulating in our bodies is actually "bioelectricity" and that our body is a "living electromagnetic field." This field is affected by our thoughts, feelings, activities, the food we eat, the quality of the air we breathe, our lifestyle, the natural energy that surrounds us, and also the unnatural energy that modern science inflicts upon us.

A Modern Definition of Qì

It is important that you know about the progress that has been made by modern science in the study of Qì. This will keep you from getting stuck in the ancient concepts and level of understanding.

In ancient China, people had very little knowledge of electricity. What they understood about acupuncture was that when a needle was inserted into acupuncture cavities, some kind of energy other than heat was produced that often caused a shock or a tingling sensation. It was not until the last few decades, when the Chinese people were more acquainted with electromagnetic science, that they began to recognize that this energy circulating in the body, which they called Qì, might be the same thing that today's science calls "bioelectricity."

It is now understood that the human body is constructed of many different electrically conductive materials, and that it forms a living electromagnetic field and circuit. Electromagnetic energy is continuously being generated in the human body through the biochemical reaction in food and air assimilation, and circulated by the electromotive forces (EMF) generated within the body.

In addition, we are constantly being affected by external electromagnetic fields such as that of the earth, or the electrical fields generated by clouds. When you practice Chinese medicine or Qìgōng, you need to be aware of these outside factors and take them into account.

Countless experiments have been conducted in China, Japan, and other countries to study how external magnetic or electrical fields affect and adjust the body's Qì field. Many acupuncturists use magnets and electricity in their treatments. They attach a magnet to the skin over a cavity and leave it there for a period of time. The magnetic field gradually affects the Qì circulation in that channel. Alternatively, they insert needles into cavities and then run an electric current through the needle to reach the Qì channels directly. Although many researchers have claimed a degree of success in their experiments, none has been able to publish any detailed and convincing proof of the results, or give a good explanation of the theory behind the experiment. As with many other attempts to explain the *how* and *why* of acupuncture, conclusive proof is elusive, and many unanswered questions remain. Of course, this theory is quite new, and it will probably take a lot more study and research before it is verified and completely understood. At present, there are many conservative acupuncturists who are skeptical.

To untie this knot, we must look at what modern Western science has discovered about bioelectromagnetic energy. Many reports on bioelectricity have been published, and frequently the results are closely related to what is experienced in Chinese Qìgōng training and medical science. For example, during the electrophysiological research of the 1960s, several investigators discovered that bones are piezoelectric; that is, when they are stressed, mechanical energy is converted to electrical energy in the form of electric current. This might explain one of the practices of Marrow Washing Qìgōng in which the stress on the bones and muscles is increased in certain ways to increase the Qì circulation.

Dr. Robert O. Becker has done important work in this field. His book *The Body Electric* reports on much of the research concerning the body's electric field. It is presently believed that food and air are the fuels that generate the electricity in the body through biochemical reaction. This electricity, which is circulated throughout the entire body by means of electrically conductive tissue, is one of the main energy sources that keep the cells of the physical body alive.

Whenever you have an injury or are sick, your body's electrical circulation is affected. If this circulation of electricity stops, you die. But bioelectric energy not only maintains life, it is also responsible for repairing physical damage. Many researchers have sought ways of using external electrical or magnetic fields to speed up the body's recovery from physical injury. Richard Leviton reports: "Researchers at Loma Linda University's School of Medicine in California have found, following studies in sixteen countries with over 1,000 patients, that low-frequency, low-intensity magnetic energy has been successful in treating chronic pain related to tissue ischemia and has also worked in clearing up slow-healing ulcers, and in 90 percent of patients tested, raised blood flow significantly."

Mr. Leviton also reports that every cell of the body functions like an electric battery and is able to store electric charge. He reports that "other bio-magnetic investigators take an even closer look to find out what is happening, right down to the level of the blood, the organs, and the individual cell, which they regard as 'a small electric battery.'" This has convinced me that our entire body is essentially a big battery that is assembled from millions of small batteries. All of these batteries together form the human electromagnetic field.

Furthermore, much of the research on the body's electrical field relates to acupuncture. For example, Dr. Becker reports that the conductivity of the skin is much higher at acupuncture cavities, and that it is now possible to locate them precisely by measuring the skin's conductivity (Figure 1-1). Many of these reports prove that the acupuncture that has been done in China for thousands of years is reasonable and scientific.

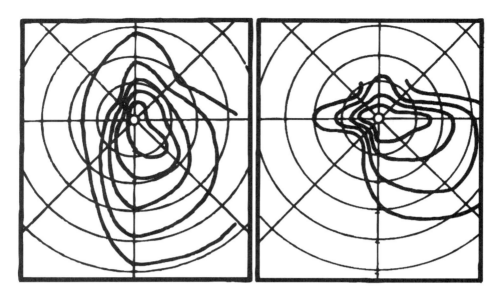

Figure 1-1. Electric Conductivity Maps of the Skin
Surface over Acupuncture Points.

Some researchers use the theory of the body's electricity to explain many of the ancient "miracles" attributed to the practice of Qìgōng. A report by Albert L. Huebner states: "These demonstrations of body electricity in human beings may also offer a new explanation of an ancient healing practice. If weak external fields can produce powerful physiological effects, it may be that fields from human tissues in one person are capable of producing clinical improvements in another. In short, the method of healing known as the laying on of hands could be an especially subtle form of electrical stimulation."

Another frequently reported phenomenon is that when a Qìgōng practitioner has reached a high level of development, a halo would appear behind or around his head during meditation. Halos are commonly seen in paintings of Jesus Christ, the Buddha, and various Oriental immortals. Frequently the light is pictured as surrounding the whole body. This phenomenon may again be explained by the body electric theory. When a person has cultivated their Qì (electricity) to a high level, the Qì may be led to accumulate in the head. This Qì may then interact with the oxygen molecules in the air and ionize them, causing them to glow.

Although the link between the theory of *The Body Electric* and the Chinese theory of Qì is becoming more accepted and better proven, there are still many questions to be answered. For example, how does the mind generate an EMF (electromotive force) to circulate the electricity in the body? Is the bioelectricity circulating in the animal body a DC or an AC current? How is the human electromagnetic field affected by the multitude of other electric fields that surround us, such as radio wiring or electrical appliances? How can we readjust our electromagnetic fields and survive in outer space or on other planets where the magnetic field is completely different from Earth's? You can see that the future of Qìgōng and bioelectric science is a challenging and exciting one. It is about time we started to use modern technology to understand the inner energy world that has for the most part been ignored by Western society.

Definition of Qìgōng

Now that you have a clear concept of Qì, let us discuss how Qìgōng is traditionally defined. Again, we will define it from both a general and a narrow point of view. Later, after you have become familiar with the modern concept of Qì, we will define the meaning of Qìgōng based on the scientific understanding of today.

A GENERAL TRADITIONAL DEFINITION OF QÌGŌNG

We have explained that Qì is energy, and that it is found in the heavens, in the earth, and in every living thing. In China, the word "Gōng" (功) is often used instead of "Gōng-fū" (or Kūng Fū, 功夫), which means energy and time. *Any study or training that requires a lot of energy and time to learn or to accomplish is called Gōngfū.* The term can be applied to any special skill or study as long as it requires time, energy, and patience. Therefore, *the correct definition of Qìgōng is any training or study dealing with Qì that takes a long time and a lot of effort.* You can see from this definition that Qìgōng is a science that studies the energy in nature. The main difference between this energy science and Western energy science is that Qìgōng focuses on the inner energy of human beings while Western energy science pays more attention to the energy outside of the human body. When you study Qìgōng, it is worthwhile to also consider the modern, scientific point of view, and not restrict yourself to only the traditional beliefs.

The Chinese have studied Qì for thousands of years. Some of the information on the patterns and cycles of nature has been recorded in books, one of which is the *Yìjīng* (易經) (*Book of Changes*; 1122 BCE). When the *Yìjīng* was written, the Chinese people believed that natural power included Heaven (Tiān, 天), Earth (Dì, 地), and Man (Rén, 人). These are "The Three Powers" (Sāncái, 三才), discussed above, that are manifested by the three Qì's: Heaven Qì, Earth Qì, and Human Qì. These three facets of nature have their definite rules and cycles. The rules never change, and the cycles are repeated regularly. The Chinese people used an understanding of these natural principles and the *Yìjīng* to calculate the changes of natural Qì. This calculation is called "The Eight Trigrams" (Bāguà, 八卦). From the Eight Trigrams the sixty-four hexagrams are derived. Therefore, the *Yìjīng* was probably the first book that taught the Chinese people about Qì and its variations in nature and man. The relationship of the Three Natural Powers and their Qì variations were later discussed extensively in the book *Theory of Qì's Variation* (Qìhuàlùn, 氣化論) by Zhuāngzi (莊子) (370–369 BCE).

Understanding Heaven Qì is very difficult, and it was especially so in ancient times when the science was just developing. But since nature is always repeating itself, the experiences accumulated over the years have made it possible to trace the natural patterns. Understanding the rules and cycles of "heavenly timing" (tiānshí, 天時) will help you to understand the natural changes of the seasons, climate, weather, rain, snow, drought, and all other natural occurrences. If you observe carefully, you can see many of these routine patterns and cycles caused by the rebalancing of the Qì fields. Among the natural cycles are those that repeat every day, month, or year, as well as cycles of twelve years and sixty years.

Earth Qì is a part of Heaven Qì. If you can understand the rules and the structure of the earth, you can understand how mountains and rivers are formed, how plants grow, how rivers move, what part of the country is best for someone, where to build a house and which direction it should face so that it is a healthy place to live, and many other things related to the earth. In China there are people, called "geomancy teachers" (dìlǐshī, 地理師) or "wind water teachers" (fēngshuǐshī, 風水師), who make their living this way. The term "wind water" (Fēngshuǐ, 風水) is commonly used because the location and character of the wind and water in a landscape are the most important factors in evaluating a location. These experts use the accumulated body of geomantic knowledge and the *Yìjīng* to help people make important decisions such as where and how to build a house, where to bury their dead, and how to rearrange or redecorate homes and offices so that they are better places to live and work in. Many people believe that setting up a store or business according to the guidance of Fēngshuǐ can make it more prosperous.

Among the three Qì's, Human Qì is probably the one studied most thoroughly. The study of Human Qì covers a large number of different subjects. The Chinese people believe that Human Qì is affected and controlled by Heaven Qì and Earth Qì, and that they in fact determine your destiny. Therefore, if you understand the relationship between nature and people, in addition to understanding "human relations" (rénshì, 人事), you can predict wars, the destiny of a country, a person's desires and temperament, and even his future. The people who practice this profession are called "calculate life teachers" (suànmìngshī, 算命師).

However, the greatest achievement in the study of Human Qì is in regard to health and longevity. Since Qì is the source of life, if you understand how Qì functions and know how to regulate it correctly, you should be able to live a long and healthy life. Remember that you are part of nature, and you are channeled into the cycles of nature. If you go against this natural cycle, you may become sick, so it is in your best interest to follow the way of nature. This is the meaning of "Dào" (道), which can be translated as "The Natural Way."

Many different aspects of affecting Human Qì have been researched, including acupuncture, acupressure, massage, herbal treatment, meditation, and Qìgōng exercises. The use of acupuncture, acupressure, and herbal treatment to adjust Human Qì flow has become the root of Chinese medical science. Meditation and moving Qìgōng exercises are widely used by the Chinese people to improve their health or even to cure certain illnesses. In addition, Daoists and Buddhists use meditation and Qìgōng exercises in their pursuit of enlightenment.

In conclusion, *the study of any of the aspects of Qì, including Heaven Qì, Earth Qì, and Human Qì, should be called Qìgōng.* However, since the term is usually used today only in reference to the cultivation of Human Qì through meditation and exercise, we will only use it in this narrower sense to avoid confusion.

A NARROW TRADITIONAL DEFINITION OF QÌGŌNG

As mentioned earlier, the narrow definition of Qì is "the energy circulating in the human body." Therefore, *the narrow definition of Qìgōng is "the study or the practice of circulating the Qì in the human body."* Because our bodies are part of nature, the narrow definition of Qìgōng should also include the study of how our bodies relate to Heaven Qì and Earth Qì. Today, Chinese Qìgōng consists of several different fields: medical Qìgōng, scholar Qìgōng, religious Qìgōng, and martial arts Qìgōng. Naturally, since all of these practices share the same root, these fields are mutually related, and in many cases cannot be separated.

In ancient times, Qìgōng was also commonly called "tǔnà" (吐納). Tǔnà means to "utter and admit," which implies *uttering and admitting the air through the nose.* The reason for this is simply that Qìgōng practice is closely related to the methods of how to inhale and exhale correctly. Zhuāngzi (莊子), during the Chinese Warring States Period (403–222 BC) (Zhànguó, 戰國), said: "Blowing puffing to breathe, uttering the old and admitting the new, the bear's natural (action) and the bird's extending (the neck), are all for longevity. This is also favored by those people living as long as Péng, Zǔ (彭祖) who practice Dǎoyǐn (i.e., Direct and Lead) (導引), and nourishing the shapes (i.e., cultivating the physical body)." Péng, Zǔ was a legendary Qìgōng practitioner during the period of Emperor Yáo (堯) (2356–2255 BCE), who was said to have lived for eight hundred years. From this saying, we can see that Qìgōng was also commonly called "Dǎoyǐn," which means *to use the mind and physical movements to direct and to lead the circulation of Qì in the correct way.* The physical movements commonly imitate the natural instinctive movements of animals such as bears and birds. A famous medical Qìgōng set passed down at this time was "The Five Animal Sports" (Wǔqínxì, 五禽戲) that imitates the movements of the tiger, deer, bear, ape, and bird.

The biggest and most popular medical Qìgōng practices are acupuncture, herbal treatment, Qìgōng massage (i.e., acupressure), and Qìgōng exercises. These Qìgōng are not only used for health maintenance, but also used for treatment of illness.

However, when Qìgōng is defined in scholarly society, it is somewhat different. The Qìgōng practice is focused on regulating the disturbed emotional mind. When the emotional mind is regulated into a peaceful and calm state, the body will be relaxed, which will assist the Qì to circulate smoothly in the body and therefore regulate itself into a more harmonious state. From this, mental and physical health can be achieved.

When Qìgōng is defined in Daoist and Buddhist society, it refers to the method or training of leading the Qì from the Real Lower Dāntián (i.e., Real Lower Elixir Field) (Zhēn Xià Dāntián, 真下丹田) to the brain for spiritual enlightenment or Buddhahood. The Real Lower Dāntián is the place at the abdominal area where one is able to store the Qì. It is considered a Qì storage area or bioelectric battery. Naturally, its training theory and methods will not be easy. In fact, religious Qìgōng is considered one of the highest levels of Qìgōng training in China.

Finally, when Qìgōng is defined in martial arts society, it refers to the theory and methods of using Qì to energize the physical body to its maximum efficiency of power manifestation. These martial Qìgōng were developed in those monasteries located in remote mountains such as Sōng Mountain (Sōngshān, 嵩山), Wǔdāng Mountain (Wǔdāngshān, 武當山), Éméi Mountain (Éméishān, 峨嵋山), Qīngchén Mountain (Qīngchénshān, 青城山), and many others. As a matter of fact, almost all of the practices followed Dharma's (Dámó, 達摩) teaching, Muscle/Tendon Changing and Marrow/Brain Washing Qìgōng (Yìjīnjīng and Xǐsuǐjīng, 易筋經、洗髓經). This classic not only taught the monks how to condition and strengthen the physical body, but also offered them a guide to achieve the final goal of spiritual enlightenment and Buddhahood. From this, it is not surprising to see that the profound level of martial arts Qìgōng training actually was the same as that of religious Qìgōng, spiritual enlightenment.

A Modern Definition of Qìgōng

If you accept that the inner energy (Qì) circulating in our bodies is bioelectricity, then we can formulate a definition of Qìgōng, based on electrical principles.

Let us assume that the circuit shown in Figure 1-2 is similar to the circuit in our bodies. Unfortunately, although we now have a certain degree of understanding of this circuit from acupuncture, we still do not know in detail exactly what the body's circuit looks like. We know that there are twelve primary Qì channels (Qì rivers) (shíèrjīng, 十二經) and eight vessels (Qì reservoirs) (bāmài, 八脈) in our body. There are also thousands of small Qì channels (luò, 絡) that allow the Qì to reach the skin and the bone marrow. In this circuit, the twelve internal organs are connected and mutually related through these channels. Finally, there is a dāntián (丹田) (elixir field) (bio-battery) that produces and stores the Qì.

If you look at the electrical circuit in the illustration, you will see that:

1. The Qì channels are like the wires that carry electric current.
2. The internal organs are like the electrical components such as resistors and solenoids.
3. The Qì vessels are like capacitors, which regulate the current in the circuit.
4. The dāntián is like a battery, which stores the charge and provides the EMF in the circuit.

How do you keep this electrical circuit functioning most efficiently? Your first concern is the resistance of the wire that carries the current. In a circuit, you want to use a wire that has a high level of conductivity and low resistance; otherwise heat may be generated

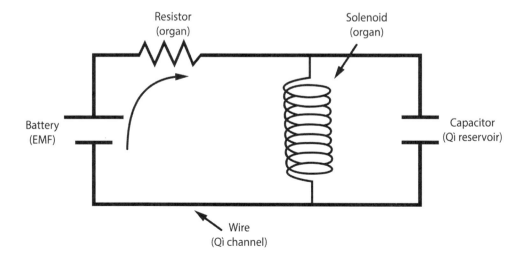

Figure 1-2. The Human Bioelectric Circuit Is Similar to an Electric Circuit.

and the wire may melt. Therefore, the wire should be of a material like copper or perhaps even gold. In your body, you want to keep the current flowing smoothly. This means that your first task is to remove anything that interferes with the flow and causes stagnation. Fat has low conductivity, so you should use diet and exercise to remove excess fat from your body. You should also learn how to relax your physical body, because this opens all of the Qì channels. This is why relaxation is the first goal in tàijíquán and many Qìgōng exercises.

Your next concern in maintaining a healthy electrical circuit is the components—your internal organs. If you do not have the correct level of current in your organs, they will either burn out from too much current (Yáng) or malfunction because of a deficient level of current (Yīn). In order to avoid these problems in a machine, you use a capacitor to regulate the current. Whenever there is too much current, the capacitor absorbs and stores the excess, and whenever the current is weak, the capacitor supplies current to raise the level. The eight Qì vessels are your body's capacitors. Qìgōng is concerned with learning how to increase the level of Qì in these vessels so that they will be able to supply current when needed and keep the internal organs functioning smoothly. This is especially important as you get older when your Qì level is generally lower.

In addition, in order to have a healthy circuit, you must be concerned with the components themselves. If any of them are not strong and of good quality, the entire circuit may malfunction. This means that the final concern in Qìgōng practice is how to maintain or even rebuild the health of your internal organs. Before we go any further, we should point out that there is an important difference between the circuit shown in the diagram and the Qì circuit in our bodies. This difference is that the human body is alive, and with the proper Qì nourishment, all of the cells can be regrown and the state of health improved. For example, if you are able to jog about three miles today, and if you keep jogging regularly and gradually increase the distance, eventually you will easily be able to jog five miles. This is because your body rebuilds and readjusts itself to fit the circumstances.

This means that if we are able to increase the Qì flow through our internal organs, they can become stronger and healthier. Naturally, the increase in Qì must be slow and gradual so that the organs can adjust to it. In order to increase the Qì flow in your body, you need to work with the EMF (electromotive force) in your body. If you do not know what EMF is, imagine two containers filled with water and connected by a tube. If both containers have the same water level, then the water will not flow. However, if one side is higher than the other, the water will flow from that container to the other. In electricity, this potential difference is called electric potential difference or electromotive force. Naturally, the higher the EMF is, the stronger the current will flow.

You can see from this discussion that the key to effective Qìgōng practice is, in addition to removing resistance from the Qì channels, learning how to increase the EMF in your body. Now let us see what the sources of EMF in the body are so that we may use them to increase the flow of bioelectricity. Generally speaking, there are six major sources:

1. Mind. The human mind is the most important and efficient source of bioelectric EMF. Any time you move you must first generate an idea (Yì, 意). This idea generates the EMF and leads the Qì through the Qì channels to the nervous system to energize the appropriate muscles to carry out the desired motion. The more you can concentrate, the stronger the EMF you can generate, and the stronger the flow of Qì you can lead. Naturally, the stronger the flow of Qì you lead to the muscles, the more they will be energized. Because of this, the mind is considered the most important factor in Qìgōng training.

2. Food and Air. In order to maintain life, we take in food and air essence through our mouths and noses. These essences are then converted into Qì through biochemical reaction in the chest and digestive system (called the Triple Burner in Chinese medicine). When Qì is converted from the essence, an EMF is generated that circulates the Qì throughout the body. Consequently, a major part of Qìgōng is devoted to getting the proper kinds of food and fresh air.

3. Exercise. Exercise converts the food essence (fat) stored in your body into Qì, and therefore builds up the EMF. Many Qìgōng styles have been created that utilize movement for this purpose.

4. Natural Energy. Since your body is constructed of electrically conductive material, its electromagnetic field is always affected by the sun, the moon, clouds, the earth's magnetic field, and by the other energies around you. The major influences are the radiation of the sun and moon, the moon's gravity, and the earth's magnetic field. From the moment you were formed, these influences have affected your Qì circulation significantly and are responsible for the pattern of your Qì circulation. We are now also being greatly affected by the energy pollution generated by modern technology, such as electromagnetic waves generated by radio, TV, microwave ovens, computers, and many other devices.

5. Converting Pre-Birth Essence into Qì. The hormones produced by our endocrine glands are referred to as "Pre-Birth Essence" or "Original Essence" (Yuánjīng, 元精) in Chinese medicine. They can be used to regulate the biochemical reaction that converts the food or fat into Qì. Hormones regulate our body's biochemical reaction process (metabolism). Thus, hormones are able to stimulate the functioning of our physical body, thereby increasing our vitality. Balancing hormone production when you are young and increasing its production when you are old are important subjects in Chinese Qìgōng.

6. Artificial Stimulation. The enhancement or the adjustment of the Qì circulation can also be done artificially. In fact, this is the basic theory of Chinese medicine such as acupuncture and Qìgōng massage. From external artificial Qì stimulation, the Qì can be brought to a state of balance, thus preventing or curing sickness.

From the foregoing, you can see that within the human body, there is a network of electrical circuitry. In order to maintain the circulation of bioelectricity, there must be a battery (or power supply) wherein to store and supply charge. Where, then, is the battery in our body?

Chinese Qìgōng practitioners believe that there are places in the body able to store Qì (bioelectricity). This place is called the dāntián (elixir field, 丹田). According to ancient practitioners, there are three dāntiáns in the human body. One is located at the abdominal area, one or two inches below the navel, called the "Lower Dāntián" (xià dāntián, 下丹田). The second is in the area of the lower sternum that is connected to the diaphragm, and is called the "Middle Dāntián" (zhōng dāntián, 中丹田). Since the Qì's status accumulated in the diaphragm affects the heart's beating and shānzhōng cavity (膻中) (Co-17) (midpoint between nipples), often the heart and shānzhōng cavity are also considered as part of Middle Dāntián. The third is the center of the brain, which connects to the lower center of the forehead (or the Third Eye), and is called the "upper dāntián" (shàng dāntián, 上丹田). In fact, often the entire brain is considered to be the upper dāntián.

The Lower Dāntián is considered to be the residence of the water Qì, or the Qì that is generated from the "Original Essence" (Yuánjīng, 元精). Therefore, Qì stored here is called "Original Qì" (Yuánqì, 元氣). According to Chinese medicine, in this same area there is a cavity called "Qìhǎi" (Co-6) (氣海), which means "Qì Ocean." This is consistent with the conclusions drawn by Qìgōng practitioners, who also call this area the "Lower Dāntián" (lower elixir field). Both groups agree that this area is able to produce Qì or elixir like a field, and that here the Qì is abundant like an ocean.

At this point, you should understand two important things. First, from a scientific point of view, even though the upper dāntián and the Middle Dāntián are able to store the Qì to an abundant level, they do not produce Qì, and thus they should be considered as capacitors instead of batteries. That means the real bio-battery is only located at the Lower Dāntián area. Second, according to a Daoist understanding, there are two Lower Dāntián, false Lower Dāntián (假下丹田) and real Lower Dāntián (真下丹田), located at the abdominal area. We will discuss the differences later in Section 1.4.

In Qìgōng practice, it is commonly known that in order to build up the Qì to a higher level in the Lower Dāntián, you must move your abdominal area (Lower Dāntián) up and down through abdominal breathing. This kind of up and down abdominal breathing exercise is called "qǐhuǒ" (起火) and means "start the fire." It is also called "back to childhood breathing" (fǎntóng hūxī, 返童呼吸). Normally, after you have exercised the Lower Dāntián for about ten minutes, you will have a feeling of warmth in the lower abdomen, which verifies the accumulation of Qì or energy. Therefore, Daoists called the abdominal area the "dānlú" (丹爐), which means the "elixir furnace."

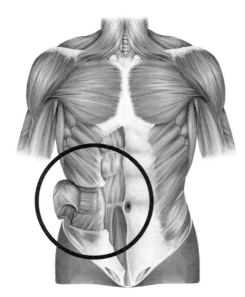

Figure 1-3. Muscles of the Abdominal Area.
(Illustration by Shutterstock)

Theoretically and scientifically, what is happening when the abdominal area is moved up and down? If you look at the structure of the abdominal area, you will see that there are about six layers of muscle and fasciae sandwiching each other in this area (Figure 1-3). In fact, what you actually see is the sandwich of muscles and fat accumulated in the fasciae layers. When you move your abdomen up and down, you are actually using your mind to move the muscles, not the fat. Whenever there is a muscular contraction and relaxation, the fat slowly turns into bioelectricity. When this bioelectricity encounters resistance from the fasciae layers, it turns into heat. From this, you can see how simple the theory might be for the generation of Qì. Another thing you should know is that, according to our understanding today, fat and fasciae are poor electrical conductors, while the muscles are relatively good electrical conductors." When these good and poor electrical materials are sandwiched together, they act like a battery. This is why, through up and down abdominal movements, the energy can be stored temporarily and warmth generated.

1.3 Important Fundamental Concepts (Zhòngyào Jīběn Gàiniàn, 重要基本概念)

Yīn and Yáng, Kǎn and Lí 陰－陽，坎－離

Kǎn (坎) and Lí (離) training has long been of major importance to Qìgōng practitioners. In order to understand why, you must understand these two words and the theory behind them. The terms Kǎn and Lí occur frequently in Qìgōng documents. In the Eight Trigrams, Kǎn represents "water," while Lí represents "fire." However, the everyday terms for water and fire are also often used.

First you should understand that though Kǎn-Lí and Yīn-Yáng are related, Kǎn and Lí are not Yīn and Yáng. Kǎn is water, which is able to cool your body and make it more Yīn, while Lí is fire, which warms your body and makes it more Yáng. *Kǎn and Lí are the methods or causes, while Yīn and Yáng are the results.* When Kǎn and Lí are adjusted or regulated correctly, Yīn and Yáng will be balanced and interact harmoniously.

Qìgōng practitioners believe that your body is always too Yáng, unless you are sick or have not eaten for a long time, in which case your body may be more Yīn. When your body is always Yáng, it is degenerating and burning out. It is believed that this is the cause of aging. If you are able to use water to cool down your body, you can slow down the process of degeneration and thereby lengthen your life. This is the main reason Qìgōng practitioners have been studying ways of improving the quality of water in their bodies and of reducing the quantity of fire. I believe that as a Qìgōng practitioner, you should always keep this subject at the top of your list for study and research. If you earnestly ponder and experiment, you can grasp the trick of adjusting them.

If you want to learn how to adjust them, you must understand that water and fire mean many things in your body. The first concern is your Qì. Qì is classified as fire or water. When your Qì is not pure and causes your physical body to heat up and your mental/spiritual body to become unstable (Yáng), it is classified as Fire Qì (Huǒqì, 火氣). The Qì that is pure and is able to cool both your physical and spiritual bodies (make them more Yīn) is considered Water Qì (Shuǐqì, 水氣). However, your body can never be purely water. Water can cool down the fire, but it must never totally quench it, because then you would be dead. It is also said that Fire Qì is able to agitate and stimulate the emotions, and these emotions generate a "mind." This mind is called Xīn (心) (i.e., heart) and is considered the fire mind, Yáng mind, or emotional mind. On the other hand, the mind that Water Qì generates is calm, steady, and wise. This mind is called Yì (意), and is considered to be the water mind or wisdom mind. If your spirit (Shén, 神) is nourished by Fire Qì, although your spirit may be high, it will be scattered and confused. This confused and excited spirit is called "Yángshén" (陽神) and means Yáng spirit. Naturally, if the spirit is nourished and raised by Water Qì, it will be firm and steady and is called "Yīnshén" (陰神), which means Yīn spirit. When your Yì is able to govern your emotional Xīn effectively, your will (strong emotional intention) can be firm.

You can see from this discussion that your Qì is the main cause of the Yīn and Yáng of your physical body, your mind, and your spirit. To regulate your body's Yīn and Yáng, you must learn how to regulate your body's Water and Fire Qì, and to do this efficiently you must know their sources.

In order to understand Kǎn and Lí clearly and to adjust them efficiently, you are urged to use the modern scientific, medical point of view to analyze the concepts. This will allow you to marry the past and present, and give birth to the future.

Yīn and Yáng Worlds (Yīn/Yáng Jiè, 陰陽界)

When the *Dàodéjīng* was written by Lǎozi about 2,500 years ago (476–221 BCE), *The Book of Changes* (*Yìjīng,* 易經) had already existed for at least seven hundred years. *The Book of Changes* has been considered the preeminent of all ancient Chinese classics (Qún-jīng Zhīshǒu, 群經之首) in Chinese history and has influenced Chinese culture heavily. Naturally, Lǎozi's mind was also influenced by this classic. Therefore, if you understand some basic concepts of *The Book of Changes*, you will see how the Yīn and Yáng spaces (Yīnjiān/Yángjiān, 陰間 / 陽間) are co-existing and related to each other. Without knowing this basic concept, you will have difficulty in understanding some of the discussion later.

According to *The Book of Changes* (*Yìjīng,* 易經), this Great Nature has two poles that balance with each other. Though there are two poles to Nature, these two are two faces of the same thing. These two poles are two spaces or dimensions, called Yīn Space (Yīnjiān, 陰間) and Yáng Space (Yángjiān, 陽間). Yīn Space is the spiritual space while Yáng Space is the material space. Yīn space is the Dào (道) while the Yáng Space, the manifestation of the Dào, is the Dé (德). These two cannot be separated but co-exist simultaneously. They mutually communicate, correspond, and influence each other. Therefore, there are two spaces, but in function, it is one. The spiritual energy of the Yīn Space can be considered the female (i.e., mother) of the myriad objects in the Yáng Space. Since humans, as well as all other objects, are formed and generated from these two spaces, a human being includes both a spiritual and material life. Since we don't actually know what the Dào (i.e., natural spirit) is, we also don't know what the human spirit is.

External Elixir and Internal Elixir (Wàidān Yǔ Nèidān, 外丹與內丹)

Chinese Qìgōng can generally be categorized into External Elixir (Wàidān, 外丹) and Internal Elixir (Nèidān, 內丹) Qìgōng. From External Elixir Qìgōng practice, a student learns how to build up the Qì to a higher level in the limbs and at the surface of the body. He then allows it to flow inward to the center of the body and the internal organs to nourish them. Through this practice, Qì circulation in the body can be improved and enhanced to achieve the goal of maintaining health. For example, physical exercise, acupuncture, acupressure, and massage are considered external elixir since the Qì is build up on skin, muscles, and limbs, then flows inward to nourish internal organs. Therefore, Eight Pieces of Brocade (Bāduànjǐn, 八段錦), Five Animal Sports (Wǔqínxì, 五禽戲), or even walking and jogging are considered external elixir.

In Internal Elixir Qìgōng practice, a practitioner will build up the Qì internally through correct breathing and meditation methods. When the Qì has been built up to an abundant level, this Qì will then be distributed outward to nourish the entire body and enhance its vital functions. For example, Small Circulation (Xiǎozhōutiān, 小周天) and Embryonic Breathing (Tāixī, 胎息) meditations are considered internal elixir.

From this information, you can see that Grand Circulation (Dàzhōutiān, 大周天) can include both External and Internal Elixirs since this category of practice may cover the movements or the tension of the physical body, but also covers still meditation for the central Qì system. As a matter of fact, a large portion of Grand Circulation practices contain both External and Internal Elixir. For example, Tàijí Ball Qìgōng (Tàijíqiú Qìgōng, 太極球氣功), Martial Qìgōng (wǔxué Qìgōng, 武學氣功), Meridian Qìgōng (jīngshāo Qìgōng, 經梢氣功), or Tàijí Qìgōng (太極氣功) are a mixture of both Internal and External Elixirs.

Experience teaches that, compared to Internal Elixir Qìgōng practice is simpler, easier, and also safer. However, the benefits that can be obtained from External Elixir practice are limited to enhancing the health of the physical body. If one wishes to reach the goal of longevity and spiritual enlightenment, Internal Elixir Qìgōng practice is essential.

Jīng, Qì, and Shén 精、氣、神

Understanding Jīng (essence, 精), Qì (internal energy, 氣), and Shén (spirit, 神) is one of the most important requirements for effective Qìgōng training. They are the root of your life and therefore also the root of Qìgōng practice. Jīng, Qì, and Shén are called "Sānbǎo" (三寶), which means "The Three Treasures," "Sānyuán" (三元), which means "The Three Origins," or "Sānběn" (三本), which means "The Three Foundations." In Qìgōng training, a practitioner learns how to "firm his Jīng" (gùjīng; 固精)—Gù means to firm, solidify, retain, and conserve—and how to convert it into Qì. This is called "liànjīng huàqì" (練精化氣), which means "to refine the Jīng and convert it into Qì." Then he learns how to lead the Qì to the head to convert it into Shén (also called nourishing Shén). This is called "liànqì huàshén" (練氣化神), which means "to refine the Qì and convert it into (nourish) the Shén." Finally, the practitioner learns to use his energized Shén to govern the emotional part of his personality. This is called "liànshén liǎoxìng" (練神了性), or "to refine the Shén to end human (emotional) nature."

These conversion processes are what enable you to gain health and longevity. As a Qìgōng practitioner, you must pay a great deal of attention to these three elements during the course of your training. If you keep these three elements strong and healthy, you will live a long and healthy life. If you neglect or abuse them, you will frequently be sick and will age prematurely. Each one of these three elements or treasures has its own root. You must know the roots so you can strengthen and protect your three treasures.

Jīng (Essence) 精

The Chinese word Jīng means a number of things depending on where, when, and how it is used. Jīng can be used as a verb, an adjective, or a noun. When it is used as a verb, it means "to refine." For example, to refine or purify a liquid to a high quality is called "jīngliàn" (精煉). When it is used as an adjective, it is used to describe or signify something which is "refined," "polished," and "pure without mixture." For example, when a piece of art work is well done, people say "jīngxì" (精細), which means "delicate and painstaking" (literally, "pure and fine") or "jīngliáng" (精良), which means "excellent quality" (literally "pure and good"). When Jīng is used to apply to personal wisdom or personality, it means "keen" and "sharp." For example, when someone is smart or wise, they are called "jīngmíng" (精明), which means "keen and clever." When Jīng is applied to a thought, it means "profound" or "astute," and indicates that the idea or plan was well and carefully considered. When used as a noun for an object, Jīng means "the essence" or "the essentials." When it is used for the energy side of a being, it means "spirit" or "ghost." Since Chinese tradition believes that the male sperm or semen is the refined and the most essential product of a man, Jīng also means sperm or semen.

When Jīng is used as "essence," it exists in everything. Jīng may be considered the primal substance or original source from which a thing is made, and which exhibits the true nature of that thing. When Jīng refers to animals or humans, it means the very original and essential source of life and growth. This Jīng is the origin of the Shén, which makes an animal different from a tree. In humans, Jīng is passed down from the parents. Sperm is called "jīngzǐ" (精子), which means "the sons of essence." When this essence is mixed with the mother's Jīng (egg), a new life is generated which, in certain fundamental respects, is an intertwinement of the Jīng of both parents. The child is formed, the Qì circulates, and the Shén grows. The Jīng that has been carried over from the parents is called "Yuánjīng" (元精), which means "Original Essence."

Once you are born, Original Jīng is the fountainhead and root of your life. It is what enables you to grow stronger and bigger. After birth you start to absorb the Jīng of food and air, converting these Jīng into the Qì that supplies your body's needs. You should understand that when Jīng is mentioned in Qìgōng society, it usually refers to Yuánjīng (Original Jīng, 元精). Qìgōng practitioners believe that Original Jīng is the most important part of you, because it is the root of your body's Qì and Shén. The quantity and quality of Original Jīng is different from person to person, and it is affected significantly by your parents' health and living habits while they were creating you. According to Chinese medicine, you probably cannot increase the amount of Jīng you have. However, it is believed that Qìgōng training can improve its quality.

In Qìgōng training, knowing how to conserve and firm your Original Jīng is of primary importance. To conserve means to refrain from abusing your Original Jīng through overuse. For example, if you are a male and overindulge in sexual activity, you will lose Original Jīng faster and your body will degenerate faster. To firm your Jīng means to keep and protect it. For example, you should know how to keep your kidneys strong. Kidneys are thought of as the residence of Original Jīng. When your kidneys are strong, the Original Jīng will be kept firm and will not be lost without reason. The firming of your Original Jīng is called "Gùjīng" (固精), which is translated "to make solid, to firm the essence."

Only after you know how to retain (meaning to conserve and firm) your Original Jīng can you start seeking ways to improve its quality. Therefore, conserving and firming your Jīng is the first step in training. You need to know the root of your Jīng, where the Original Jīng resides, and how Original Jīng is converted into Qì.

The root of your Original Jīng before your birth is in your parents. After birth, this Original Jīng stays in its residence, the kidneys, which are now also its root. When you keep this root strong, you will have plenty of Original Jīng to supply your body.

Here, you should know that the Chinese define kidneys as internal kidneys (nèishèn, 內腎) and also external kidneys (wàishèn, 外腎). Internal kidneys are the same kidneys as defined by Western medicine. However, the external kidneys mean testicles or ovaries. All of these places (i.e., glands) are capable of producing "Original Essence" (Yuánjīng, 元精) (i.e., hormones).

Qì (Inner Energy) 氣

Since we have already discussed Qì at the beginning of this chapter in general terms, we will now discuss Qì in the human body and in Qìgōng training. Please note that as of yet, there is no clear explanation of the relationship between all of the circulatory systems and the Qì circulatory system. The Western world knows of the blood system, nervous system, and lymphatic system. Now, there is the Qì circulation system from China. How are, for example, the Qì and the nervous system related? If the nervous system does not match the Qì system, where does the sensing energy in the nervous system come from? How is the lymphatic system related to the Qì system? All of these questions are still waiting for study by modern scientific methods and technology. Here, we can only offer you some theoretical assumptions based on the currently available research.

Chinese medical society believes that the Qì and blood are closely related. Where Qì goes, blood follows. That is why the term "Qìxuě" (Qì-blood, 氣血) is commonly used in Chinese medical texts. It is believed that Qì provides the energy that keeps the blood cells alive. As a matter of fact, it is believed that blood is able to store Qì and that it helps to transport Air Qì to every cell of the body.

If you look carefully, you can see that the elements of your physical body such as the organs, nerves, blood, and even every tiny cell are all like separate machines, each with their own unique function. Just like electric motors, if there is no current in them, they are dead. If you compare the routes of the blood circulatory system, the nervous system, and the lymphatic system with the course of the Qì channels, you will see that there is a great deal of correspondence. This is simply because Qì is the energy needed to keep them all alive and functioning.

Now, let us look at your body as an entire system. Your body is composed of two major parts. The first is your physical body, and the second is the energy supply your body needs to function. Your body is like a factory. The organs in your body correspond to the machines required to process raw materials into the finished product. Some of the raw materials brought into a factory are used to create the energy with which other raw materials will be converted into finished goods. The raw materials for your body are food and air, and the finished product is life.

The Qì in your body is analogous to the electric current that the factory obtains from coal or oil via a power plant. The factory has many wires connecting the power plant to the machines and other wires connecting telephones, intercoms, and computers. There are also many conveyer belts, elevators, wagons, and trucks to move material from one place to another. It is no different in your body, where there are systems of intestines, blood vessels, complex networks of nerves, and Qì channels to facilitate the supply of blood, sensory information and energy to the entire body. However, unlike the digestive, circulatory, and central nervous systems—all of whose supportive vessels can be observed as material structures in the body—Qì channels cannot be observed as physical objects. The circulatory, nervous, and Qì systems all possess similar configurations within the body and are distributed rather equally throughout the body.

In a factory, different machines require different levels of electrical current. It is the same for your organs, which require different levels of Qì. If a machine is supplied with an improper level of power, it will not function normally and may even be damaged. In the same way, when the Qì level supplied to your organs is either too positive or too negative, they will be damaged and will degenerate more rapidly.

In order for a factory to function smoothly and productively, it will not only need high quality machines, but also a reliable power supply. The same goes for your body. The quality of your organs is largely dependent on what you inherited from your parents. To maintain your organs in a healthy state and to ensure that they function well for a long time, you must have an appropriate Qì supply. If you don't have it, you will become sick.

Qì is affected by the quality of air you inhale, the kind of food you eat, your lifestyle, and even your emotional make-up and personality. Food and air are like the fuel or power supply, and their quality affects you. Your lifestyle is like the way you run the machine, and your personality is like the management of the factory.

The above metaphor clarifies the role Qì plays in your body. However, it should be noted that it is an oversimplification, and that the behavior and function of Qì is much more complex and difficult to handle than the power supply in a factory. You are neither a factory nor a robot; you are a human being with feelings and emotions. These feelings also have a major influence on your Qì circulation. For example, when you pinch yourself, the Qì in that area will be disturbed. This Qì disturbance will be sensed through the nervous system and interpreted by your brain as pain. No machine can do this. Moreover, after you have felt the pain, unlike a machine, you will react either as a result of instinct or conscious thought. Human feelings and thought affect Qì circulation in the body, whereas a machine cannot influence its power supply. In order to understand your Qì, you must use your feelings, rather than just the intellect, to sense its flow and make judgments about it.

Now a few words as to the source of Human Qì. As mentioned, Chinese doctors and Qìgōng practitioners believe that the body contains two general types of Qì. The first type is called Pre-Birth Qì or Original Qì (Yuánqì, 元氣). Original Qì is also called "Xiāntiān Qì" (先天氣) which, translated literally, means "Pre-Heaven Qì." Heaven here means the sky, so Pre-Heaven means before the baby sees the sky. In other words, before birth. Original Qì comes from converted Original Jīng (Yuánjīng, 元精), which you received before your birth. This is why Original Qì is also called Pre-Birth Qì. Once the Qì is converted, it will stay at its residence, the Lower Dāntián.

The second type is called Post-Birth Qì or "Hòutiān Qì" (後天氣), which means "Post-Heaven Qì." This Qì is drawn from the Jīng (i.e., essence) of the food and air we take in. As mentioned, the residence of the Post-Birth Qì is the Middle Dāntián. This Qì then circulates and mixes with the Pre-Birth or Dāntián Qì (Original Qì) (Yuánqì, 元氣). Together, they circulate down, passing into the Conception Vessel (Rènmài, 任脈) and Governing Vessel (Dūmài, 督脈), from where they are distributed to the entire body.

Pre-Birth Qì is commonly called "Water Qì" (Shuǐqì, 水氣) because it is able to cool down the Post-Birth Qì, which is called "Fire Qì" (Huǒqì, 火氣). Fire Qì usually brings the body to a positive (Yáng) state, which stimulates the emotions and scatters and confuses the mind. When the Water Qì cools your body down, the mind will become clear, neutral, and centered. It is believed in Qìgōng society that Fire Qì supports the emotional part of the body, while Water Qì supports the wisdom part.

After the Fire Qì and Water Qì mix, this Qì will not only circulate to the Conception Vessel (Rènmài, 任脈) and Governing Vessel (Dūmài, 督脈), but will also supply the "Thrusting Vessel" (Chōngmài, 衝脈), which will lead the Qì directly up through the spinal cord to nourish the brain and energize the Shén and soul. As will be discussed later, energizing the brain and raising the Shén are very important in Qìgōng practice.

Qì can be divided into two major categories, according to its function. The first is called "Yíngqì" (Managing Qì, 營氣), because it manages or controls the functioning of the body. This includes the functioning of the brain and the organs, and even body movement. Yíngqì is again divided into two major types. The first type circulates in the channels and is responsible for the functioning of the organs. The circulation of Qì to the organs and the extremities continues automatically as long as you have enough Qì in your reservoirs and you maintain your body in good condition. The second type of Yíngqì is linked to your Yì (mind, intention). When your Yì decides to do something, for example to lift a box, this type of Yíngqì will automatically flow to the muscles needed to do the job. This type of Qì is directed by your thoughts and is therefore closely related to your feelings and emotions.

The second major category of Qì is "Wèiqì" (Guardian Qì, 衛氣). Wèiqì forms a shield on the surface of the body to protect you from negative outside influences. Wèiqì is also involved in the growth of hair, the repair of skin injuries, and many other functions on the surface of the skin. Wèiqì comes from the Qì channels and is led through millions of tiny channels to the surface of the skin. This Qì can even extend beyond the body. When your body is positive (Yáng), this Qì is strong, and your pores will be open. When your body is negative (Yīn), this Qì is weak, and your pores will close up to preserve Qì.

In the summertime, your body is Yáng and your Qì is strong, so your Qì shield will be bigger and extend beyond your physical body, and the pores will be wide open. In the wintertime, your body is relatively Yīn (negative), and you must conserve your Qì in order to stay warm and keep pathogens out. The Qì shield is smaller and doesn't extend out much beyond your skin.

Wèiqì functions automatically in response to changes in the environment, but it is also influenced significantly by your feelings and emotions. For example, when you feel happy or angry, the Qì shield will be more open than when you are sad.

In order to keep your body healthy and functioning properly, you must keep the Yíngqì functioning smoothly and, at the same time, keep the Wèiqì strong to protect you from negative outside influences such as the cold. Chinese doctors and Qìgōng practitioners believe that the key to doing this is through Shén. Shén is considered to be the headquarters that directs and controls the Qì. Therefore, when you practice Qìgōng you must understand what your Shén is and know how to raise it. When people are ill and facing death, very often the ones with a strong Shén, which is indicative of a strong will to live, will survive. The people who are apathetic or depressed will generally not last long. A strong will to live raises the Shén, which energizes the body's Qì and keeps you alive and healthy.

In order to raise your Shén, you must first nourish your brain with Qì. This Qì energizes the brain so that you can concentrate more effectively. Your mind will then be steady, your will strong, and your Shén raised.

As a Qìgōng practitioner, in addition to paying attention to the food and air you take in, it is important for you to learn how to generate Water Qì and how to use it more effectively. Water Qì can cool down the Fire Qì and, therefore, slow down the degeneration of the body. Water Qì also helps to calm your mind and keep it centered. This allows you to judge things objectively. During Qìgōng practice, you can sense your Qì and direct it effectively.

In order to generate Water Qì and use it efficiently, you must know how and where it is generated. Since Water Qì comes from the conversion of Original Jīng, they have both the kidneys for their root. Once Water Qì is generated, it resides in the Lower Dāntián below your navel. In order to conserve your Water Qì, you must keep your kidneys firm and strong.

Shén (Spirit) 神

It is very difficult to find an English word to exactly express Shén. As in so many other cases, the context determines the translation. Shén can be translated as spirit, god, immortal, soul, mind, divine, and supernatural.

When you are alive, Shén is the spirit that is directed by your mind. When your mind is not steady it is said that "Xīnshén Bùníng" (心神不寧), which means "the (emotional) mind and spirit are not at peace." The average person can use his emotional mind to energize and stimulate his Shén to a higher state, but at the same time he must restrain his emotional mind (Xīn, 心) with his wisdom mind (Yì, 意). If his Yì can control the Xīn, the mind as a whole will be concentrated and the Yì can govern the Shén. When someone's Shén is excited, however, it is not being controlled by his Yì, so we say, "Shénzhì Bùqīng" (神志不清), which means "the spirit and the will (generated from Yì) are not clear." In Qìgōng it is very important for you to train your wisdom Yì to control your emotional Xīn effectively. In order to reach this goal, Buddhists and Daoists train themselves to be free of emotions. Only in this way are they able to build a strong Shén that is completely under their control.

When you are healthy you are able to use your Yì to protect your Shén and keep it at its residence: the Upper Dāntián. Even when your Shén is energized, it is still controlled. However, when you are very sick or near death, your Yì becomes weak and your Shén will leave its residence and wander around. When you are dead, your Shén separates completely from the physical body. It is then called a "Hún" (魂) (soul). Often the term "Shénhún" (神魂) is used, since the Hún originated with the Shén. Sometimes "Shénhún" is also used to refer to the spirit of a dying person since his spirit is between "Shén" and "Hún."

The Chinese believe that when your Shén reaches a higher and stronger state, you are able to sense and feel more sharply, and your mind is cleverer and more inspired. The world of living human beings is usually considered a Yáng world (Yángjiān, 陽間), and the spirit world after death is considered a Yīn world (Yīnjiān, 陰間). When your Shén has reached its higher, more sensitive state, you can transcend your mind's normal capacity. Ideas beyond your usual grasp can be understood and controlled, and you may develop the ability to sense or even communicate with the Yīn world. This supernatural Shén is called "Líng" (靈). "Líng" describes someone who is sharp, clever, nimble, and able to quickly empathize with people and things. It is believed that when you die this supernatural Shén will not die with your body right away. It is this supernatural Shén (Língshén, 靈神) that still holds your energy together as a "ghost" (Guǐ, 鬼). Therefore, a ghost is also called "Língguǐ" (靈鬼) meaning "spiritual ghost" or "Línghún" (靈魂) meaning "spiritual soul."

From this you can see that Líng is the supernatural part of the spirit. It is believed that if this supernatural spiritual soul is strong enough, it will live for a long time after the physical body is dead and have plenty of opportunity to reincarnate. Chinese people believe that if a person has reached the stage of enlightenment and Buddhahood when he is alive, after he dies this supernatural spirit will leave the cycle of reincarnation and live forever. These spirits are called "Shénmíng" (神明), which means "spiritually enlightened beings," or simply "Shén" (神), which here implies that this spirit has become divine. Normally, if you die and your supernatural spiritual soul is not strong, your spirit has only a short time to search for a new residence in which to be reborn before its energy disperses. In this case, the spirit is called "Guǐ" (鬼), which means "ghost."

Buddhists and Daoists believe that when you are alive you may use your Jīng and Qì to nourish the Shén (Yǎngshén, 養神) and make your Líng strong. When this "Língshén" (靈神) is built up to a high level, your will is able to lead it to separate from the physical body even while you are alive. When you have reached this stage, your physical body is able to live for many hundreds of years. People who can do this are called "Xiān" (仙), which means "immortal," "god," or "fairy." Since "Xiān" originated with the Shén, the "Xiān" is sometimes called "Shénxiān" (神仙), which means "immortal spirit." The "Xiān" is a living person whose Shén has reached the stage of enlightenment or Buddhahood. After his death, his spirit will be called "Shénmíng" (神明).

The foundation of Buddhist and Daoist Qìgōng training is to firm your Shén, nourish it, and grow it until it is mature enough to separate from your physical body. In order to do this, the Qìgōng practitioner must know where the Shén resides and how to keep, protect, nourish, and train it. It is also essential for you to know the root or origin of your Shén.

Your Shén resides in the Upper Dāntián (i.e., brain). When you keep your Yì (i.e., attention) in the Limbic System at the center of your head, the Shén can be firmed. This center is called "Shén Dwelling" (Shénshì, 神室) or Mud Pill Palace (Níwángōng, 泥丸宮) in Chinese Qìgōng. Firm here means to keep and to protect. When someone's mind is scattered and confused, his Shén wanders. This is called "Shén Bù Shǒushè" (神不守舍), which means "the spirit is not kept at its residence."

According to Qìgōng theory, though your Xīn (Emotional Mind, 心) is able to raise up your spirit, this mind can also make your Shén confused, so that it leaves its residence. You must constantly engage your Yì (Wisdom Mind) to restrain and control your Shén at its residence.

In Qìgōng, when your Qì can reach and nourish your Shén efficiently, your Shén will be energized to a higher level and, in turn, conduct the Qì in its circulation. Shén is the force that keeps you alive, and it is also the control tower for the Qì. When your Shén is strong, your Qì is strong and you can lead it efficiently. When your Shén is weak, your Qì is weak and the body will degenerate rapidly. Likewise, Qì supports the Shén, energizing it and keeping it sharp, clear, and strong. If the Qì in your body is weak, your Shén will also be weak.

Once you know the residence of your Shén, you must understand the root of your Shén and learn how to nourish it and make it grow. We have already discussed Original Essence (Yuánjīng, 元精), which is the essential life inherited from your parents. After your birth, this Original Essence is your most important energy source. Your Original Qì (Yuánqì, 元氣) is created from this Original Essence, and it mixes with the Qì generated from the food you eat and the air you breathe to supply the energy for your growth and activity. Naturally, this mixed Qì is nourishing your Shén as well. While the Fire Qì will energize your Shén, Water Qì will strengthen the wisdom mind to control the energized Shén. The Shén that is kept in its residence by the Yì, that is nourished by the Original Qì, is called Original Shén (Yuánshén, 元神). Therefore, the root of your Original Shén is traced back to your Original Essence. When your Shén is energized but restrained by your Yì it is called "Jīngshén" (精神), literally "Essence Shén," which is commonly translated "Spirit of Vitality."

Original Shén is thought of as the center of your being. It is able to make you calm, clear your mind, and firm your will. When you concentrate your mind on doing something, it is called "Jùjīng Huìshén" (聚精會神), which means "gathering your Jīng to meet your Shén." This implies that when you concentrate, you must use your Original Essence to meet and lift up your Original Shén, so that your mind will be calm, steady, and concentrated. Since this Shén is nourished by your Original Qì, which is considered Water Qì, Original Shén is considered Water Shén.

For those who have reached a higher level of Qìgōng practice, cultivating the Shén becomes the most important subject. For Buddhists and Daoists the final goal of cultivating the Shén is to form or generate a Holy Embryo (Xiāntāi, 仙胎) from their Shén and nourish it until the spiritual baby is born and can be independent. For the average Qìgōng practitioner, however, the final goal of cultivating Shén is to raise up the Shén through Qì nourishment while maintaining control with the Yì. This raised-up Shén can direct and govern the Qì efficiently to achieve health and longevity.

In conclusion, we would like to point out that your Shén and brain cannot be separated. Shén is the spiritual part of your being and is generated and controlled by your mind. The mind generates the will, which keeps the Shén firm. The Chinese commonly use Shén (spirit) and Zhì (will) together as "Shénzhì" (神志) because they are so related. In addition, you should understand that when your Shén is raised and firm, this raised spirit will firm your will. They are mutually related and assist each other. From this you can see that the material foundation of the spirit is your brain. When it is said "nourish your Shén," it means "nourish your brain." As we discussed previously, the original nourishing source is your Jīng. This Jīng is then converted into Qì, which is led to the brain to nourish and energize it. In Qìgōng practice, this process is called "Fǎnjīng Bǔnǎo" (返精補腦), which means "to return the Jīng to nourish the brain."

About Muscle/Tendon Changing and Marrow/Brain Washing Qìgōng

It is extremely important, before you read any further, to have a general concept of the Muscle/Tendon Changing and Marrow/Brain Washing Qìgōng (*Yìjīnjīng/Xǐsuǐjīng*, 易筋經/洗髓經). These two ancient Qìgōng practices have significantly influenced Chinese religious and martial arts Qìgōng society. Furthermore, these two practices provide you the crucial keys to health, longevity, and enlightenment. Without knowing these two practices, your understanding of Grand Circulation in this book will be shallow. In this section, we will briefly explain these two Qìgōng practices. If you wish to know more about history, theory, and training of these two Qìgōngs, please refer to the book, *Qìgōng, The Secret of Youth*, published by YMAA Publication Center.

In this subsection, we will first introduce Dámó (達摩), the Indian monk who brought these practices to China. After that, we will summarize the meaning of *Yìjīnjīng* and *Xǐsuǐjīng* and characterize the purposes of these two trainings. Finally, we will point out the Kǎn (坎) and Lí (離) training in these two Qìgōng practices.

Dámó 達摩

Dámó (Dharma) (達摩), whose last name was Sārdìlì (Kshatriya) (剎帝利) and who was also known as Bodhidarma, was once a prince of a small tribe in southern India. He was of the Mahayana school of Buddhism and was considered by many to have been a bodhisattva, or an enlightened being who had renounced nirvana in order to save others. From the fragments of historical records, it is believed he was born about 483 CE. At that time, India was considered a spiritual center by the Chinese, since it was the source of Buddhism, which was still very influential in China. Many of the Chinese emperors either sent priests to India to study Buddhism and bring back scriptures, or else they invited Indian priests to come to China to preach. It is believed that Dámó was the second Indian priest to be invited to China.

Dámó was invited to China to preach by Emperor Liáng in 527 CE (Liángwǔdì, Dàtóng first year, 梁武帝大同一年 or Wèixiàomíngdì Xiàochāng third year, 魏孝明帝孝昌三年). When the emperor decided he did not like Dámó's Buddhist theory, the monk withdrew to the Shàolín Temple (Shàolínsì, 少林寺). When Dámó arrived, he saw that the priests were weak and sickly, so he shut himself away to ponder the problem. When he emerged after nine years of seclusion, he wrote two classics: *Yìjīnjīng* (易筋經) (Muscle/Tendon Changing Classic) and *Xǐsuǐjīng* (洗髓經) (Marrow/Brain Washing Classic).

What Are Yìjīnjīng and Xǐsuǐjīng?

Yì (易) means "to change, to replace, or to alter," Jīn (筋) means "muscles and tendons," and Jīng (經) means "classic or bible." Therefore, it is commonly translated as "Muscle Changing Classic, Tendon Changing Classic," or "Muscle/Tendon Changing Classic." "Muscles and tendons" do not refer only to the literal muscles and tendons. It actually refers to all of the physical system that is related to the muscles and tendons, including the internal organs. The *Yìjīnjīng* describes Qìgōng theory and training methods that are able to improve your physical body and change it from weak to strong. Naturally, these methods are also very effective in maintaining your physical health.

Xǐ (洗) means "to wash" or "to clean." Suǐ (髓) includes "Gǔsuǐ" (骨髓), which means "bone marrow," and "Nǎosuǐ" (腦髓), which refers to "the brain, including limbic system, cerebrum, cerebellum, and medulla oblongata." Jīng (經) means "classic or bible." This work is commonly translated "Marrow Washing Classic," but "Marrow/Brain Washing Classic" is a more accurate translation. The first translation probably became less popular because of a misunderstanding of the scope of the work, which had been kept secret for a long period of time. Also, the goal of "brain washing" is enlightenment or Buddhahood, which, in addition to being difficult to understand, is less interesting to laymen. It was not until recently, when many of the secret documents were made available to the general public, that a clearer and more complete picture of the training emerged. A correct translation shows that *Xǐsuǐjīng* training deals with the bone marrow and the brain. However, the training does not actually focus on the physical matter of the bone marrow and the brain. Instead, it emphasizes how to lead the Qì to the bone marrow and brain to nourish them and keep them functioning at an optimal level. The final goals are to obtain longevity and reach spiritual enlightenment. However, the most important part of *Xǐsuǐjīng* is learning how to wash the negative thoughts from our genetic memory, such as domination, killing, enslaving, raping, greediness, and selfishness. These memories have been instilled from oft repeated and constantly occurring incidences throughout human history, and they continue to obstruct our spiritual evolution.

The major difference between these two classics and the traditional Chinese method was Dámó's teaching that the training of the physical body was just as important as the spiritual cultivation. Without a strong and healthy body, the final goal of spiritual cultivation was hard to reach. This is called "dual cultivation of temperament and physical life" (Xìngmìng Shuāngxiū, 性命雙修) in Qìgōng society. Though his new training theory was resisted by many Buddhists, many others believed his theory and started to train. The Shàolín Temple (Shàolínsì, 少林寺) became a center for teaching his theories, and soon after his death they had spread to every corner of China. His Chán (禪) meditation was exported to Japan, where it became known as Rěn (忍).

THE PURPOSES OF THE YÌJĪNJĪNG AND XǏSUǏJĪNG

There is a section in the documents that talks about the general purposes of the *Yìjīnjīng* and *Xǐsuǐjīng*. It is translated here for your reference.

> *Yìjīn Gōngfū is able to change the tendons and shape, Xǐsuǐ Gōngfū is able to change the marrow and Shén (spirit). (They are) especially capable of increasing spiritual bravery, spiritual power, spiritual wisdom, and spiritual intelligence. Its training methods, compared with the Daoist family's Liànjīng (train Essence), Liànqì (train Qì), and Liànshén (train Spirit), are repeatedly mutually related in many ways, and its Yì (i.e., goal or intention) of practice is completely the same.*

易筋功夫，可換筋換形；洗髓功夫，可換髓換神；尤可增加神
勇、神力、神智、神慧。其功法與道家之練精、練氣、練神，亦
復脈脈相通，而用意則全同。

THE PURPOSE OF THE YÌJĪNJĪNG

The main purpose of *Yìjīnjīng* training is to change the physical body from weak to strong and from sick to healthy. In order to reach this goal, the physical body must be stimulated and exercised, and the Qì in the energy body must be regulated. The main goals of the training are:

A. To open up the Qì channels and maintain the appropriate level of smooth Qì circulation in the twelve primary Qì channels or meridians (Shíèrjīng, 十二經). This maintains the health and proper functioning of the related organs. Smooth Qì circulation also makes it possible to greatly strengthen the physical body.

B. To fill up the Qì in the two main Qì reservoirs—the Conception and Governing Vessels (Rènmài and Dūmài, 任脈 · 督脈) (i.e., *Yìjīnjīng* Small Circulation) (*Yìjīnjīng* Xiǎozhōutiān, 易筋經小周天). The Conception Vessel is responsible for regulating the six Yīn channels, while the Governing Vessel governs the six Yáng channels. When an abundant supply of Qì is stored in these two vessels, the twelve primary channels can be regulated effectively.

C. To open the small Qì branches from the primary channels to the surface of the skin and maintain healthy conditions for the muscles and skin.

D. For those who also wish to train *Xǐsuǐjīng* and reach a higher level, to build up the necessary level of Qì.

THE PURPOSE OF THE XǏSUǏJĪNG

The main purposes of *Xǐsuǐjīng* training are to use the abundant Qì generated from *Yìjīnjīng* training to wash the marrow, to nourish the brain, and to fill up the Qì in the other six vessels. The main goals of the training are:

A. To keep the Qì at an abundant level and continue to build up the Qì to a higher level from other sources. An abundant Qì supply is the key to successful Marrow Washing and nourishing of the brain for raising the spirit. Experience has shown that the genitals can be an important source of extra Qì. Therefore, one of the main goals of *Xǐsuǐjīng* training is learning how to increase the production of semen Essence and improving the efficiency of its conversion into Qì.

B. In order to keep an abundant supply of Qì, the fuel (Original Essence, 元精) must be conserved, protected, and firmed. Therefore, the second purpose of *Xǐsuǐjīng* is to regulate the usage of Original Essence.

C. Learning how to lead Qì to the marrow to keep the marrow fresh and to lead Qì to the brain to raise the Spirit of Vitality. Marrow is the factory which produces your red and white blood cells; when the marrow is fresh and clean, the blood will be healthy. As this blood flows to every part of your body, the metabolism of your body will be carried out healthily and smoothly. Practicing *Xǐsuǐjīng* can therefore slow down the aging process. When the brain has plenty of Qì to nourish it, you are able to maintain the normal functioning of your brain and also raise up the Spirit of Vitality. When the spirit is raised, the Qì in the body can be governed effectively.

D. For a sincere Buddhist or Daoist monk, the final goal of *Xǐsuǐjīng* is reaching enlightenment or Buddhahood. For them, the training purposes listed above are considered temporary. They are only steps in the process of building up their "spiritual baby" (Língtái, 靈胎) and nurturing it until it is independent and has eternal life. The crucial step of reaching this goal is to wash off or control those evil genetic memories that are hanging in our subconscious mind continuously. Without knowing how to govern the continuous development of these thoughts, the conscious and emotional mind will continue to dominate our being and obstruct our spiritual evolution.

From this brief summary, it is clear that the *Yìjīnjīng* and *Xǐsuǐjīng* can change both your physical and spiritual qualities and lead you to a higher level of physical and spiritual life.

Kǎn and Lí in Yìjīnjīng and Xǐsuǐjīng (Yìjīnjīng Hé Xǐsuǐjīng Zhī Kǎn-Lí, 易筋經和洗髓經之坎離)

Yìjīnjīng and *Xǐsuǐjīng* trainings are based on the concept of Yīn and Yáng. The *Yìjīnjīng* is Lí (fire) because it generates Qì and manifests it as physical strength (Muscle/Tendon Changing), thus generating Yáng. The *Xǐsuǐjīng* is Kǎn (water), because it utilizes and stores the Qì in the marrow/brain and generates Yīn. The *Yìjīnjīng* deals with the muscles/tendons and skin, which are visible externally, while the *Xǐsuǐjīng* deals with the marrow and brain, which must be felt internally. While the *Yìjīnjīng* training emphasizes the physical body, the *Xǐsuǐjīng* training focuses on the spiritual body. Therefore, Yīn and Yáng are balanced and coexist harmoniously.

In the *Yìjīnjīng*, the physical stimulation and exercises are considered Lí and cause the body to become Yáng, while the still meditation of the Small Circulation is Kǎn, which counterbalances the Lí and makes the body more Yīn. Again, in the physical stimulation Lí training, external strength is Lí while internal mental strength is Kǎn. In still meditation, the physical body is still and is Kǎn, while the Qì moving inside and led by the mind is Lí.

The same theory prevails in *Xǐsuǐjīng* training. The physical stimulation to increase the Original Essence production is Lí, while the techniques of internal cultivation that are used to lead the Qì to the marrow and brain are Kǎn.

You can see from this discussion that the basic key to successful Qìgōng training is Yīn and Yáng balance, and the trick to reaching this goal is Kǎn and Lí adjustment. Once you understand this fundamental theory, you will not have too much difficulty understanding the foundation of Qìgōng practice.

1.4 Body's Qì Network—Qìgōng Science (Réntǐ Qìwǎng—Qìgōng Kēxué, 人體氣網－氣功科學)

In this section, I would like to summarize the essential structures of the human Qì network. Without knowing these crucial structures, you will encounter many questions when you read the following chapters of this book. In this section, we will cover the following topics:

1. Two Poles in a Human Body 人身兩儀 (Rénshēn Liǎngyí)
2. Qì Channels and Vessels 經絡與氣脈 (Jīngluò Yǔ Qìmài)
3. Upper and Lower Bodies 上半身與下半身 (Shàngbànshēn Yǔ Xiàbànshēn)
4. Qì Cavities 氣穴 (Qìxuè)
5. Two Chambers and Two Pumps of Life 人體二會聽與二泵 (Réntǐ Èr Huìtīng Yǔ Èr Bèng)
6. False and Real Lower Dāntián 假/真下丹田 (Jiǎ/Zhēn Xiàdāntián)
7. Guardian Qì and Marrow Qì 衛氣與髓氣 (Wèiqì Yǔ Suǐqì)
8. Spiritual Triangle 練神三角塔 (Liànshén Sānjiǎotǎ)

Two Poles in a Human Body

As discussed earlier, we have three Dāntiáns. The top (Upper Dāntián) (Shàng Dāntián, 上丹田) and the bottom (Real Lower Dāntián) (Zhēn Xiàdāntián, 真下丹田) ones establish a two-pole system which constitute a human central energy line (i.e., Human Qì polarity). These two poles, one Yīn and one Yáng, synchronize and harmonize with each other. They are just like the polarities of a magnet which cannot be separated. The Real Lower Dāntián (human gut or second brain) is the north pole that stores Qì and supplies it for the functioning of the entire body. The Upper Dāntián (brain) is the south pole that directs and governs the quality of Qì manifestation.

When we compare these two poles with the Tàijí Yīn-Yáng symbol, we can easily see that the spirit (Shén, 神) residing in the Upper Dāntián is classified as Yáng since it manifests the Qì into action. That is why the spirit is called "Yángshén" (陽神) in Chinese Qigong society. The area located in the Real Lower Dāntián or Huìyīn (Co-1) (會陰) (perineum) is called "Sea Bottom" (Hǎidǐ, 海底) and is classified as Yīn, where it is able to store Qì to an abundant level. The Qì stored in the Real Lower Dāntián is thus called "Yīnshuǐ" (陰水), which means "Yīn water" (Figure 1-4). It was believed that this Yīn water originates from the Original Essence (Yuánjīng, 元精) stored in the internal kidneys (Nèishèn, 內腎) and external kidneys (Wàishèn, 外腎). External kidneys are testicles or

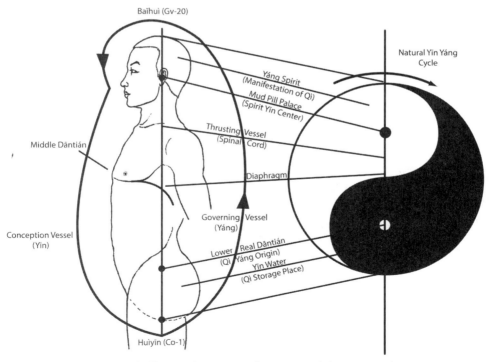

Figure 1-4. The Body's Yīn and Yáng, and the Two Poles.

ovaries. In fact, it is understood that the Original Essence is actually the hormones produced from the adrenals of the internal kidneys and also from the gonads of the testicles and ovaries. For this reason, the water (Qì) produced in these glands is often called "kidneys' water" (Shènshuǐ, 腎水).

However, from another point of view, we can see that since the Real Lower Dāntián supplies the quantity of Qì, it can be considered to be Yáng, while the spirit that governs the quality of Qì manifestation can thus be considered to be Yīn. From this, you can see how Yīn and Yáng are defined according to different points of view. If we take a closer look, we can see this viewpoint clearly.

Again, if you observe the Tàijí Yīn-Yáng symbol closely, you can see that there is a hidden Yáng fountain (Yángquán, 陽泉) in the center of the Yīn water while there is a concealed Yīn spirit (Yīnshén, 陰神) in the center of the Yáng spirit. In fact, in Qìgōng Embryonic Breathing training, you train these two centers (i.e., poles of human polarity) of hidden Yáng and concealed Yīn. For example, if you are able to keep your mind at the center of the hidden Yáng in the Yīn water, the Qì at the Real Lower Dāntián will continue to be stored and preserved. It is just like a spring or a fountain that is able to produce water continuously.

The spirit Yīn Center (i.e., upper pole) is just like a steering wheel that is able to govern the status of the Shén's actions. If the Shén can stay at this center, then it can be focused and centered. That means if you know how to keep the spirit condensed at its center (i.e., concealed Yīn), then the quality of Qì manifestation will reach a higher level of efficiency. If the Shén is away from this center, then it is scattered. When this happens, even if the Shén is high, it is not focused. In order to bring the Shén to this Yīn center, first your mind must be calmed. To keep your mind calm, you must avoid any emotional disturbance and desires. This is one of the main focus points in Qìgōng Embryonic Breathing.

The lower pole is at the Real Lower Dāntián located at the center of the Large and Small Intestines (i.e., second brain). This area acts as a biobattery that is able to store the Qì (bioelectricity). It is in this area that the food essence is absorbed and converted into energy (Qì). In order to keep the Qì at its residence, you must also learn how to keep your mind at this Qì Yáng Origin (i.e., Real Lower Dāntián or Center of Gravity). Here is the place where the Qì can be preserved and stored to an abundant level (Yáng).

In summary, these are two concealed poles, one at the center of the head (Mud Pill Palace) (Níwángōng, 泥丸宮) (Shén residence) (Shénshì, 神室) and the other at the center of the gut (Qì dwelling) (Qìshè, 氣舍). Though they are two, they function as one. If you are able to keep your mind at these two poles, the spirit and the Qì will stay in their residences. This process is called "Embracing Singularity" (Bàoyī, 抱一).

Qì Channels and Vessels (Jīngluò Yǔ Qìmài, 經絡與氣脈)

PRIMARY AND SECONDARY QÌ CHANNELS (JĪNG YǓ LUÒ, 經與絡)

The Chinese have discovered that the human body has twelve primary Qì channels (Shíèrjīng, 十二經) (also called Meridians) that branch out with countless secondary channels (Luò, 絡). This is similar to the blood circulatory system in the body. The primary channels are like arteries and veins while the secondary channels are like capillaries. The twelve primary channels are like rivers and the secondary channels are like streams which branch out from rivers. From this network, the Qì is distributed throughout the entire body, connecting the extremities (fingers and toes) to the internal organs and also the skin to the bone marrow. Here you should understand that *the "internal organs" of Chinese medicine do not necessarily correspond to the physical organs as understood in the West, but rather to a set of clinical functions similar to each other and related to the organ system.*

When a person is sick, his Qì level tends to be either too positive (excessive, Yáng, 陽) or too negative (deficient, Yīn, 陰). A Chinese physician would either use a prescription of herbs to adjust the Qì, or else he would insert acupuncture needles at various spots on the channels to inhibit the flow in some channels and stimulate the flow in others, so that balance could be restored. However, there is another alternative, and that is to use certain physical and mental exercises to adjust the Qì. In other words, to use Qìgōng exercises.

You should also know the Yīn/Yáng classifications of the organs. There are six Yáng organs and six Yīn organs. Each Yáng organ is associated with a Yīn organ by a special Yīn/Yáng relationship. Pairs of Yīn and Yáng organs belong to the same phase in the Five Phases (Wǔxíng, 五行); their channels are sequential to each other in the circulation of Qì, their functions are closely related, and disease in one usually affects the other. In Chinese medicine, the channel corresponding to the Yáng organ is often used to treat disorders of its related Yīn organ.

In the limbs, the Yáng channels are on the external side of the limbs while the Yīn channels are on the internal side. Generally speaking, the outsides of the limbs are more Yáng and are more resistant and prepared for an attack, while the internal sides are more Yin and weaker.

The organs are further subdivided in order to distinguish the different levels of the Yīn/Yáng characteristics. The Yáng organs are divided into Greater Yáng (Tàiyáng, 太陽), Lesser Yáng (Shàoyáng, 少陽), and Yáng Brightness (Yángmíng, 陽明). The Yīn organs are divided into Greater Yīn (Tàiyīn, 太陰), Lesser Yīn (Shàoyīn, 少陰), and Absolute Yīn (Juéyīn, 厥陰).

These Twelve Primary Qì Channels are:

The Lung Channel of Hand—Greater Yīn 手太陰肺經 (Shǒu Tàiyīn Fèijīng)

The Large Intestine Channel of Hand—Yáng Brightness 手陽明大腸經 (Shǒu Yáng-míng Dàchángjīng)

The Stomach Channel of Foot—Yáng Brightness 足陽明胃經 (Zú Yángmíng Wèijīng)

The Spleen Channel of Foot—Greater Yīn 足太陰脾經 (Zú Tàiyīn Píjīng)

The Heart Channel of Hand—Lesser Yīn 手少陰心經 (Shǒu Shàoyīn Xīnjīng)

The Small Intestine Channel of Hand—Greater Yáng 手太陽小腸經 (Shǒu Tàiyáng Xiǎochángjīng)

The Urinary Bladder Channel of Foot—Greater Yáng 足太陽膀胱經 (Zú Tàiyáng Pángguāngjīng)

The Kidney Channel of Foot—Lesser Yīn 足少陰腎經 (Zú Shàoyīn Shènjīng)

The Pericardium Channel of Hand—Absolute Yīn 手厥陰心包絡經 (Shǒu Juéyīn Xīnbāoluòjīng)

The Triple Burner Channel of Hand—Lesser Yáng 手少陽三焦經 (Shǒu Shàoyáng Sānjiāojīng)

The Gall Bladder Channel of Foot—Lesser Yáng 足少陽膽經 (Zú Shàoyáng Dǎnjīng)

The Liver Channel of Foot—Absolute Yīn 足厥陰肝經 (Zú Juéyīn Gānjīng)

If you are interested to know more about these twelve primary Qì channels, please refer to acupuncture books.

THE EIGHT VESSELS (BĀMÀI, 八脈)

The first brief mention of some of these eight vessels is found in the second part of the *Nèijīng* (內經) chapter of the book *Huángdì Nèijīng Sùwèn* (*Plain Questions: Yellow Emperor's Internal Canon of Medicine*, 黃帝內經素問) (Hàn Dynasty, circa 100–300 BCE) by Líng Shū (靈樞) (*Miraculous Pivot*). Also, some of the vessels were mentioned in Biǎn Què's (扁鵲) classic *Nànjīng* (*Classic on Disorders*, 難經) (Qín and Hàn Dynasties, 221 BCE–220 CE, 秦、漢). It was not until the sixteenth century that all eight vessels were deeply studied by Lǐ, Shí-Zhēn (1518–1593 CE, 李時珍) and revealed in his book *Qíjīng Bāmài Kǎo* (奇經八脈考) (*Deep Study of the Extraordinary Eight Vessels*). From then until only recently, very few documents have been published on this subject. Although there has been more research published in the last few years, there is still no single document that is able to define this subject systematically and in depth.

The eight vessels are called "Qíjīng Bāmài" (奇經八脈). "Qí" (奇) means "odd, strange, or mysterious." "Jīng" (經) means "meridian or channels." "Bā" (八) means "eight" and "Mài" (脈) means "vessels." Qíjīng Bāmài is then translated as "Odd Meridians and Eight Vessels" or "extraordinary meridian (EM)." Odd has a meaning of strange in Chinese. It is used simply because these eight vessels are not well understood yet. Many Chinese doctors explain that they are called "Odd" simply because there are four vessels that are not paired. Since these eight vessels also serve the function of homeostasis, sometimes they are called "Homeostatic Meridians." French acupuncturists call them "Miraculous Meridians" because they were able to create therapeutic effects when all other techniques had failed. In addition, because each of these channels exerts a strong effect upon psychic functioning and individuality, the command points are among the most important psychological points in the body. For this reason, they are occasionally called "The Eight Psychic Channels."

These vessels are: 1. Governing Vessel (Dūmài, 督脈); 2. Conception Vessel (Rènmài, 任脈); 3. Thrusting Vessel (Chōngmài, 衝脈); 4. Girdle (or Belt) Vessel (Dàimài, 帶脈); 5. Yáng Heel Vessel (Yángqiāomài, 陽蹻脈); 6. Yīn Heel Vessel (Yīnqiāomài, 陰蹻脈); 7. Yáng Linking Vessel (Yángwéimài, 陽維脈); and 8. Yīn Linking Vessel (Yīnwéimài, 陰維脈).

The general functions of the eight vessels are:

A. Serve as Qì Reservoirs. Because the eight vessels are so different from each other, it is difficult to generalize their characteristics and functions. However, one of the most common characteristics of the eight vessels was specified by Biǎn Què (扁鵲) in his *Nàn-jīng* (*Classic on Disorders*, 難經). He reported that the twelve organ-related Qì channels constitute rivers, and the eight extraordinary vessels constitute reservoirs. The reservoirs, especially the Conception and Governing Vessels (Rènmài/Dūmài, 任脈/督脈), absorb excess Qì from the main channels, and then return it when they are deficient.

You should understand, however, that because of the limited number of traditional documents, as well as the lack of modern, scientific methods of Qì research, it is difficult to determine the precise behavior and characteristics of these eight vessels. The main difficulty probably lies in the fact that they can be taken at different levels, because they perform different functions and contain every kind of Qì such as Yíngqì (營氣), Wèiqì (衛氣), Jīngqì (精氣), and even blood.

When the twelve primary channels are deficient in Qì, the eight vessels will supply it. This store of Qì can easily be tapped with acupuncture needles through those cavities that connect the eight vessels with the twelve channels. The connection cavities behave like the gate of a reservoir, which can be used to adjust the strength of the Qì flow in the rivers and the level of Qì in the reservoir. Sometimes, when it is necessary, the reservoir will release Qì by itself. For example, when a person has had a shock, either physically or mentally, the Qì in some of the main channels will be deficient. This will cause particular organs to be stressed, and Qì will accumulate rapidly around these organs. When this happens, the reservoir must release Qì to increase the deficient circulation and prevent further damage.

B. Guarding Specific Areas against "Evil Qì" (Xiéqì, 邪氣). The Qì that protects the body from outside intruders is called "Wèiqì" (衛氣) (Guardian Qì). Among the eight vessels, the Thrusting Vessel (Chōngmai 衝脈), the Governing Vessel (Dūmài, 督脈), the Conception Vessel (Rènmài, 任脈), and the Girdle Vessel (Dàimài, 帶脈) play major roles in guarding the abdomen, thorax, and the back.

C. Regulating the Changes of Life Cycles. According to Chapter 1 of *"Sùwèn"* (素問) (*Plain Questions*), the Thrusting Vessel (Chōngmai 衝脈) and the Conception Vessel (Rènmài, 任脈) also regulate the changes of the life cycles that occur at seven-year intervals for women and eight-year intervals for men.

D. Circulating Jīngqì to the Entire Body, Particularly the Five "Ancestral Organs." One of the most important functions of the eight vessels is to deliver Jīngqì (Essence Qì, 精氣) that has been converted from Original Essence and sexual Essence to the entire body, including the skin and hair. They must also deliver Jīngqì to the five ancestral organs: the brain and spinal cord, the liver and gall bladder system, the bone marrow, the uterus, and the blood system.

Upper and Lower Bodies (Shàngbànshēn Yǔ Xiàbànshēn, 上半身與下半身)

The Chinese Qìgōng concept of upper body and lower body is somewhat different from the Western concept. Usually, to a Westerner, the dividing point of the upper and lower body is the waist area where the center of gravity is. This is from a physical view point since the waist area is where the physical center is located. However, to a Chinese medical doctor or Qìgōng practitioner, the dividing line is actually the diaphragm. This is from the Qì distribution point of view.

The diaphragm is composed of good electric conductive material while the top and the bottom of it are covered and insulated by fasciae, a poor conductive material. From this structure, you can see it as the structure of a battery since the Qì or bioelectricity can be stored at the diaphragm. The diaphragm is considered to be the Middle Dāntián (Zhōng Dāntián, 中丹田). It is believed that the Qì stored here is related to the food and air you absorb. For example, if you eat a lot of hot spicy food, the Middle Dāntián will be on fire and trigger heartburn and cause the heart to beat faster. As matter of fact, the heart is often considered as part of the Middle Dāntián in Qìgōng.

Above the diaphragm, there are three organs, heart, lungs, and pericardium, that are protected by the ribs. These three Yīn organs were evolved over eons as neighbors. They help and harmonize with each other like neighbors. For examples, the pericardium functions as a cooler that leads the over-Fire Qì (i.e., excess Qì) of the heart to the center of the palm and middle fingers to release it. Whenever your heartbeat is on fire and faster than normal, you may also take a few deep breaths to cool down the heart fire and slow down your heartbeat effectively. This Qìgōng exercise is called "use the lung metal to subdue the heart fire." Lungs are considered as metal while the heart is considered as fire in the Chinese medical "five elements" (Wǔxíng, 五行) theory.

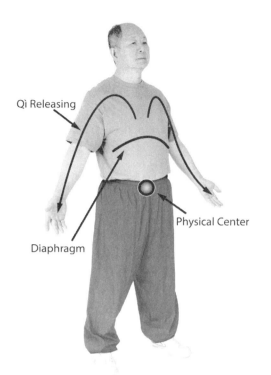

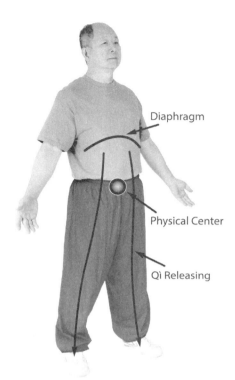

Figure 1-5. Releasing Qi to the Arms.

Figure 1-6. Releasing Qì to the Legs.

However, if all three Yīn organs (lungs, heart, and pericardium) are on fire and cannot handle too much Qì and harmonize with each other, the excess Qì will be led through the arms to the finger tips: thumb (lungs), middle finger (pericardium), and pinky (heart). In order to release excess Qì so the body can be cooled down more efficiently, their matching Yáng organs, large intestine, triple burners, and small intestine, will also release the Qì from the fingers: second finger (large intestine), ring finger (triple burner), and pinky (small intestine) (Figure 1-5).

For the same reason, if the three Yīn organs' Qì status, liver, kidneys, and spleen positioned under the diaphragm, is too Yáng, the excess Qì must be released from the toes: liver (big toe), kidneys (small toe), and spleen (big toe). Naturally, their Yáng matching organs, gall bladder (fourth toe), bladder (small toe), and stomach (second toe), will also release excess Qì as well. (Figure 1-6) From this structure, you can understand why the diaphragm is considered as the dividing line of the upper and lower body.

From this Qì distribution network, it is understood that in order to reduce the excess Qì of the lungs, heart, and breast area, we should exercise our arms. For example, the exercise of swinging arms is an effective Qìgōng to prevent breast cancer and reduce the risk of heart attack. Naturally, in order to keep the Qi's circulation smooth in the liver, kidneys, and spleen, we should exercise our legs. From theoretical and logical points of view, the structure of both our Qì and our physical bodies was evolved from our most common daily activity: walking, the exercise of arms and legs. Therefore, exercising the arms and legs are the crucial Qìgōng to maintain smooth and healthy Qi circulation in the body's twelve meridians. Unfortunately, due to the invention of cars, we don't walk as much as we used to, and this has triggered all kinds of problems such as problems with the knee and hip joints and abnormal function of the liver and kidneys.

Qì Cavities (Qìxuè, 氣穴)

Before we go further, you should first understand that there are two different definitions of "cavity" (Xuè, 穴) defined in Chinese Qìgōng society. One is the acupuncture cavity (Zhēnjiǔxuè, 針灸穴) and the other is the Qì field cavity (Qìchǎngxuè, 氣場穴).

A. Acupuncture Cavities (Acupoints) (Zhēnjiǔxuè, 針灸穴)

During the Shāng Dynasty (1600–1046 BCE) (Shāngcháo, 商朝), the Chinese discovered that there are many special tiny areas in the body that are sensitive, and through stimulating these cavities, different illnesses could be treated. Later during the Chinese Hàn Dynasty (202 BCE–220 CE) (Hàncháo, 漢朝), a clearer chart of the cavities was compiled.

During the 1980s, it was discovered that Qì was actually bioelectricity and these cavities were the small areas where the electricity conductivity was higher than the surrounding area. Therefore, these areas formed Qì cavities or holes where, through needles or moxibustion, the Qi's circulation status in Qì channels could be manipulated and corrected. These cavities are just like the windows or doors of a house that allow the body's Qì to circulate and communicate with the outside.

It was discovered that there were more than seven hundred cavities that could be used to treat imbalanced Qì circulation of internal organs through a needle's penetration or moxibustion. Among these cavities, 108 are bigger ones compared with others. Since these cavities can be stimulated through finger pressing without using needles, these cavities are commonly used for acupressure (cavity press massage) (Diǎnxué Ànmó, 點穴按摩) or martial arts. Among them, seventy-two are considered not vital while thirty-six are vital since if any one of these thirty-six cavities is struck (Diǎnxuè, 點穴) with correct position and timing, the Qi's normal circulation in the meridians can be interrupted and the associated organs can be shocked, thus causing death. This is because the Qi's circulation in these cavities is related to the time of day. Finally, among these thirty-six cavities, there are seven matching pairs of cavities that are considered most important since these they build up the body's major Qì network structure:

1. Huìyīn (Co-1, 會陰) and Bǎihuì (Gv-20, 百會); 2. Yìntáng (M-HN-3, 印堂) and Qiángjiān (Gv-18, 強間) [or Nǎohù (Gv-17, 腦戶)]; 3. Rénzhōng (Gv-26, 人中) and Fēngfǔ (Gv-16, 風府); 4. Tiāntū (Co-22, 天突) and Dàzhuī (Gv-14, 大椎); 5. Jiūwěi (Co-15, 鳩尾) and Língtái (Gv-10, 靈臺); 6. Yīnjiāo (Co-7, 陰交) and Mìngmén (Gv-4, 命門); and 7. Lóngmén (M-CA-24, 龍門) [or Xiàyīn (下陰)] and Chángqiáng (Gv-1, 長強) [or Wěilú (尾閭)]. Among these seven, two pairs are the most important: Huìyīn (Yīn) and Bǎihuì (Yáng), and Yīnjiāo (Yīn) and Mìngmén (Yáng). Huìyīn is connected to Bǎihuì through the Thrusting Vessel (Chōngmài, 衝脈), which establishes the central balance of Qì distribution in the body. Yīnjiāo is also connected to Mìngmén through the Thrusting Vessel and joins the Conception Vessel (Rènmài, 任脈) in front and the Governing Vessel (Dūmài, 督脈) behind, providing front and rear Qì balance to the body. These four are the main Qì gates (Figure 1-7).

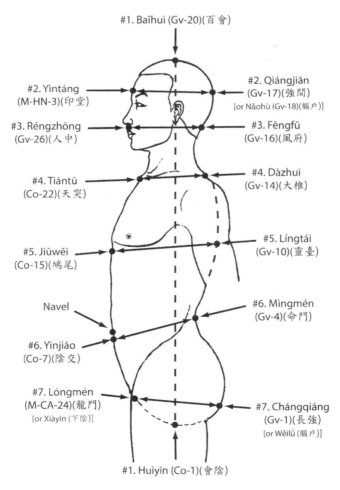

Figure 1-7. Seven Pairs of Corresponding Qì Gates.

Tiāntū controls vocal vibrations and generates the sounds of Hēng (哼) (Yīn) and Hā (哈) (Yáng) for manifestation of Qì. It is a gate of expression, and though it matches with Dàzhuī, its energy also corresponds with Yìntáng, where the spirit resides. When spirit is high in Yìntáng, the energy manifested is strong, and alertness and awareness are high. Jiūwěi and Língtái connect to the heart (emotional mind) and offer a strong driving force to raise the spirit.

B. Qì Field Cavities—Qì Resonant Center (Qìchǎngxuè, 氣場穴)

In any space, there are one or more energy centers. These energy centers emit and collect energy and resonant the entire space. For example, in a sphere, the center of the sphere is the center of energy or Qì. If you make even a tiny sound, it can resonate throughout the entire sphere space and the energy will also bounce back to you (Figure 1-8). However, in an ellipse shape, there are two centers, one on each side of the ellipse (Figure 1-9). The

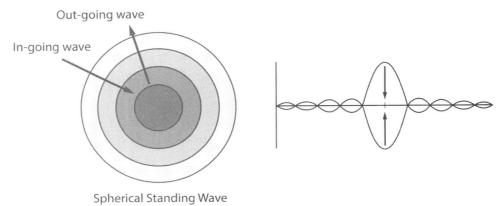

Figure 1-8. Resonance of a Sphere.

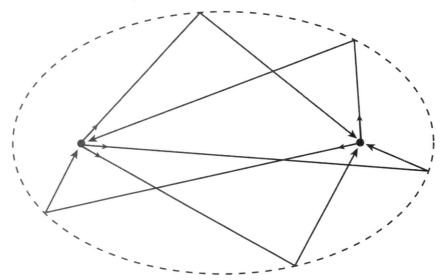

Figure 1-9. Resonance of an Ellipse.

energy or Qì emitted from one center will correspond, synchronize, and resonate with the other and vibrate the entire ellipse. These centers of the Qì field are the cavities of the space and the places where Qìgōng practitioners can cultivate their Qì and spirit. It is believed that if you meditate or live in one of these energy centers, you will be able to exchange and collect Qì for nourishment more efficiently. These energy or Qì field cavities are also the centers that the Fēngshuǐ masters (Fēngshuǐshī, 風水師) are looking for.

Now, if we look at how a human life is developed, we can see that when a sperm enters an egg and becomes the first cell, it is a sphere though there are two poles. Positive and negative charges already exist, thus forming a tiny battery that can be charged and discharged. Each individual cell carries all the DNA information needed for life. This cell has its own memory and life. It has long been recognized by Chinese medicine that the blood cells store Qì and release Qì.

When this first cell begins to divide into two, four, eight, and so on, a life form is developing (Figure 1-10). When this cell has developed for eight weeks, it is called an embryo. It has a shape of a bean or a pea (i.e., ellipse). The first stage of human construction is forming two physical pole centers that are connected by the spinal cord (Figure 1-11). You can also see this two-pole structure by looking at the development of a chicken egg (Figure 1-12). After this stage, four limbs begin to develop and the human shape can be seen. From this point of development until birth, it is called a fetus. You can see that a life is forming from singularity into two poles (i.e., polarity) and then four phases (four limbs) and finally eight Qì vessels.

If the Yīn/Yáng derivation theory is correct, then eight vessels will continue to develop to sixteen Qì channels. However, as we mentioned earlier there are twelve primary Qì channels recognized in Chinese medicine. Does this mean that we still don't know what the other four internal organs are and about their Qì circulation network? Is it possible that the limbic system (Yīn) at the center of head and brain (Yáng) are a pair of Yīn and Yáng matching organs with different Qì channels? Can the last remaining pair of organs and Qì channels be the pancreas (Yīn) and vermiform appendix (Yáng)? It will be

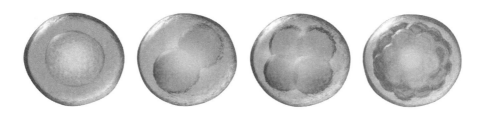

Figure 1-10. Cell's Multiplication.
(Illustration by Shutterstock)

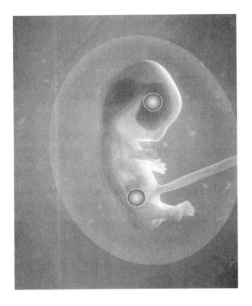

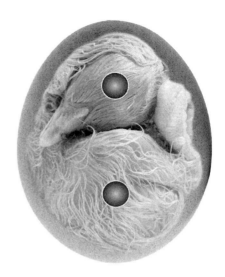

Figure 1-11. Two-Week-
Old Human Embryo.
(Illustration by Shutterstock)

Figure 1-12. A Chick Is
Forming in the Shell.
(Illustration by Shutterstock)

interesting to know more once science has advanced to a level where we can understand the body's Qì circulatory system more clearly.

What is very clear even now is that there are two poles (human polarity) that exist in our body from the beginning of development. One pole is in the head, the brain and limbic system (first brain) (i.e., Upper Dāntián) (Shàng Dāntián, 上丹田), and the other in the center of gravity area, the guts (second brain) (i.e., Real Lower Dāntián) (Zhēn Xiàdāntián, 真下丹田). These two brains are connected by the spinal cord (i.e., Thrusting Vessel) (Chōngmài, 衝脈), which is constructed of highly conductive tissue. While there are two brains physically, in function it is only one since they synchronize with each other simultaneously. These two brains form the two energy centers of a human body. From these two poles, the entire body is developed continuously, the Qì is stored, and the memory is stored.

From over more than two thousand years of study, the Chinese recognized that the top brain is a spiritual center that connects with nature spirit (the Dào or the God) while the lower brain provides the Qì or energy to maintain physical life. In order to achieve a proficient level of physical health, longevity, and spiritual enlightenment, you need both the right quantity of Qì and a high quality of Qì. While the top brain (i.e., Upper Dāntián) allows you to focus, the lower brain (i.e., Real Lower Dāntián) provides the quantity of Qì and stores it.

Two Chambers and Two Pumps of Life

In order to have Qì circulating in your body smoothly and efficiently, you must know the location of the pumps to make the Qì circulate. Just as the heart is the pump for blood circulation in the body, there are two other pumps that pump the Qì, circulating it for your life. You must also know where the chambers are that store Qì in your body. Without recognizing these chambers and pumps and knowing how to manipulate them, your Qìgōng practices will be shallow.

The lungs are the first chamber. Through breathing, the Air Qì can be absorbed and expelled. In this exchange, oxygen can be distributed to the body and carbon dioxide can be collected and removed from the body. The diaphragm is the pump that makes this oxygen and carbon dioxide exchange happen. As you know, without this chamber and the healthy functioning of the diaphragm, you will sicken and die. Therefore, to practice Qìgōng, you must know how to condition your lungs and keep them healthy. You must also know how to regulate your breathing so the function of the lungs can be carried out smoothly. No wonder many people believe the major goal of Qìgōng practice is regulating the breathing.

However, there are very few people in lay society who recognize that there is another chamber that is as important as the lungs. In Chinese Qìgōng practice, Air Qì is considered as external Qì (Wàiqì, 外氣) while the bioelecticity circulation in the body is considered as internal Qì (Nèiqì, 內氣). From the previous discussion, you may have already figured out that this second chamber is where the internal Qì or bioelectricity can be led in for storage and out for usage. The second chamber is the Real Lower Dāntián (i.e., guts or the second brain). But where is the pump that leads the Qì out and in from this chamber? You need

to know that the place from where you are able to manipulate the in-and-out movement of Qì is the Huìyīn (Co-1) (會陰) (i.e., perineum). When the Huìyīn is pushed out the Qì is released and when the Huìyīn is held upward, the Qì is retained. Traditionally, the Huìyīn is called "Qiàomén" (竅門) and means "knack gate" since it is the crucial gate to manipulate Qì function in the body (Figure 1-13).

In order to use these two pumps effectively and efficiently, you should not manipulate them through the diaphragm and

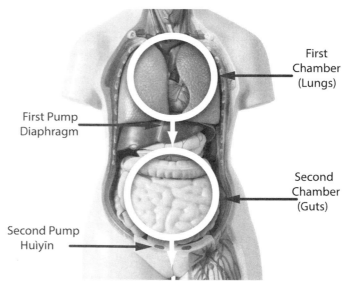

First Chamber (Lungs)

First Pump Diaphragm

Second Chamber (Guts)

Second Pump Huìyīn

Figure 1-13. Two Chambers and Two Pumps.
(Illustration by Shutterstock)

perineum. If you do so, these areas will be tensed and consequently restrict the chambers' function. It is just like if you wanted to loosen up your wrist, you should not use the muscles around the wrist since then the wrist will be tensed. Instead, you should use your elbow to manipulate the movement of the wrist.

It is the same for manipulating the diaphragm and Huìyīn. If you use your abdominal muscles to manipulate the diaphragm's up-and-down movement and use the anus to handle the in-and-out movement in the Huìyīn, then both chambers will be able to relax. This is the crucial key to manipulating these two pumps. We will discuss this more later.

False and Real Lower Dāntián (Jiǎ/Zhēn Xiàdāntián, 假/真下丹田)

Through nearly two thousand years of experience, Daoists say that the front abdominal area is not the Real Dāntián, but is in fact a "False Dāntián" (Jiǎ Dāntián, 假丹田). Their argument is that, although this Lower Dāntián is able to generate Qì and accumulate it to a higher level, it cannot be stored there for a long time. This is because it is located on the path of the Conception Vessel (Rènmài, 任脈), and whenever Qì is built up to a higher energy state, it will circulate in the Conception and Governing Vessels (Rèn/Dūmài, 任/督脈) and will be distributed to the entire body for consumption. This Lower Dāntián, therefore, cannot be a real battery. A real battery should be able to store the Qì to an abundant level. Where then, is the "Real Lower Dāntián" (Zhēn Xiàdāntián, 真下丹田)? We will discuss the Real Lower Dāntián later. For now, let us first clarify the function of the False Lower Dāntián (Jiǎ Xiàdāntián, 假下丹田).

False Lower Dāntián (Jiǎ Xiàdāntián, 假下丹田)

As mentioned earlier, through abdominal movement in coordination with the breathing, the fat accumulated at the abdominal area can be converted into Qì. This kind of abdominal exercise is called "back to childhood breathing" (Fǎntóng Hūxī, 返童呼吸). Consequently, the amount of Qì can be increased in the body. From this, we see something at variance with the ancient teachings. It is said that through abdominal breathing, the Original Essence (Yuánjīng, 元精) can be converted into Original Qì (Yuánqì, 元氣). Today, we know that Original Essence refers to hormones. If we look closely, we can see that the Qì is actually converted from the fat stored in the abdominal area. Fat is the extra food essence stored in our bodies for an emergency. Fat is a material that has been filtered by the liver and has a very high content of calories. Therefore, it can be converted into Qì efficiently.

Look at the evolution of humans. Before humans knew how to raise cattle and grow food, we were no different from other animals. When we had food, we ate a lot and when we did not have food, we starved. However, like animals, we did not die from a short time of starvation. This is because the body has different places to store the extra food essence (fat) in the body. When we lack food, this extra food essence is converted naturally into energy to supply our needs. The abdominal area is the main area for the storage of fat. There are six layers of muscles and six layers of fasciae mutually sandwiched between each other. Wherever there are fasciae, there is a stagnation of Qì and blood circulation, and consequently fat can be deposited. Through abdominal exercises, this fat can be converted into Qì efficiently. Remember, muscles are good conductors while fasciae and fat are poor conductors. When these good and poor conductors are sandwiched together, it forms a battery. That is why the False Dāntián is able to store Qì to a certain level.

From this we can see that it is not Original Essence (hormones) that is converted into Qì. However, due to the function of hormones, the Qì can be converted from food essence or fat stored in the body more efficiently. This is because hormones are your body's chemical messengers. They travel in your bloodstream to tissues or organs to help them do their work. They affect many different processes of the body, including growing and development, metabolism, sexual function, reproduction, and mood.

One of the possible causes of increasing hormone (glucagon and insulin) production through the abdominal up-and-down exercise is the stimulation of islets of Longerhans in the pancreas. The other one is that, through the up-and-down movement of the diaphragm, the adrenal glands are massaged and thus the secretion of dehydroepiandrosterone (DHEA) (an endogenous steroid hormone) increases.

REAL LOWER DĀNTIÁN (ZHĒN XIÀDĀNTIÁN, 真下丹田)

Daoists teach that the Real Lower Dāntián is at the center of the abdominal area, at the physical center of gravity located in the large and small intestines (Figure 1-14). Let us analyze this from two different points of view.

As we mentioned earlier, life starts with a sperm from the father entering an egg from the mother, thus forming the original human cell. This cell next divides into two cells, then four cells, etc. When this group of cells adheres to the internal wall of the uterus, the umbilical cord starts to develop. Nutrition and energy for further cell multiplication is absorbed through the umbilical cord from the mother's body. The baby keeps growing until it develops a more mature body. During this nourishing and growing process, the baby's abdomen is moving up and down, acting like a pump drawing in nutrition and energy into his or her body. Immediately after birth, air and nutrition are taken in from the nose engaging the lungs in oxygen

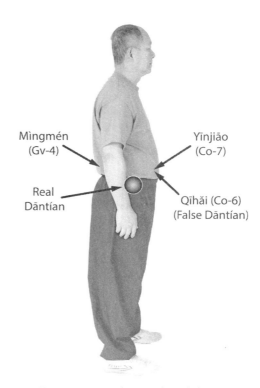

Mìngmén (Gv-4)

Yīnjiāo (Co-7)

Real Dāntián

Qìhǎi (Co-6) (False Dāntián)

Figure 1-14. The Real and the False Lower Dāntián.

exchange and the sucking action of the mouth to take in nutrition. As the child grows, it slowly forgets the natural movements of the abdomen. This is why the abdomen's up-and-down movement is called "back to childhood breathing."

Think carefully: if your first human cell were still alive, where would it be? Naturally, this cell has already died a long time ago. It is understood that approximately one trillion (10^{12}) cells die in a human body each day. However, if we assume that this first cell is still alive, then it should be located at our physical center, that is, our center of gravity. If we ponder carefully, we can see that it is from this center that the cells could multiply evenly outward until the body was fully constructed. In order to maintain this even multiplication physically, the energy or Qì must be centered at this point and radiate outward. When we are in an embryonic state, this is the center of gravity and also the Qì center. As we grow after birth, this center remains.

The above argument adheres solely to the traditional point of view of the physical development of our body. Next, let us analyze this center from another point of view.

If we look at the physical center of gravity, we can see that the entire area is occupied by the large and small intestines (Figure 1-15). We know that there are three kinds of muscles existing in our body, and we can examine them in ascending order of our ability to control them. The first kind includes the heart muscle, in which the electrical conductivity among muscular groups is the highest. The heart beats all the time, regardless of our attention, and through practice and discipline, we are only able to regulate its beating, but not start and stop it. If we supply electricity to even a small piece of this muscle, it will pump like the heart. The second category of muscles are those

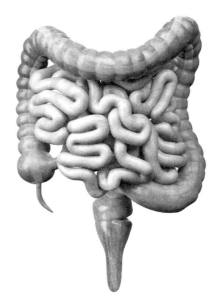

Figure 1-15. Large and Small Intestines.

that contract automatically but over which we can exert significant control if we make the effort. Our eyelids, certain sexual responses, and the diaphragm that controls breathing are examples of this muscle type, and their electrical conductivity is lower than the first type. The third kind of muscles are those directly controlled by our conscious mind. The electric conductivity of these muscles is the lowest of the three groups.

If you look at the structure of the large and small intestines, the first thing you notice is that their total length is approximately six times your body's height (Figure 1-16). With such long electrically conductive tissues sandwiched between all of the mesenteries, water, and linings (which it is reasonable to believe are poor electrical conductive tissues), the intestines act like a huge battery in our body (Figure 1-17).

Like the brain, your gut contains more than one hundred million neurons (also called nerve cells and nerve fibers) and like the brain, the gut has memories. Neurons are excitable cells in the nerve system. Their main function is to process and transmit information. Actually, the gut talks to the brain, releasing hormones into the bloodstream, for example, to tell the brain how hungry you are. Recent

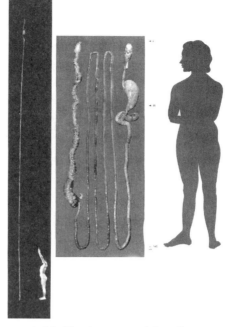

Figure 1-16. The Large and Small Intestines Are About Six Times Your Height.

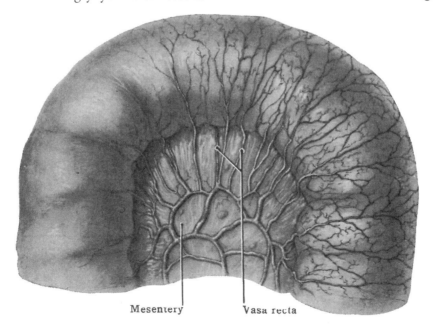

Figure 1-17. Low Electrically Conductive Material Such as Mesentery, Outer Casing, and Water in and Around the Intestines Makes the Entire Area Act Like a Battery.
(Used with permission: James E. Anderson, M.D., Grant's Atlas of Anatomy, 7th ed., ©Williams and Wilkins)

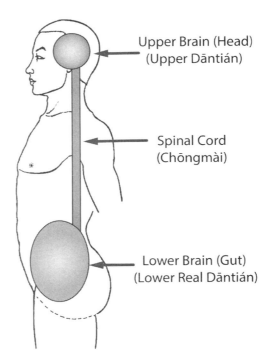

Upper Brain (Head)
(Upper Dāntián)

Spinal Cord
(Chōngmài)

Lower Brain (Gut)
(Lower Real Dāntián)

Figure 1-18. Two Polarities (Brains) of a Human Body.

studies have confirmed that the gut actually has a direct connection to the brain through a neural circuit that allows it to transmit signals in mere seconds. Memory allocation is a process that determines which specific synapses and neurons in a neural network will store a given memory. Although multiple neurons can receive a stimulus, only a subset of the neurons will induce the necessary plasticity for memory encoding. From this, you can see that it makes sense both logically and scientifically that the center of gravity, rather than the False Dāntián, is the real battery in our body.

Furthermore, according to a 1996 article in *The New York Times*, a human being can be thought of as having two brains. One brain is in the head, and the other is in the gut (i.e., the digestive system). Though these two brains are separated physically, through the connection of the spinal cord (high electrically conductive tissue) (Thrusting Vessel, 衝 脈), they actually function as one (Figure 1-18).

The article explains that the upper brain is able to think and has memory. It is able to store data, utilizing electrochemical charges. The lower brain has memory, but does not have the capability of thought. This discovery offers confirmation of the Chinese belief that the Real Lower Dāntián (Large and Small Intestines) is able to store Qì, while the Upper Dāntián governs thinking and directs the Qì. Theoretically speaking, if the upper brain is able to think, then it should be able to generate an EMF (electromotive force) while the lower brain should have a large capacity for storing charge. In other words, the lower brain is the human battery in which the life force resides. Once the brain has generated an idea (EMF), the charge will immediately be directed from the lower brain, through the spinal cord and nervous system, to the desired area in order to activate the physical body.

According to Ohm's Law in physics,

$$\Delta V = I\,R$$

where ΔV is potential difference or EMF, I is current, and R is resistance. From this formula, we can see that if R is a constant (i.e., resistance), then the higher the potential or EMF, the stronger will be the current that is generated. That means the more we are able to concentrate (higher EMF), the stronger the Qì flow will be. This parallels the Chinese Qìgōng concept that *the more you concentrate, the higher your energy circulation will be.* From Chinese Qìgōng, higher levels of concentration can be trained through still meditation. In addition, if we assume the EMF to be constant, that means the mind's concentration remains the same. Then, the lower the R (resistance), the higher the current flow will be. According to past Qìgōng experience, the more relaxed you are, the more Qì (current) can flow.

At this point you should also know that Qì can also be produced directly from food or herbs and then stored at the Real Lower Dāntián. That means different foods can produce a different quantity and quality of Qì. This is the reason that herbs that can produce more Qì in the body were researched and studied in Chinese herbalism. For example, ginseng has long been recognized as one of the many herbs able to produce more Qì.

Guardian Qì and Marrow Qì (Wèiqì Yǔ Suǐqì, 衛氣與髓氣)

As mentioned earlier, there are eight Qì vessels (Mài, 脈) that function like reservoirs, and twelve primary Qì channels (Shíèr-jīng, 十二經), which function like rivers in your body. In addition, there are millions of tiny secondary channels called "Luò" (絡) branching out from the twelve primary Qì channels to the surface of the skin to generate a shield of Guardian Qì (Wèiqì, 衛氣) (Figure 1-19). When the Guardian Qì is

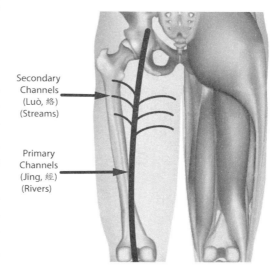

Secondary Channels (Luò, 絡) (Streams)

Primary Channels (Jīng, 經) (Rivers)

Figure 1-19. Secondary Qì Channels Leads the Qì to Skin and Marrow.
(Illustration by Shutterstock)

strong, your body is more Yáng and your immune system will function efficiently, thus you will not get sick easily.

These tiny secondary channels also lead the Qì inward from the primary Qì channels into the bone marrow (Suǐqì, 髓氣) (i.e., Marrow Qì), and make the body more Yīn. This Yīn is to balance the Yáng manifested by the Guardian Qì. When the Marrow Qì is strong, the blood cell production will be normal and healthy, which is the key to slowing down the aging process. This is because the blood cells are carriers of the Qì, nutrients, oxygen, and any other material required for the body's metabolism.

Spiritual Triangle (Liànshén Sānjiǎotǎ, 練神三角塔)

When the Qì storage at the Real Dāntián is abundant, the Qì in the Girdle Vessel (Dàimài, 帶脈) is also abundant. Therefore, the Guardian Qì will be strong and make the function of the immune system more effective. From this, we can see that the function of the Girdle Vessel (extreme Yáng in eight vessels) is to manifest the Qì so the physical body can be strong. When the Qì is led upward to nourish the brain (i.e., Upper Dāntián) from the Real Lower Dāntián, more brain cells will be activated and the functioning of the brain will be improved. Through Embryonic Breathing Meditation, the Qì stored at the brain can be focused at the spiritual residence (i.e., limbic system) (Níwángōng, 泥丸宮) and then led forward through the Spiritual Valley (i.e., space between two lobes of brain) to reopen the Third Eye (Tiānmù/Tiānyǎn, 天目/天眼). The Thrusting Vessel (Chōngmài, 衝脈) keeps your mental and physical body at the centerline while the Girdle Vessel expands Qì horizontally to maintain your mental and physical balance. *When you are centered, you have balance and when you have balance, you will be centered. That is why both the Thrusting Vessel and Girdle Vessel, though they are physically two, in function they are actually only one.* Together they build a so-called "spiritual triangle." (Figure 1-20) When the Qì in your Real Lower Dāntián is abundant, your Guardian Qì will be able to expand farther, your immune system will be stronger, and you will be more balanced and stronger physically. Consequently, your physical life will be strong. Not only that, if you lead the Qì up to activate more brain cells and know how to focus the Qì forward, you may reopen the Third Eye so you are able to reconnect with the natural spirit. This is the stage of "Unification of Heaven and Human" (Tiānrén Héyī, 天人合一).

1.5 Quantity of Qì and Quality of Qì's Manifestation (Qìliàng Yǔ Qìxiǎnzhí, 氣量與氣顯質)

In order to reach the final goal of Qìgōng practice successfully, all Qìgōng practitioners must pay attention to two important elements: build up an abundant level of Qì and also manifest the Qì efficiently. Without these two elements, it will be like you don't have money in the bank and also don't know how to use your money efficiently.

Increase the Quantity of Qì

There are various ways of producing the extra Qì at the Lower Dāntián. For example, you may use herbs to increase the quantity of Qì in the body. You may also use massage to loosen up the fat at the Lower Dāntián area so it can be converted into Qì. You may also use the abdomen's up-and-down movements in coordination with the breathing.

First, I would like to introduce the two most commonly known methods of breathing that are able to increase the quantity of Qì in your body. These methods have often been used by Buddhist and Daoist monks in the past. As long as you practice patiently and know the theory, with these two methods you will be able to convert the fat stored at the abdominal area into the extra Qì in your body.

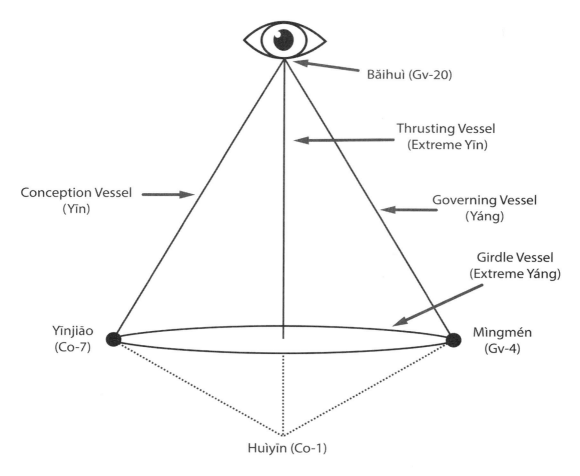

Figure 1-20. Spiritual Triangle.

After these two breathing concepts are explained, I will briefly introduce how to condition your bio-battery so it can store the Qì to an abundant level. Finally, in the section on enhancing the quality of your Qi's manifestation, I will summarize Embryonic Breathing Meditation, which allows you to conserve your Qì and manifest it efficiently.

Remember, in all the exercises your tongue should touch the palate of your mouth to bridge the Conception Vessel (Rènmài, 任脈) and Governing Vessel (Dūmài, 督脈).

Normal Abdominal Breathing (Buddhist Breathing) (Zhèng Fùhūxī, 正腹呼吸) (Fójiā Hūxī, 佛家呼吸)

In Normal Abdominal Breathing, when you inhale, your abdomen and Huìyīn (Co-1) (會陰) (perineum or anus) are gently pushed out, and when you exhale, the abdomen is withdrawn and you gently hold up your Huìyīn (Figures 1-21 and 1-22). When you do so, you are converting the food essence (fat) into Qì through the abdominal movements. Not only that, through the movements of the abdomen and the Huìyīn cavity, the Original Essence (Yuánjīng, 元精) (Hormone) in the pancreas (islets of Langerhans) and gonads (sex glands) will also be produced. It was also discovered that through the up-and-down movement of the diaphragm in abdominal breathing, the diaphragm actually could push the adrenal glands down at least two centimeters and massage them. This massage can stimulate and enhance the production of the hormone DHEA. After you have practiced

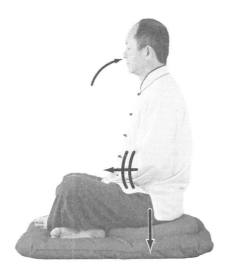

Figure 1-21. Normal Abdominal Breathing. (Inhalation)

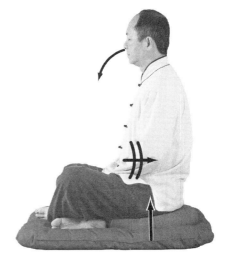

Figure 1-22. Normal Abdominal Breathing. (Exhalation)

for a few weeks, you will start to experience some warm feeling and even some trembling at the abdominal area. This signals the increase of the Qì in this area.

As a beginner, you should practice Normal Abdominal Breathing for at least six months until your mind is able to control the muscles around the abdominal area efficiently. Remember, this kind of breathing is more relaxing and natural, and so will not cause any troublesome tension at the stomach area.

REVERSE ABDOMINAL BREATHING (DAOIST BREATHING) (FǍN FÙHŪXĪ, 反腹呼吸) (NÌ FÙHŪXĪ, 逆腹呼吸) (DÀOJIĀ HŪXĪ, 道家呼吸)

After you have practiced Normal Abdominal Breathing for at least six months, then you may proceed to Reverse Abdominal Breathing. In Reverse Abdominal Breathing, when you inhale, the abdomen and Huìyīn are gently pulled inward, and when you exhale, the abdomen and Huìyīn are gently pushed outward (Figures 1-23 and 1-24).

Often, a Qìgōng or martial arts beginner encounters the problem of tightness in the abdominal area. The reason for this is that in Reverse Abdominal Breathing, when you inhale, the diaphragm is pulling downward while the abdominal area is withdrawing. This can generate tension in the stomach area. To reduce this problem, you must already have mastered the skill of Normal Abdominal Breathing and be able to control the abdominal

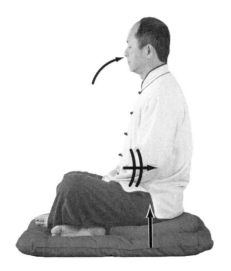 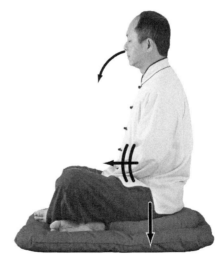

Figure 1-23. Reverse Abdominal Breathing. (Inhalation)

Figure 1-24. Reverse Abdominal Breathing. (Exhalation)

muscles efficiently. In addition, you may start on a small scale with Reverse Abdominal Breathing. When you can control the abdominal muscles efficiently, only then should you increase to a larger scale of abdominal movement. Naturally, this will take time.

CONDITIONING THE BIOBATTERY (REAL LOWER DĀNTIÁN)

In order to store a large quantity of Qì in the Real Lower Dāntián, the first step is to condition this bio-battery to improve the Qì storage capacity. Remember, the ability to store Qi to a high level is essential for reaching profounds levels of Small Circulation and Grand Circulation and the ultimate goal of opening the Third Eye.

From the ancient classic, *Muscle/Tendon Changing and Marrow/Brain Washing Qìgōng* (*Yìjīnjīng/Xǐsuǐjīng*, 易筋經 · 洗髓經), it is recognized that the most efficient way of conditioning this bio-battery (False and Real Lower Dāntiáns) is through massage and stimulation. Massage gets rid of the fat hidden within so the circulation ca be smoother, and stimulation will condition the sensitivity of the nerves in the area so they are able to handle a larger quantity of Qì stored there. The entire conditioning process is long and needs a great deal of training and patience. You must understand the theory behind the conditioning clearly. If you wish to know more about this training, please refer to my book, *Qìgōng, The Secret of Youth* and the video *Neigong*, both published by YMAA.

A. ENHANCE THE QUALITY OF QÌ'S MANIFESTATION

In order to reach a profound level of both Internal Elixir or External Elixir Qìgōng (Nèidān/Wàidān Gōng, 內丹/外丹功) practice, you should first understand and practice Embryonic Breathing (Tāixī Jìngzuò, 胎息靜坐), especially if you are interested in Small and Grand Circulation Meditation practices.

EMBRYONIC BREATHING (CAVITY BREATHING) (WÚJÍ BREATHING) (TĀIXĪ, 胎息) (XUÈWÈIXĪ, 穴位息) (WÚJÍXĪ, 無極息)

Purposes of Embryonic Breathing 胎息靜坐之目的 (Tāixī Jìngzuò Zhī Mùdì)

1. **To Regulate the Mind.** From this practice, you will be able to minimize the domination or activities of your conscious mind and thus allow your subconscious mind to wake up and grow. When this happens, you will be able to reconnect with nature and develop your divine feeling. This is crucial especially for Spiritual Enlightenment Grand Circulation (Shéntōng Dàzhōutiān Jìngzuò, 神通大周天靜坐). In addition, once you have regulated your mind to a certain stage, your regulated mind will be able to communicate your Qì and lead it efficiently and effectively. This is the stage of "the harmonization of mind and Qì" (Yìqì Xiānghé, 意氣相合). This is especially critical for Small and Grand Circulation Meditation practices. *Remember that once you have a regulated mind, you will have "quality" for leading and manifestation of Qì.*

2. **To Lead Qì to the Real Lower Dāntián and Store It There at an Abundant Level.** To reach a profound achievement of both Small and Grand Circulations, you need an abundant level of Qì storage in your bio-battery (Zhēn Xiàdāntián, 真下丹田). Embryonic Breathing teaches you how to generate more Qì, conserve it, and store it to an abundant level. This will provide you the "quantity" of Qì for your practice.

Practice of Embryonic Breathing

1. **Locate the Spiritual Center** (Figure 1-25). In practice, you must first be able to feel your Limbic System at the center of your head. If you cannot feel this center, how can you lead the Qì there and keep your spirit (Shén, 神) in its residence (Shéshì, 神室)? Once you are able to keep your spirit in its residence and lead the Qì from the brain to the Limbic System, you will minimize the conscious mind's activities and awaken your subconscious mind that is connected to your spirit. This will increase the sensitivity of your spiritual feeling. Consequently, your alertness and awareness will be higher.

Naturally, it is harder for a beginner to locate this center. One of the keys to finding this center is making a Hēng (哼) sound, the sound of crying and sighing. This sound is generated from this center. Once you are able to feel it, then just make a sound in your mind without actually making sound. Otherwise, you will not be able to lead the Qì to the center. As we mentioned before, the key to leading the Qi is inhaling longer than exhaling and near the end, just hold your breath for five seconds. Then exhale.

When this happens, due to the mind concentrating at the Yīn center of the Upper Dāntián, the production of melatonin (pineal gland) and growth hormone (pituitary gland) will also

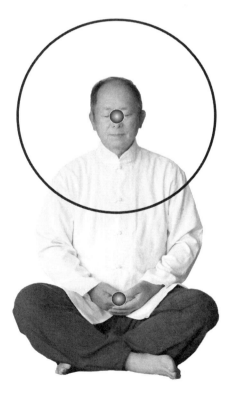

Figure 1-25. Locate Your Limbic System. (Spiritual Residence)

be regulated and increased. With these hormones, all of the biochemical reactions will become smooth and the metabolism of the body can be regulated and improved.

2. **Store the Qì in Real Lower Dāntián** (Figure 1-26). In order to store the Qì in the human bio-battery, you must first recognize the center of the Real Lower Dāntián through feeling and then practice to keep your mind there. When your mind is in the Real Lower Dāntián, the Qì will not be led away from its residence. Keeping the mind at the Real Lower Dāntián (Yìshǒu Dāntián, 意守丹田) is the crucial key to successfully conserving Qi.

The way to keep the mind at the Real Lower Dāntián so the Qì can be led there is through moving the front abdominal area and the lower back area at the same time. The front abdominal area (navel or Yīnjiāo cavity, 陰交) is called "Shēngmén" (生門) and means "the door of life," while the rear lower back area is called "Bìhù" (閉戶) and means "the closed door," which implies the Mingmén (Gv-4) (命門) cavity between L2 and L3 (Figure 1-27). Through this balanced front and back movement, you are able to easily locate the center (Yáng water). Naturally, in the beginning, your mind will be at these two places. However, after you have practiced for a period of time and have reached the stage of "regulating without regulating," the mind will easily be at the center.

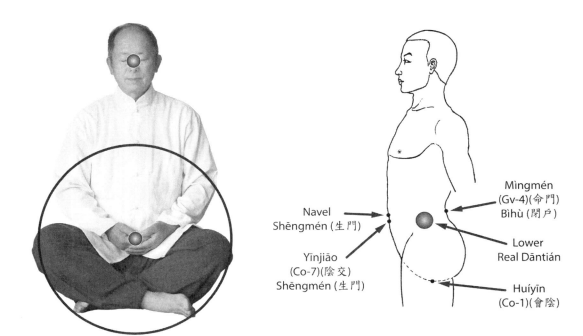

Figure 1-26. Locate Qì Center. (Qì Dwelling)

Figure 1-27. Yīnjiāo (陰交), Mìngmén (命門), and Huìyīn (會陰).

That means when you practice Embryonic Breathing, the first step is to find the two doors and move them in and out at the same time. Naturally, extra Qì will be produced at both the front and the rear. While you are doing so, you must also coordinate with the up-down movements of the Huìyīn (Co-1) (會陰) or anus. Soon you will feel the Qì in the entire Girdle Vessel (Dàimài, 帶脈) expanding and withdrawing at the same time (Figure 1-28).

The most amazing part of the practice is that, through these movements, the production of insulin hormone from the islets of Langerhans in the pancreas, DHEA (dehydroepiandrosterone) in the adrenal glands, and testosterone (male) and estrogen and progesterone (female) in the sex glands can be regulated and possibly increased. This is due to the stimulation of the glands through the exercises.

3. **Synchronize Both Centers** (Figure 1-29). Once you have located the two centers, then you need to synchronize the two centers with the breathing. Remember, these two poles simultaneously correspond with each other. In function, it is one system, but physically there are two poles. One provides the Qi and the other governs Qi manifestation. As a beginner, you must understand the theory and then practice until you can feel for yourself how to synchronize them and make them work together.

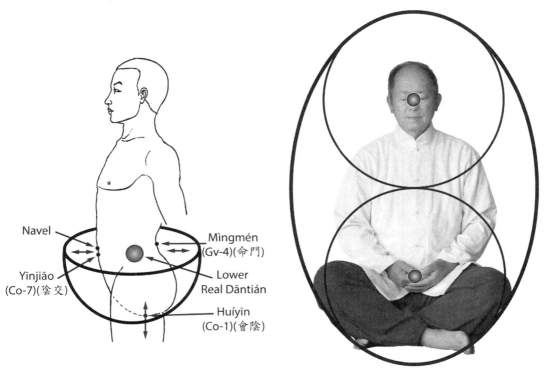

Figure 1-28. Girdle Vessel Breathing.

Figure 1-29: Synchronize Two Centers.

4. **Lead the Mind and Qì Down to the Real Lower Dāntián** (Figure 1-30). Once you have taken a few minutes to synchronize the two poles, then bring your subconscious mind down to the Real Lower Dāntián. Naturally, your spirit will also be led downward.

5. **Unification of Spirit and Qì (Embryonic Breathing)** (Figure 1-31). This is the final stage of Embryonic Breathing. It is called "unification of spirit and Qì" (Shénqì Xiānghé, 神氣相合) or "unification of mother and son" (Mǔzǐ Xiānghé, 母子相合). The mother is the Qì that nourishes the spirit, the son. In the *Dào Dé Jīng* book this is called "embracing the singularity" (Bàoyī, 抱一).

If you are interested in Embryonic Breathing Meditation, please refer to the books: *Qìgōng Meditation: Embryonic Meditation* and *Dào Dé Jīng: A Qìgōng Interpretation*, by YMAA Publication Center.

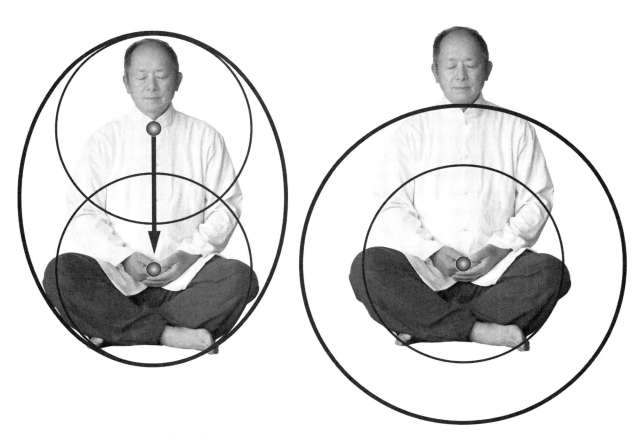

Figure 1-30. Leading the Mind and Qì Down.

Figure 1-31. Embryonic Breathing.

1.6 FIVE REGULATINGS (WŬTIÁO, 五調)

No matter what kind of Qìgōng you practice, either Internal Elixir (Nèidān, 內丹) or External Elixir (Wàidān, 外丹), there are normally five regulating processes (Wŭtiáo, 五調) involved in reaching the final goal of practice. These regulating processes are: regulating the body (Tiáoshēn, 調身), regulating the breathing (Tiáoxí, 調息), regulating the emotional mind (Tiáoxīn, 調心), regulating the Qì (Tiáoqì, 調氣), and regulating the spirit (Tiáoshén, 調神).

Before discussing them you should first understand the word Tiáo (調) that I translate as "regulating." Tiáo (調) is constructed of two words: Yán (言), which means "speaking" or "negotiating," and Zhōu (周), which means "to be complete," "to be perfect," or "to be round." Therefore, the meaning of Tiáo means to adjust or tune up until it is complete and harmonious with others. It is just like tuning a piano so the keyboard is harmonized. Tiáo means to coordinate, to cooperate, and to harmonize with others by continuing adjustment. That means all of the five items—body, breathing, mind, Qì, and spirit—need to be regulated with each other until the final harmonious stage is reached.

Regulating the Body (Tiáoshēn, 調身)

If the postures in Qìgōng practice are incorrect, the practice will not be effective. Regulating the body is done with stationary or moving Qìgōng. Some popular Qìgōng forms with movements are The Eight Pieces of Brocade (Bāduànjǐn, 八段錦), Tàijí Qìgōng (太極氣功), and Five Animal Sports (Wŭqínxì, 五禽戲) Qìgōng. Regulating is also involved with standing still (Zhànzhuāng, 站椿) or sitting meditations such as Embryonic Breathing (Tāixí, 胎息) and Small Circulation (Xiǎozhōutiān, 小周天) meditations. The practice of regulating the body for moving Qìgōng involves:

A. **Correct Postures and Movements.** The beginning stage of practicing moving Qìgōng is learning how to move the body correctly. All the effective Qìgōng movements were created by experienced Qìgōng masters. From their knowledge and experience, they found that a specific movement had its special purpose in regulating the body's Qì. If the movements are not done correctly, the purposes of training will be meaningless. Remember, every Qìgōng movement has its reason and consequence. Naturally, only those who have abundant knowledge and profound understanding of Qìgōng are able to create effective Qìgōng exercises.

B. **Center, Balance, and Rooting.** Usually, in order to have a smooth and freely flowing Qì circulation, practitioners must have their body centered, balanced, and rooted. Otherwise, the body will be tensed. Tension is one of the biggest obstacles for smooth Qì circulation. However, you should understand that some Muscle/Tendon Changing Qìgōng exercises intentionally tense some specific area of the physical body for conditioning. When you practice these Hard Qìgōng (Yìng Qìgōng, 硬氣功), your body should still be centered, balanced, and rooted.

C. **Relaxation and Softness.** If you practice Soft Qìgōng (Ruǎn Qìgōng, 軟氣功), then you must be relaxed and as soft as possible, otherwise the Qì circulation will be stagnant. Naturally, if you are not relaxed, this will defeat the purpose of practice.

If you practice still Qìgōng such as Standing Meditation (Zhànzhuāng, 站樁) or Sitting Meditation (Jìngzuó, 静坐) (Dǎzuò, 打坐), then regulating the body can be somewhat different than those with movements.

A. **Find the Most Natural, Relaxed, Balanced, and Comfortable Posture for Meditation.** This will allow the Qì to flow freely, help you to breathe naturally and smoothly, and help the mind remain relaxed and focused so the spirit can be raised to a higher level. However, you should understand that if you practice Standing Meditation with or without specific arm postures, your body will be partially tensed. For example, in Wújí Standing Meditation (Wújí Qìgōng, 無極 氣功), though your arms are relaxed, your legs are tense because you are standing and also because of the slightly forward-leaning angle of your body (Figure 1-32). You should keep all other parts of the body natural and relaxed as much as possible. In some Standing Meditations such as Éméi Big Roc Gōng (Éméi Dàpéng Gōng, 峨眉大鵬功), in which the arms are lifted in front of the body, some arm muscles are tensed due to the lifting of the arms (Figure 1-33). You should know that the tension of parts of the body was purposely designed into these Standing Meditations for special reasons.

B. **To Provide the Best Conditions for Internal Feeling.** When your physical body is regulated correctly, your feeling can reach to a deep and profound level. Your judgment will be more accurate. The efficiency of your mind-body communication will increase to a high level. It is through this profound feeling that your mind is able to lead the Qì to circulate effectively in the body.

C. **To Coordinate and Harmonize the Physical Center and Mental Center.** By using the Yì (意) (i.e., wisdom mind) and correct feeling, you can bring your physical center and mental center to a high level of coordination and harmony.

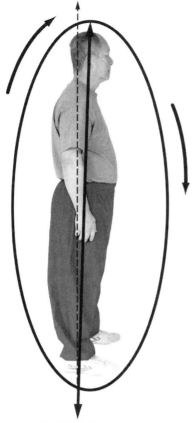
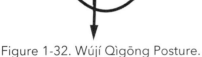

Figure 1-32. Wújí Qìgōng Posture.

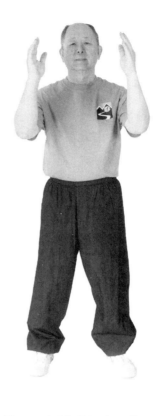

Figure 1-33. Dàpéng Gōng.

Regulating the Breathing (Tiáoxí, 調息)

When you have regulated your body to the stage of *regulating without regulating* (Tiáoér Wútiáo, 調而無調), then you should pay attention to the breathing. Regulating without regulating means that you have reached the stage of regulating the condition naturally and subconsciously. It is just like learning to drive. After you have driven for some time, your conscious mind does not have to be there to regulate your operation and you are able to drive the car naturally and subconsciously.

Breathing is considered to be the central strategy in Qìgōng practice. When the breathing methods are correct, the mind can lead the Qì efficiently and effectively. Therefore, Qìgōng breathing methods have been studied and practiced since ancient times. In many cases, the methods were kept top secret in each style.

The purposes of regulating the breathing are:

1. **To Take in Oxygen Sufficiently and Smoothly and Also to Expel the Carbon Dioxide Efficiently.** Approximately one trillion (10^{12}) cells die every day in a healthy person. In order to slow down the aging process, the same number of new healthy cells must be produced each day. We know that oxygen is one of the necessary elements in the production of the new cells. Without an ample supply of oxygen, the new cells constructed will be deformed or unhealthy. In addition, dead cells in the body must be excreted to prevent problems in the body. The whole job of supplying sufficient oxygen and bringing out the dead cells (i.e., carbon) falls to our respiratory system. Therefore, if you are able to inhale and exhale deeply, you will have reached this goal that allows the smooth replacement of the cells.

2. **To Serve the Strategic Purpose in Qìgōng Practice of Regulating the Body's Yīn and Yáng.** Breathing is both Kǎn (water, 坎) and Lí (fire, 離), and by using breathing strategies you are able to adjust the Yīn and Yáng condition of your body. Inhalation can make the body more Yīn, while exhalation can make the body more Yáng. Therefore, the methods of how to breathe correctly have become one of the major subjects of study in Chinese Qìgōng society.

From past experience, it is known that there are four crucial and fundamental keys to manipulate the body's Yīn and Yáng condition through breathing.

A. **The Length of Respirations.** When your inhalation is longer than your exhalation, the body's Qì is led inward. If your exhalation is longer than your inhalation, the body's Qì is led outward. This phenomena can be seen in our laughing and crying. When we laugh, we subconsciously exhale longer than we inhale and the body's Qì expands outward; consequently, we feel warm and hot. However, if we are sad or frightened, we inhale longer than we exhale and the body's Qì condenses inward. Consequently, we feel chilly. This is the main crucial key to Skin/Marrow Breathing or Muscle/Tendon Changing and Marrow/Brain Washing.

B. **Sounds.** When you practice and make a Hā (哈) sound (i.e., laughing) in coordination with the exhalation, you are able to more strongly expand the Qì outward. However if you make a Hēng (哼) sound (i.e., sad sound) with the inhalation, you can lead the Qì inward more strongly. You can see these phenomena occurring naturally.

C. **Holding the Breath.** We know that each cell in our body is like a small battery that can be charged and discharged. However, these batteries cannot be charged instantly. It will take time to reach a high level or the full charge. When you practice Qìgōng, once you hold your breath, the Qì circulation becomes stagnant and thus allows the cell to be charged continuously to a higher level. Notice that when you push or lift something heavy, after you exhale to a certain point, you hold your breath. This allows the cells to be charged to a higher level; consequently, the power manifested will be stronger.

D. Coordinating and harmonizing with the Body, the Mind, the Qì, and the Spirit. Since breathing is one of the five important regulatings for which a Qìgōng practitioner must reach a profound level of practice, it plays an important role in coordination and harmonization. For example, concentrating during a deep profound inhalation can make you calmer and the spirit can be more condensed. If you focus during exhalation, the body's energy can be raised, the mind will be more aroused, and spirit can be raised. In addition, with correct breathing, the Qì can be led by the mind to the desired place more efficiently.

Regulating the Mind (Tiáoxīn, 調心)

Regulating the mind means to regulate and control the emotional mind (Xīn, 心). This practice has always been the most difficult subject to understand and train in Internal Elixir Qìgōng (Nèidān Qìgōng, 內丹氣功) practice. Here you are dealing with your own mind. Everyone has his own thinking and variety of emotional disturbance. Thus, it is also the most difficult subject to explain.

The methods of regulating the mind have been widely studied, discussed, and practiced in all Chinese Qìgōng societies, which include scholar, medical, religious, and martial arts groups. Before we continue to the purposes of regulating the mind, first you should understand the difference between Xīn (心) (i.e., emotional mind) and Yì (意) (i.e., wisdom mind).

Two Minds—Emotional and Wisdom Minds (Xīn, Yì, 心 · 意)

In Chinese society, it is commonly recognized that we have two minds. The mind that is related to our emotional feeling is called "Xīn" (心) (i.e., heart). This mind is Yáng and makes you confused, scattered, depressed, and excited. The other mind, which is related to our rational and logical thinking, is called "Yì" (意) (i.e., intention or wisdom mind). This mind is Yīn and makes you calm, able to concentrate, and able to feel and ponder deeply. The Chinese word "Yì" (意) is constructed of three words: "立" (Lì) on the top means "to establish," "曰" (Yuē) in the middle means "to speak," and "心" (Xīn) at the bottom means the "heart." From this you can see that the meaning of Yì is "to establish communication (an opinion) with the emotional mind under control." This means logical thinking and judgment. To regulate the mind is actually to regulate the "heart" (Tiáoxīn, 調心) or emotional mind.

Two Other Minds—Conscious and Subconscious Minds (Yìshì, Qiǎnyìshì, 意識 · 潛意識)

There are two other different categories of the mind, the conscious mind (Yìshì, 意識) and the subconscious mind (Qiǎnyìshì, 潛意識). The conscious mind is generated from brain cells located at the cerebrum while the subconscious mind is generated from the limbic system at the center of the head. The conscious mind thinks and has memory while the subconscious does not think but has memory. The conscious mind is related to the type of thoughts and behavior humans typically exhibit after they're born and socialized: emotional, playing tricks, and not truthful. The subconscious mind is related to the natural instinct we are born with and is more truthful. We live in a duplicitous society, and we all lie and wear a mask on our face. From a Chinese Qìgōng understanding, it is believed that the spirit resides at the limbic system and connects to our subconscious mind. The limbic system is called the "spirit dwelling" (Shénshì, 神室) or Mud Pill Palace (Níwángōng, 泥丸宮) in Chinese Qìgōng society. It is believed that, in order to reconnect with the natural spirit, we must downplay our conscious mind to allow the subconscious mind to awaken and grow. In order to reconnect to the natural spirit, we must reopen our Third Eye. The Third Eye is called "heaven eye" (Tiānyǎn/Tiānmù, 天眼/天目), and through it we are able to connect with Nature (Figure 1-34).

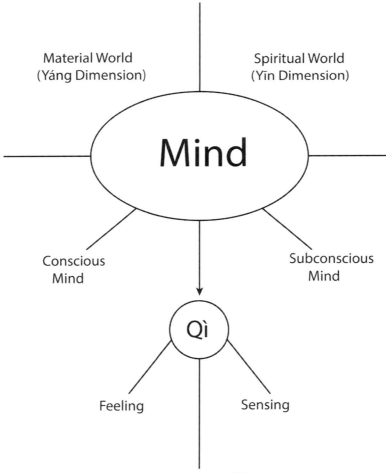

Figure 1-34. Yīn/Yáng Worlds and Mind.

PURPOSES OF REGULATING THE MIND

There are many different purposes or goals for regulating the mind. These purposes can be varied from one school to another. For example, the Qìgōng practitioners in scholar and medical Qìgōng societies are aiming for a calm, peaceful, and harmonious mind so the emotional mind will not disturb the body's Qì circulation. It is believed that our thinking can seriously influence the normal healthy Qì circulation of the body. For instance, if you are happy and excited, the Qì status in your heart will be too Yáng and can trigger a heart attack. If you are angry, the Qì level in your liver will be abnormal and affect the healthy function of the liver. In the same way, the Qì circulation in the kidneys is related to fear, while that of the lungs is related to sadness. Therefore, if you are able to regulate your emotional mind to a harmonious and peaceful state, you will be healthy.

However, for Daoist and Buddhist religious groups, in addition to regulating the emotional mind to a calm and peaceful state, they are also aiming for Buddhahood and enlightenment. Therefore, once they have controlled the emotional mind and developed their wisdom mind to a profound stage, they will minimize the activities of the conscious mind and awaken or enhance the subconscious mind's development. They believe that in order to reconnect their spirits with the natural spirit, they must develop their subconscious mind so the Third Eye can be reopened.

Finally, the martial arts Qìgōng practitioners aim to raise the Spirit of Vitality and build up a highly concentrated mind to develop a sense of enemy. This is critical in battle. While your mind is calm and clear, your spirit must be raised to a state of high alertness and awareness. They also recognize that in order to reach a high level of natural reflex, a crucial key to surviving in battle, you must develop your subconscious mind.

However, it does not matter what the goals of each school are; the basic training rules and principles remain the same. In order to reach their goals, they must follow the same training path.

To conclude, the purposes of regulating the mind are:

1. **To Harmonize the Body and the Mind.** In order to have a calm meditative mind, you must first regulate the condition of your physical body. When your body is tense and energized, your mind will be excited and your breathing will be faster. Therefore, the body and the mind must coordinate and harmonize with each other. This is called "the balance of the body and the Xīn" (Shēnxīn Pínghéng, 身心平衡).

2. **To Harmonize the Breathing and the Mind.** As mentioned earlier, to regulate the emotional mind is to learn how to use the wisdom mind to control the function of the emotional mind. In Chinese Qìgōng society, it is commonly said, "Xīn (is) an ape, Yì (is) a horse" (Xīnyuán Yìmǎ, 心猿意馬). An ape is not powerful, is unsteady and disturbing, and generates confusion and excitement. However, a horse, though powerful, can yet be calm, steady, and controllable.

In Chinese Qìgōng society, through thousands of years of studying the method of regulating the mind, it is understood that in order to lead an ape into a cage and restrain it, you need a banana. This banana is the control of the breathing. As long as you are able to concentrate your mind on your breathing, sooner or later your emotional mind will be restrained and will calm down. That means when your breathing is long, slender, soft, and calm, your mind will be calm. Naturally, in order to make your breathing long, slender, soft, and calm, you must also keep your mind calm. Both the mind and breathing mutually affect each other. They must work together harmoniously in order to reach a high mental state of meditation. Therefore, it is said that "the Xīn and the breathing mutually rely on each other" (Xīnxí Xiāngyī, 心息相依).

3. **To Use the Mind to Build Up, to Store, and to Lead the Qì's Circulation.** In religious and martial arts Qìgōng groups, one of the main goals of practicing Qìgōng is using the mind to build up the Qì, to store it, and also to lead its circulation. In order to build up and store Qì in the Real Lower Dāntián (Zhēn Xiàdāntián, 真下丹田), you must practice Embryonic Breathing (Tāixī, 胎息). The crucial key to this breathing is keeping your mind in this Qì residence and center. Once your mind is away from this center, your Qì will be led away from it and consumed. Therefore, the Qì will never build up and be stored in the body to a higher level. That is why it is said: "Keep the Yì at the Dāntián" (Yìshǒu Dāntián, 意守丹田). This is the practice of storing the Qì. Once you have stored Qì to an abundant level, you can learn how to use your mind to lead the Qì. It is said: "Use the Yì to lead the Qì" (Yǐyì Yǐnqì, 以意引氣).

4. **To Raise the Spirit of Vitality for Enlightenment.** To Buddhists and Daoists, the final goal of Qìgōng practice is to reach enlightenment or Buddhahood. Once you have learned how to store the Qì at the Real Lower Dāntián, you then lead it upward following the Thrusting Vessel (spinal cord) (Chōngmài, 衝脈) to the brain to nourish the Shén. The goal is to reopen the Third Eye. It is believed that since, through thousands of years, we learned to lie and cheat in order to protect our secrets behind a mask, we closed our Third Eye so that other people are unable to see the truth. Therefore, we have lost the power of telepathy and communication with natural Qì and spirit. In order to reopen this Third Eye (Tiānyǎn, 天眼) (Tiānmù, 天目), we must develop our truthful subconscious mind and be truthful to the point where there is nothing to hide. Then, we learn how to accumulate the Qì in the front of the brain. From past experience, the Third Eye can be reopened. In practice, in order to raise the Shén to an enlightened level, you must first regulate your Xīn until it has reached an extremely calm state. When you are in this state, your mind is clear and not wandering.

Regulating the Qì (Tiáoqì, 調氣)

There are two main purposes of regulating the Qì. One is to increase the quantity of Qì and store it in the Real Lower Dāntián. The other one is to improve the quality of Qì's manifestation so Qì consumption can be more efficient. Here, we will list the general purposes for regulating Qì.

1. **Increasing the Qì storage at the Real Lower Dāntián.** When the Qì is stored to an abundant level in the Real Lower Dāntián, you will always have plenty of Qì for applications. This has always been the first main concern in all Qìgōng practices.

2. **Increasing the Qì Storage Level in the Eight Qì Vessels.** The eight vessels are the Qì reservoirs that can be used to regulate the Qì quantity circulating in twelve primary Qì channels. When the Qì storage in the vessels is abundant, you will have plenty of Qì to regulate the primary channels.

3. **Improving the Qì Circulation, Thereby Maintaining Health.** Smooth Qì circulation in the body is the crucial key to maintaining health. Therefore, how to improve your Qì circulation is always a concern.

4. **Removing the Existing Qì Stagnation in the Body (i.e., Healing).** If there is a Qì stagnation in your body, you will be sickened. Removing the stagnation of Qì (Qì knot) (Qìjié, 氣結) is the main key to healing.

5. **Bringing the Qì Circulation in the Internal Organs to a Harmonious and Balanced State.** When all internal organs are balanced and harmonized with each other, you will be healthy.

6. **Enhancing the Qì Circulation in the Conception and Governing Vessels (i.e., Small Circulation).** There are two main purposes of Small Circulation (Xiǎozhōutiān, 小周天) Qìgōng meditation. One is to improve the Qì storage and the other is to enhance the Qì circulation in these two vessels. When the Qì circulation is strong and abundant and the twelve primary Qì channels' circulation are regulated adequately, not only can your twelve internal organs be healthy, you will also build a foundation for Muscle/Tendon Changing Qìgōng practice.

7. **Strengthening Guardian Qì to Make the Immune System Stronger.** When the Qì is circulating in the Girdle Vessel (Dàimài, 帶脈) abundantly and smoothly, your Guardian Qì (Wèiqì, 衛氣) can be strengthened and the immune system enhanced.

8. **Washing the Bone Marrow to Maintain Healthy Function of the Bone Marrow (i.e., Longevity).** When the marrow has plenty of Qì nourishment, it will function efficiently to produce healthy blood cells. Blood cells are carriers of Qì and all other required ingredients such as oxygen and nutrients for cell replacement in the body. Bone Marrow Washing is the key to longevity.

9. **Achieving Various Grand Circulations.** The final goal of Qìgōng practice is to apply the Qì for conditioning the body and for spiritual cultivation in Grand Circulation (Dàzhōutiān, 大周天). For example, you can lead the Qì to an injured area for healing or to a special area such as the wrist for conditioning. You may also lead the Qì following the spinal cord (Chōngmài, 衝脈) to nourish your brain for spiritual enlightenment.

10. **Reunifying the Human Spirit and Qì with the Natural Spirit and Qì.** This is the final goal of spiritual cultivation and is called "unification of heaven and human" (Tiānrén Héyī, 天人合一).

In order to reach a highly efficient level of Qì regulation, you must already have regulated the body, breathing, and mind to a profound level. As mentioned earlier, regulating the body, regulating the breathing, and regulating the mind—these three cannot be separated. They are mutually related and interact with each other. Only when these three are harmoniously coordinated can the Qì be led by the clear and calm mind.

Since regulating the Qì is the main goal of Qìgōng practice, each purpose of regulating the Qì mentioned is a huge subject for discussion. For example, it would take a few books just to cover regulation of Qì in any of the schools such as medical Qìgōng, scholar Qìgōng, and also martial Qìgōng societies. The coverage of regulating the Qì in the religious group is even larger and deeper than any of the other three groups. Therefore, you should keep your mind open and continue to search for the right training theory and methods.

Regulating the Spirit (Tiáoshén, 調神)

In general, there are four major goals in regulating your spirit (Shén, 神): Learning A.) how to raise your spirit, B.) how to keep it at its residence and strengthen it, C.) how to coordinate it with your breathing, and finally D.) how to use your spirit to direct and manifest your Qì effectively. All of these are called "Liànshén" (練神) by Daoist Qìgōng practitioners. Liàn (練) means to refine, to train, or to discipline. In religious Qìgōng, there is another ultimate goal in regulating the spirit, and that is to train it to be independent enough to leave the physical body for spiritual Immortality or Buddhahood (Chéngxiān/Chéngfó, 成仙/成佛).

1. **Raising the Spirit** (Yǎngshén, 養神). Yǎng (養) means to nourish, to raise, or to nurse. Raising the spirit has been the main task for scholars and Buddhists in their practices. Spirit needs to be nourished by Qì. Normally, the Fire Qì that comes from food and air is able to raise the spirit easily; however, this Fire Qì also increases emotional disturbance and therefore leads the spirit away from its residence. Using your Yì, which is nourished by the Water Qì, to raise your spirit is harder. However, if you are able to do it, this spirit can be stronger and more concentrated than when you use the Fire Qì. In Qìgōng practice, you are learning how to adjust your Xīn and Yì to raise your spirit. If you are able to use your Xīn and Yì properly, your spirit will be raised but not excited, and it can remain at its residence.

Learning how to raise the spirit the correct way is almost like raising a child. You need a great amount of patience and perseverance. One way to raise a child is to help him restrain his attraction to emotions and desires. Another way is to let him maintain contact with his human nature, yet educate him and help him to develop his wisdom so that he can make clear judgments. It is a long process and demands a lot of understanding and patience. *In Qìgōng, raising the spirit is not to increase your emotional excitement. This would scatter the Yì, and your spirit would become confused and lose its center.*

2. **Keeping Spirit in Its Residence and Training It** (Shǒushén Yǔ Liànshén, 守神 與練神). After raising your Shén, you must learn how to keep it at its residence and train it. As with a child of a certain age, you must be able to keep his mind in the family instead of straying outside and running wild. Then you can educate him. In Qìgōng training, to keep and train the spirit includes four major steps:

   A. **To Protect the Spirit** (Shǒushén, 守神). "Shǒu" (守) means "to keep and to protect." While it is relatively easy to raise your spirit, it is much harder to keep it in its residence. In this training, in order to keep the spirit in its residence you must use your regulated mind to direct, to nurse, to watch, and to keep the spirit there. You must be patient and control your temper (regulate your mind). You can see, therefore, that the first step in regulating your spirit is to regulate your emotional mind (Xīn, 心) and wisdom mind (Yì, 意). If you lose your patience and temper, you will only make the child want to leave home again. Only when you have regulated your emotional and wisdom minds will you be able to guard and keep your spirit effectively.

   B. **To Firm the Spirit** (Gùshén, 固神). "Gù" (固) means "to solidify and to firm." After you can keep your spirit in its residence, you then learn how to firm and solidify it. To firm the spirit means to train your spirit to stay at its residence willingly. After you are able to control your child in the house, you must make him want from his heart to stay. Only then will his mind be steady and calm. Naturally, in order to reach this stage, you will need a lot of love and patience to educate him until he understands how important it is for him to stay home and grow up normally and healthily. Qìgōng training operates on the same principle. In order to do this, your mind must be able to regulate all emotional thoughts. Only then will your spirit be able to stay in its residence in peace.

C. **To Stabilize the Spirit** (Dìngshén, 定神). "Dìng" (定) means "to stabilize and to calm." When you have brought your child into the stage of peace, he will not be as excited and attracted to outside emotional distractions. In regulating your spirit, you must learn to calm down the spirit so that it is energized but not excited. Then the mind will be peaceful and steady.

D. **To Focus the Spirit** (Níngshén, 凝神). "Níng" (凝) means "to concentrate, to condense, to refine, to focus, and to strengthen." You can see from the above three processes that keeping, firming, and stabilizing are the foundations of the cultivation of your spirit. It is like a child who is able to stay at home willingly with a calm and steady mind. Only then will you be able to teach and train him. In Qìgōng, once you have passed these three initial steps, you will learn to condense and to focus your spirit in a tiny spot. The "condensing the spirit" stage is where you can train the spirit to a higher and more focused state. When the spirit is focused in a tiny point, it is like a sunbeam that is focused through a lens; the smaller the point, the stronger its beam. The crucial key to make this practice successful is cultivating your subconscious mind.

Important Keys to Regulating Spirit

1. **Mutual Dependence of Spirit and Breathing** (Shénxí Xiāngyī, 神息相依). After the spirit has been trained to a high degree, you can put it to work. The first assignment for your spirit is coordination with your breathing. Remember, in Qìgōng training your breathing carries out your strategy. When this strategy is directed by your spirit, it can obtain maximum results. This is called "Shénxí Xiāngyī" (神息相依), which means "the spirit and the breathing are mutually dependent." In Qìgōng training, this is called "Shénxí" (神息) which means "spirit breathing." At this stage, your spirit and breathing have united into one. When you have accomplished this, your Qì will be led most efficiently. Naturally, this is not an easy task. In order to reach this stage, you must have regulated your body, breathing, and mind.

2. **Harmonization of Spirit and Qì** (Shénqì Xiānghé, 神氣相合). The last stage of regulating spirit involves learning to use the spirit to direct the circulation and distribution of Qì in the most efficient way. In Qìgōng society, this stage is called "Shénqì Xiānghé" (神氣相合), which means "the spirit and Qì combine together." In a battle, if the spirit of the soldiers is kept high, their fighting ability and efficiency will be increased, and the strategy will be carried out more thoroughly.

1.7 GENERAL DIFFERENCES BETWEEN BUDDHIST AND DAOIST QÌGŌNG (FÚJIĀ YÙ DÀOJIĀ QÌGŌNG ZHĪ BÙTÓNG, 佛家與道家氣功之不同)

Often Qìgōng practitioners are confused by the differences between Buddhist and Daoist Qìgōng. Both of them share the same fundamental theory and similar practices. However, according to the purposes of your practice, one style can be more effective than the other. If you wish to adopt the style that is most effective and efficient for you, you should first understand these differences.

1. The Buddhist monks believed that the goal of Buddhahood could be accomplished simply through spiritual cultivation. However, according to the available documents this overemphasis on spiritual cultivation resulted in their ignoring their physical bodies. They considered the physical body of only temporary use because it served as a ladder to reach Buddhahood. They even scoffed that the physical body was only a "Chòupínáng" (臭皮囊), which means "notorious skin bag." They believed that since it was the spirit that would reach Buddhahood, why should they spend time training the physical body? Therefore, still meditation was emphasized and physical Qìgōng exercise was ignored. Naturally, except those monks who also trained martial arts, most of the monks were weak and unhealthy. This problem was aggravated by a non-nutritious, protein-deficient diet.

2. From the point of view of training philosophy, Buddhism is conservative while Daoism is open minded. Because religious Daoism was formed by absorbing the imported Buddhist culture into the traditional scholar Daoism (Dàoxué, 道學), their doctrine, generally speaking, is open minded. Whenever the Daoists could find any training method or theory that could help their training and cultivation proceed faster and more effectively, they adopted it. This was almost impossible for the Buddhists, who believed that any philosophy other than Buddhism was not accurate. In Buddhist society, new ideas on cultivation would be considered a betrayal. For example, the sixth Chán ancestor Huì-Néng (禪宗六祖慧能), who lived during the Táng dynasty (618–907 BCE) (唐朝), changed some of the meditation methods and philosophy and was considered a traitor for a long period of time. Because of this, the Chán (禪) style divided into Northern (Běizōng, 北宗) and Southern (Nánzōng, 南宗) styles. This is well known among Buddhists and is called "Sixth Ancestor Disrupting the Passed Down Method" (Liùzǔ Shuō Chuánfǎ, 六祖說傳法). Because of this attitude, the Daoists have had more opportunities to learn, to compare, and to experience. Naturally, in many aspects they have advanced faster than the Buddhists. For example, in health and longevity Qìgōng training, Daoist theory and training methods are more systematically organized and more effective than those of the Buddhists.

3. Though both Buddhists and Daoists kept their training secret for a long time, the Buddhists were stricter than the Daoists. This is especially true for the Tibetan Buddhists. Before the Qīng dynasty (清朝), although both Buddhist and Daoist Qìgōng were kept from laypeople, at least the Daoist monks were able to learn from their masters more easily than the Buddhists. In Buddhist society, only a few trusted disciples were selected to learn the deeper aspects of Qìgōng training.

4. Daoists and Buddhists have different training attitudes. Generally, the Buddhist practices are more conservative than those of the Daoists. For example, in Qìgōng practice the Buddhists emphasize "cultivating the body" (Xiūshēn, 修身) and "cultivating the Qì" (Xiūqì, 修氣). Cultivation here implies to maintain and to keep. However, Daoists will focus on "training the body" (Liànshèn, 練身) and "training the Qì" (Liànqì, 練氣). Training means to improve, to build up, and to strengthen. They are looking for ways to resist destiny, to avoid illness, and to extend the usual limits on the length of one's life. This means Buddhists' training is more passive while Daoists' training is more aggressive.

5. The main emphasis of Buddhist Qìgōng is on becoming a Buddha, while Daoist Qìgōng focuses on longevity, enlightenment, and spiritual immortality. While striving for Buddhahood, most Buddhist monks concentrate all their attention on the cultivation of their spirit. The Daoists, however, feel that in order to reach the final goal you need to have a healthy physical body. This may be the reason why more Daoists than Buddhists have had very long lives. In their more than two thousand years of research, they found many ways to strengthen the body and to slow down the degeneration of the organs, which is the key to achieving a long life. There have been many Daoists who lived more than 120 years. In Daoist society it is said: "One hundred and twenty means dying young." This does not mean that the Buddhists did not do any physical training. They did, but unfortunately it was limited to those who were doing Buddhist martial arts, such as Shàolín priests. Therefore, generally speaking, today's Buddhists can be divided into two major groups. One is Buddhist martial artists (Sēngbīng, 僧兵) and some Buddhist non-martial artists who train both the physical body and the spirit, while the other group consists of those who still ignore the physical training and emphasize only spiritual cultivation.

6. Because of their emphasis, the Buddhists' spiritual cultivation has generally reached a higher level than that of the Daoists. For example, even though Chán meditation is only a branch of Buddhist spiritual cultivation, it has reached the stage where the Daoists can still learn from it.

7. Almost all of the Buddhist monks are against such training methods as "dual cultivation" (Shuāngxiū, 雙修) or "picking herbs from outside of the Dào" (Dàowài Cǎiyào, 道外採藥) through sexual partner practices. They believe that using someone else's Qì to nourish your cultivation can lead to emotional involvement and may disturb your cultivation. The mind will not be pure, calm, and peaceful, which is necessary for spiritual cultivation. However, because many Daoists are training mainly for health and longevity instead of enlightenment, they consider these methods to be beneficial.

1.8 Brief Background of Daoist Qìgōng Practice (Dàojiā Qìgōng Liànxí Zhī Bèijǐng, 道家氣功練習之背景)

In Daoism, there are generally three ways of practice: Golden Elixir Large Way (Jīndān Dàdào, 金丹大道), Dual Cultivation (Shuāngxiū, 雙修), and Herb Picking Outside of the Dào (Dàowài Cǎiyào, 道外採藥). Golden Elixir Large Way teaches the ways of Qìgōng training within yourself. This approach believes that you can find the elixir of longevity or even enlightenment within your own body.

In the second approach, Dual Cultivation, a partner or multiple partners are used to nourish each other so the Qì can be built up to a higher abundant level. In addition, through this practice, the imbalanced Qì can be smoothed out and balanced more quickly. Normally, most people's Qì is not entirely balanced. Some people are a bit too positive, others too negative. If you know how to exchange Qì with your partner, you can help each other and speed up your training. Your partner can be either the same sex or the opposite. Some people are able to exchange Qì with animals such as cats, dogs, and horses. This Qì exchange practice is also the fundamental practice for Qì healers who heal patients using Qì exchange. As a matter of fact, to many Daoists who are looking for spiritual enlightenment, Dual Cultivation has been considered a crucial key to achieve the goal. They believe that through Dual Cultivation, they are able to build up the Qì circulation to a level abundant enough to reopen the Heaven Eye (Tiānyǎn, 天眼) (Tiānmù, 天目) (i.e., Third Eye).

The third way, Herb Picking Outside of the Dào, uses herbs to speed up and control the cultivation. Herbs can be plants such as ginseng or animal products such as musk from the musk deer. To many Daoists, herbs also mean the Qì that can be obtained from the sexual Qì exchange practices.

According to the training methods used, Daoist Qìgōng can again be divided into two major schools: Peaceful Cultivation Division (Qīngxiūpài, 清修派) and Plant and Graft Division (Zāijiēpài, 栽接派). This division was especially clear after the Sòng and Yuán dynasties (960–1367 CE) (宋 · 元). The meditation and the training theory and methods of the Peaceful Cultivation Division are close to those of the Buddhists. They believe that the only way to reach enlightenment is the Golden Elixir Large Way, according to which you build up the elixir (i.e., Qì) within your body. Using a partner for the cultivation is immoral and will cause emotional problems that may significantly affect the cultivation.

However, the Plant and Graft Division claims that their approach of using Dual Cultivation and Herb Picking Outside of the Dào in addition to Golden Elixir Large Way makes the cultivation faster and more practical. For this reason, Daoist Qìgōng training is also commonly called "Dāndǐng Dàogōng, 丹鼎道功," which means "the Dào Training in the Elixir Crucible." The Daoists originally believed that they would be able to find and purify the elixir from herbs. Later, they realized that the only real elixir (i.e., Qì) was in your body.

Next, let us look more fully over the background of Daoist Qìgōng training.

Two Major Styles of Daoist Qìgōng

Peaceful Cultivation Division (Qīngxiūpài, 清修派)

Qīng (清) means clear, clean, peaceful; Xiū (修) means cultivation, study, training; and Pài (派) means style or division. The basic rules of Peaceful Cultivation Division Daoists are to follow the traditions from the Daoist bibles. All of the training and study are based on the fundamental principles that Lǎo Zi (老子) stated: "Objects are many, each returns back to its root. When it returns to its root, (it) means calmness. It (also) means repeating life." This means that all things have their origins, and ultimately return to these origins. When things return to their origin, they are calm and peaceful. Then, from this state, life again originates. He also stated: "Concentrate the Qì to reach softness, are you able to be like a baby?" You can see from these two sayings from Lǎo Zi the emphasis on cultivating calmness, peace, harmony, and softness. These are the basic rules of traditional Chinese Daoism, which originated from the observation of natural growth and cycles. It is believed that all life originated from and grows out of the roots of calmness and peace.

All of the Peaceful Cultivation Daoists emphasize "the method of Yīn and Yáng, harmony of the numbers (according to the *Yìjīng*, 易經; *Book of Changes*), and the shape will follow the spirit and combine." This means that Yīn and Yáng must be harmonious and balance each other naturally, and the appearance of the physical body will ultimately follow the lead of the spirit. This division believes that purely spiritual cultivation is able to lead them to the final goal of enlightenment. Therefore, a strong physical body is not the main target of the training. The body is only temporarily used as a ladder to reach the final goal of spiritual enlightenment. Consequently, they emphasize sitting meditation, from which they learn to "regulate the body" (Tiáoshēn, 調身), "regulate the breathing" (Tiáoxí, 調息), "regulate the emotional mind" (Tiáoxīn, 調心), "condense the spirit" (Níngshén, 凝神), "tame the Qì" (Fúqì, 伏氣), "absorb the Essence" (Shèjīng, 攝精), and "open the crux" (Kāiqiào, 開竅). These are known as the seven steps of "internal Gōngfū" (Nèigōng, 內功), by which they cultivate, study, train, trace back to their root and origin (find the point of calmness and peace within themselves), and finally cultivate an eternal spiritual life. Through this cultivation, they endeavor to reach the level of immortality and enlightenment.

We can see that the principles and training methods of the Peaceful Cultivation Division are similar to those of Chán (禪) (Rěn, 忍) meditation in Buddhism. Their training and cultivation are based on calmness and peace. Once their mind is calm and peaceful, they look for the root and the real meaning of life, and finally learn to be emotionally neutral and reach the final goal of enlightenment.

Plant and Graft Division (Zāijiēpài, 栽接派)

Zāi (栽) means to plant or to grow. Jiē (接) means to join, to connect, or to graft. Pài (派) means style or division. In training, Plant and Graft Division Daoists walk in the opposite direction of the Peaceful Cultivation Division Daoists. They maintain the methods used by the Peaceful Cultivation Division, such as still meditation, breathing, and swallowing saliva, using the Yì (意) to lead the Qì to pass through the gates (Qì cavities) and open the Qì vessels; however, they believe that just relying on these methods is less effective and impractical. This viewpoint was expressed in the document *Wǔ Zhēn Piān* (悟真篇) (*Book on Awakening to the Truth*): "Within Yáng, the quality of Yīn essence is not tough (strong); to cultivate one thing alone is wasteful; working on the shape (body) or leading (the Qì) (only) is not the Dào; to tame the Qì (through breathing) and dining on the rosy clouds are emptiness after all." The first sentence implies that still meditation is the Yīn side of cultivation. The Yīn essence found in the Yáng world is not pure. You must also have Yáng training methods that are different from purely still meditation. This criticizes some of the Peaceful Cultivation Division Daoists and Buddhists for seeking longevity and enlightenment only through meditation. It again says that trying to lead the Qì by controlling the breathing in meditation is like trying to make a meal of rosy clouds—it is empty and in vain.

The Daoist document *Bào Pǔ Zi* (抱朴子) (*Embracing Simplicity*, which is also the Daoist name of the author Gé Hóng, 葛洪) also says: "The Top Ultimate (i.e., the emperor) knows Daoist layman techniques, (which he) carefully keeps up and respects, of thoroughly studying the ultimate emptiness, enlivening all things, then viewing its repetition, finally obtaining the Dào and entering heaven." Layman techniques are those that were used by the Plant and Graft Daoists. When the ultimate emptiness is reached, all things start again from the beginning and are enlivened. When you understand that this cycle occurs continually throughout nature, you will comprehend the real Dào. This sentence emphasizes that even the emperor, who practiced Daoist layman techniques, was able to reach the final enlightenment.

What then are the layman techniques of the Plant and Graft Division? They said: "(If) the tree is not rooted, the flowers are few; (if) the tree is old and you join it to a fresh tree, peach is grafted onto willow, mulberry is connected to plum; to pass down examples to people who are looking for the real (Dào), (these are) the ancient immortal's plant-grafting method; (then you will find that) the man who is getting old has the medicine to cure after all. Visit the famous teacher, ask for the prescriptions, start to study and immediately cultivate, do not delay." This says that when you are getting old, you can gain new life from a training partner. Mutual dual Qì transportation can be done through particular sexual practices or through special types of meditation.

They also say: "(When) clothes are torn, use cloth to patch; (when the) tree (is) senile, use (good) soil to cultivate; when man is weakening, what (should be used) to patch? (Use) Heaven and Earth to create the opportunity of variations." This sentence asks, how can a weakened person regain his energy if not from another person?

You can see that the purpose of the Plant and Graft training is "similar types working together, spiritual communication between separate bodies. Similar types of people who are working on the same training can help each other. Spiritual communication (Shénjiāo, 神交) means using your feelings and your partner's to guide your spirits to stimulate the production of hormones or Essence. This is the original source of the Qì that can be exchanged with and used to communicate with your partner. In the sexual practices, sexual feelings are used to stimulate hormone production, and particular sexual activities are used to protect and store the Qì, which can be used as the herb to cure aging. When the sexual practices are done correctly, neither side will lose Qì, and both will obtain the benefit of longevity.

You can see that this style of Daoism encourages a proper sex life. If the correct methods are practiced, both sides are able to benefit. However, with this approach it is difficult to achieve emotional neutrality, and so it is very difficult to reach the goal of enlightenment. As a result, this style mainly emphasizes a long and happy life. *Hàn Shū Yì Wén Zhì* (漢書藝文志) (*Han's Book of Art and Literature*) says: "The activity in the (bed) room is the ultimate of the personality and emotions, is the ultimate of reaching the Dào; to restrain the external joy, to forbid the internal emotion. Harmony between husband and wife is the scholarship of longevity." This clearly implies that a correct sexual life is the way to longevity, because it enables you to balance your Qì and spirit.

In addition to sexual dual cultivation, they also emphasize nonsexual dual cultivation (Shuāngxiū, 雙修). According to this theory, every person has a different level of Qì, and no one's Qì is completely balanced. For example, in the teenage years your Qì is stronger and more sufficient than at any other age. Once you pass forty, your Qì supply tends to weaken and become deficient. To be healthy, your Qì must be neither excessive nor deficient. Therefore, if you and your partner learn Dual Cultivation Meditation or other techniques, you will be able to help each other balance your Qì. The Qì balance can be done by two males, two females, or male and female. It is said: "Yīn and Yáng are not necessarily male and female, the strength and the weakness of Qì in the body are Yīn and Yáng." It is also said: "Two men can plant and graft and a pair of women can absorb and nourish."

The Plant and Graft Daoists claim that there are four requirements for reaching the Dào: "money, partner, techniques, and place (Cái, Bàn, Fǎ, Dì, 財、伴、法、地)." Without money you have to spend time earning a living, and you will not have time to study and cultivate. Without a partner, you will not be able to find the "herb" and balance your Qì. Without the right techniques, you will be wasting your time. Finally, without the right place to train, you will not be able to meditate and digest the herb you have taken.

As a Plant and Graft Daoist, after you have balanced your Qì with your partner, you must also know the techniques of retaining semen, converting this semen into Qì, and using the Qì to nourish your Shén. If you are able to reach this level, you will be able to use your energized Shén to direct the Qì into your five Yīn organs (heart, lung, liver, kidney, and spleen) so that they can function more efficiently. This is called "five Qìs toward their origins" (Wǔqì Cháoyuán, 五氣朝元). The Qì with which the organs carry out their functions is called Managing Qì (Yíngqì, 營氣). Your Shén can also direct the Qì to the skin, where it can reinforce the energy field that protects you against negative outside influences. This Qì is the Guardian Qì (Wèiqì, 衛氣). Your Shén can also lead Qì into your bone marrow. This keeps the marrow fresh and clean so that the blood cells manufactured there will be fresh and healthy. When your blood is healthy, you are healthy, and the aging process will slow down. Daoists who reach this level have long and healthy lives. However, a Daoist who desires to reach even higher and attain enlightenment needs more than just this.

The Plant and Graft Daoists also use herbs to help in their Qì cultivation, believing that they offer significant help. The Peaceful Cultivation Daoists and the Buddhists also use herbs, but usually only for healing purposes.

1.9 Some Notes about Learning Qìgōng (Guānyú Zhèběnshū, 關於這本書)

After you have read this book, you will realize that all Grand Circulation Qìgōng practices are actually the branches and flowers of a Qìgōng tree. The root of this tree is the Embryonic Breathing. From this root, two big trunks are grown and developed. One of the trunks is Muscle/Tendon Changing (Yìjīnjīng, 易筋經), the Yáng side of physical Qìgōng training. The other one is the Marrow/Brain Washing (Xǐsuǐjīng, 洗髓經), the Yīn side of spiritual Qìgōng practice. Finally, from these two trunks, numerous Grand Circulation applications, like branches and flowers, are derived. In this last section of this chapter, I would like to remind you of a few keys to reading this book.

1. Always put a question mark on what you read and learn. Naturally, it includes this book. Remember, what you read or learn is only a personal understanding and opinion. The information in this book is provided to you for pondering and inspiration. It is you who must comprehend the meaning deeply in your heart and agree or disagree with it. Then build your confidence from study and practice.

2. You must recognize that the science we have developed today is still very shallow. Though the more we understand the science, the more we are able to interpret and verify ancient Qìgōng practices, we cannot completely trust the results. After all, we are still in the infancy in the development of this science. You should continue to search and collect new information from science and ponder the new answers and analysis of these ancient practices.

3. Qìgōng is a science and also an art. It was developed from deep exploration and searching into nature and the self. In order to reach a high level of Qìgōng practice, you must know *what, why, and how.* Always keep in your mind: What is it? Why do I want it? Why is it this way? How do I apply it effectively and efficiently? Without this fundamental learning attitude, your understanding and achievement will be shallow.

4. To understand the root of Qìgōng practice, you should also study Embryonic Breathing Meditation (Tāixí Jìngzuò, 胎息静坐). Without this root, you will never be able to grow your Qìgōng tree to a successful stage.

5. After you have comprehended and practiced the root, then you must also learn the theory and practice of Muscle/Tendon Changing and Marrow/Brain Washing Qìgōngs, the two major trunks of the Qìgōng tree. One trunk is for your physical life and the other for your spiritual life.

6. Once you have understood the root and trunks, you will learn how to grow branches and flowers. Branches and flowers are the applications derived from the root and trunk.

References

1. Albert L. Huebner, "Life's Invisible Current" (*East West Journal*, June 1986).
2. Albert L. Huebner, "Life's Invisible Current" (*East West Journal*, June 1986).
3. Robert O. Becker, M.D. and Gary Selden, *The Body Electric* (New York: William Morrow, 1985).
4. Richard Leviton, "Healing with Nature's Energy" (*East West Journal*, June 1986).
5. Leviton, "Healing with Nature's Energy" (*East West Journal*, June 1986).
6. Albert L. Huebner, "Life's Invisible Current" (*East West Journal*, June 1986).
7. 《莊子刻意》：〝吹呴呼吸，吐故納新，熊經鳥伸，為壽而已矣。此導引之士，養形之人，彭祖壽考者之所好也。〞
8. Albert L. Huebner, "Life's Invisible Current" (*East West Journal*, June 1986).
9. Robert O. Becker, M.D. and Gary Selden, *The Body Electric* (New York: William Morrow, 1985).
10. Richard Leviton, "Healing with Nature's Energy" (*East West Journal*, June 1986).
11. 肺金克心火。
12. Robert O. Becker, M.D. and Gary Selden, *The Body Electric* (New York: William Morrow, 1985).
13. Lennart Nilsson, *A Child Is Born* (New York : DTP/Seymour Lawrence, 1990).
14. *A Study of Anatomic Physiology* (解剖生理學)，李文森編著。華杏出版股份有限公司。(Taipei, 1986).

15. James E. Anderson, *Grant's Atlas of Anatomy*, 7th ed. (Baltimore: Williams & Wilkins, 1978) 9–92.

16. Sandra Blakeslee, "Complex and Hidden Brain in the Gut Makes Stomachaches and Butterflies," Science, *New York Times*, January 23, 1996.

17. Michael D. Gershon, *The Second Brain: The Scientific Basis of Gut Instinct and a Groundbreaking New Understanding of Nervous Disorders of the Stomach and Intestine* (New York: Harper Collins Publications, 1998).

18. David Holliday and Robert Resnick, *Fundamentals of Physics* (Hoboken, NJ : Wiley, Inc., 1972), 512–514.

19. *A Study of Anatomic Physiology* (解剖生理學)，李文森編著。華杏出版股份有限公司。(Taipei, 1986).

20. 一百二十謂之天。

21. 老子云：〝夫物芸芸，各復歸其根，歸根曰靜，是謂復命。〞

22. 老子云：〝專氣至柔，能嬰兒乎。〞

23. 法於陰陽，和於術數，形與神俱。

24. 悟真篇云：〝陽裡陰精質不剛，獨修一物轉羸尪。勞形按引皆非道，服氣餐霞總是狂。〞

25. 抱朴子云：〝太上知玄素之術，守敬篤，致虛極，萬物並作，以觀其復而得道飛昇。〞

26. 無根樹，花正微，樹老將新接嫩枝，桃寄柳，桑接梅，傳於修真作樣兒，自古神仙栽接法，人老原來有藥醫。訪名師，問方兒，下手速修莫太遲。

27. 衣破用布補，樹衰以土培，人損將何補，乾坤造化機。

28. 同類施工，隔體神交。

29. 漢書藝文誌云：〝房中者，性情之極，至道之極，制外藥，禁內情，和夫婦，及壽考之學也。〞

30. 陰陽不必分男女，體氣強弱即陰陽。

31. 兩個男人可栽接，一對女人能採補。

CHAPTER 2

Fundamental Concepts of Small and Grand Circulations

2.1 INTRODUCTION (JIÈSHÀO, 介紹)

It is impossible to list or discuss all of the Grand Circulation (Dàzhōutiān, 大周天) practices developed from various schools in the past. There are simply too many. However, you should know that the root of any Internal Elixir (Nèidān, 內丹) Qìgōng is Embryonic Breathing Meditation (Tāixí Jìngzuò, 胎息靜坐). This is because Embryonic Breathing Meditation teaches a Qìgōng practitioner how to regulate the mind to a highly focused state so the circulation and manifestation of Qi can be done efficiently. Not only that, Embryonic Breathing also teaches a practitioner how to conserve the Qì, build up the Qì to an abundant level, and store it in the Real Lower Dāntián (Zhēn Xiàdāntián, 真下丹田). These skills provide you two of the most important requirements for a successful Qìgōng practice: the quantity of Qì's storage and the quality of Qì's manifestation. Without these two prior conditions, all the Qìgōng practices will be shallow.

From this Embryonic Breathing Meditation (Tāixí Jìngzuò, 胎息靜坐) root, two trunks, Muscle/Tendon Changing Qìgōng (Yìjīnjīng Qìgōng, 易筋經氣功) and Marrow/Brain Washing Qìgōng (Xǐsuǐjīng Qìgōng, 洗髓經氣功), are established. Muscle/Tendon Changing Qìgōng is considered as a Yáng practice that focuses on the conditioning of the physical body's health, strength, immune system, and endurance. Marrow/Brain Washing Qìgōng is classified as Yīn training that aims for spiritual enlightenment and also cleansing the bone marrow for longevity. Here you should understand that though marrow is considered a part of the physical body, the techniques used in the practice are Yīn, and so it is considered a Yīn practice.

The foundation of Muscle/Tendon Changing Qìgōng (i.e., Yáng) is the Conception/Governing Vessel Small Circulation (Rèn/Dū Mài Xiǎozhōutiān, 任 / 督脈小周天) while the base of Marrow/Brain Washing Qìgōng (i.e., Yīn) is Two Poles Small Circulation (Liǎngyí Xiǎozhōutiān, 兩儀小周天). From these fundamental foundations (i.e., trunks), all branches of Grand Circulations are derived (Tables 2-1 and 2-2).

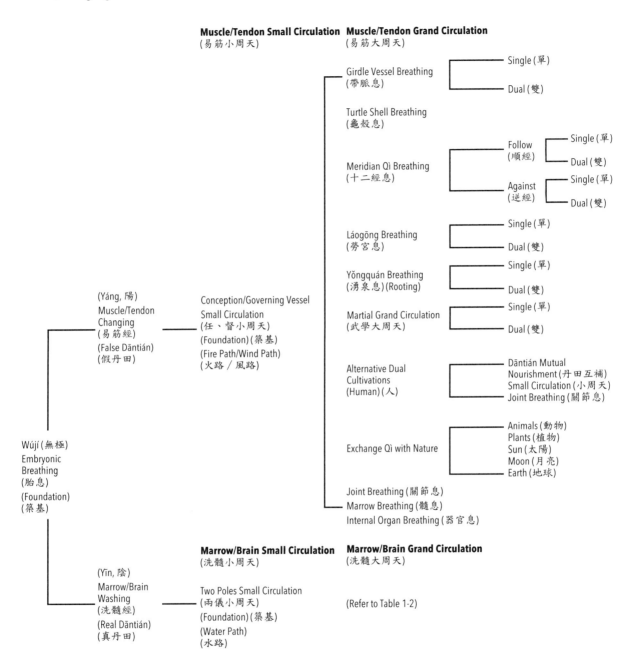

Table 1-1. Muscle/Tendon Changing Small and Grand Circulation.

Marrow/Brain Small Circulation
(洗髓小周天)

Marrow/Brain Grand Circulation
(洗髓大周天)

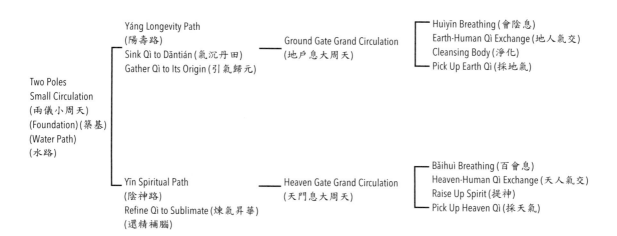

Two Poles
Small Circulation
(兩儀小周天)
(Foundation) (築基)
(Water Path)
(水路)

Yáng Longevity Path
(陽壽路)
Sink Qì to Dāntián (氣沉丹田)
Gather Qì to Its Origin (引氣歸元)

Ground Gate Grand Circulation
(地戶息大周天)

Huìyīn Breathing (會陰息)
Earth-Human Qì Exchange (地人氣交)
Cleansing Body (淨化)
Pick Up Earth Qì (採地氣)

Yīn Spiritual Path
(陰神路)
Refine Qì to Sublimate (煉氣昇華)
(還精補腦)

Heaven Gate Grand Circulation
(天門息大周天)

Bǎihuì Breathing (百會息)
Heaven-Human Qì Exchange (天人氣交)
Raise Up Spirit (提神)
Pick Up Heaven Qì (採天氣)

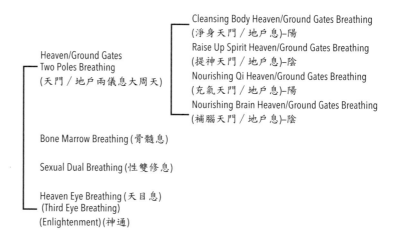

Heaven/Ground Gates
Two Poles Breathing
(天門／地戶兩儀息大周天)

Cleansing Body Heaven/Ground Gates Breathing
(淨身天門／地戶息)–陽
Raise Up Spirit Heaven/Ground Gates Breathing
(提神天門／地戶息)–陰
Nourishing Qi Heaven/Ground Gates Breathing
(充氣天門／地戶息)–陽
Nourishing Brain Heaven/Ground Gates Breathing
(補腦天門／地戶息)–陰

Bone Marrow Breathing (骨髓息)

Sexual Dual Breathing (性雙修息)

Heaven Eye Breathing (天目息)
(Third Eye Breathing)
(Enlightenment) (神通)

Table 1-2. Marrow/Brain Washing Small and Grand Circulation.

When you practice Internal Elixir Qigong meditation or applications, in order to acquire the best result, you must have a calm and peaceful mind, and also a relaxed and balanced body both physically and mentally. Without these prior conditions, your mind will be scattered and may cause Qì stagnation or misleading of Qi. There are a few suggestions or rules that you should follow to prevent some problems.

1. If your mind is disordered and disturbed emotionally, you should not practice. When the mind is not calm and under your control, this unstable mind can generate fantasy or illusion and lead the Qì to the wrong path. When this happens, it is called "waking into the fire and entering into the devil" (Zǒuhuǒ Rùmó, 走 火入魔) in Qìgōng practice. The mind can be disturbed from an uncomfortable feeling of the physical body such as full stomach, hunger, tight clothes, improper room temperature, wrong sitting posture, or many other things. The emotional instability can be from anger or being in an excited condition.

2. If you are fatigued and extremely tired, you must be careful in your meditation. You may fall asleep during meditation and cause Qì stagnation or cause Qi to enter the wrong path. If you are tired, choose a meditation practice in which you are not leading the Qi with your mind, but instead paying attention to your relaxation with deep breathing. In a relaxation meditation, even if you fall asleep, there is no harm. Actually, falling sleep is the best way of fatigue recovery.

3. At the beginning of your meditation session, always practice a few minutes of Embryonic Breathing so you are able to find your spiritual and Qì centers, and gather Qì at the Real Lower Dāntián. This will establish a firm root of your meditation session.

4. Once you finish your Small and Grand Circulations, always bring Qì back to the Real Lower Dāntián for a few minutes before you quit. This will prevent dispersed Qì from causing problems.

5. Immediately after meditation, you should conduct some recovery exercises to help the blood and Qì circulation. Stretching and movement are the keys for circulation. I will introduce some recovery exercises in Section 6.7.

6. After you finish your practice, you should practice the Three Sounds (Sānshēng, 三聲) to vibrate the Qì at the central line and lead it down to the Real Lower Dāntián. This will also help your mind be calm and allow the Qì to settle down. These recovery Three Sounds will be introduced in Section 6.7.

7. This book is aimed at experienced practitioners. You should already understand that meditation periods vary greatly. In the beginning you might want to set small goals like five minutes of focused breathing and increase your length of time to anywhere from thirty minutes to hours depending on how much time you have to meditate. When you have reached the stage where you can maintain a focused

meditation for thirty minutes you are probably at the stage where you can immediately drop into a deep meditation and at this stage even a few minutes of meditation will bring deep benefits.

Two Categories of Small Circulation

There are two kinds of Small Circulation practice in Qigong society. The first one is Conception/Governing Vessel Small Circulation (Rèn/Dū Mài Xiǎozhōutiān, 任／督脈小周天), also called Muscle/Tendon Changing Small Circulation (Yìjīnjīng Xiǎozhōutiān, 易筋經小周天). This Small Circulation is classified as Yáng meditation and is used to build a foundation for Yáng Muscle/Tendon Changing (i.e., physical life) Grand Circulation practices. This Small Circulation is commonly known in both Buddhist and Daoist monasteries and often practiced in Chinese martial arts society. This Small Circulation practice is also called Microcosmic Meditation in Indian Yoga.

The other one is Two Poles Small Circulation (Liǎngyí Xiǎozhōutiān, 兩儀小周天), also called Marrow/Brain Washing Small Circulation (Xǐsuǐ Xiǎozhōutiān, 洗髓小周天). This Small Circulation is classified as Yīn and is used to establish a firm root of Yīn Marrow/Brain Wishing (i.e., spiritual life) Grand Circulation practices. All of these Yīn side practices have seldom been shared because, traditionally, they were kept secret in monasteries. Some information became available to lay society only in the late 1980s.

Here, I will briefly review these two practices. If you wish to know more about Conception/Governing Vessel Small Circulation, please refer to the book: *Qigong Meditation—Small Circulation*, by YMAA.

Since there is no publication available in Two Poles Small Circulation, I will discuss its theory and practice more detail later in this book.

Four Categories of Grand Circulation Practices

Based on practicing methods, generally speaking, Grand Circulations can be categorized into four types.

1. **Self-Grand Circulation.** (Zìwǒ Dàzhōutiān, 自我大周天). In this practice, you practice alone to circulate the Qì in your body either for Muscle/Tendon Changing or Marrow/Brain Washing. I would like to point out that if Qì is led outward from the Twelve Qì Meridians to the physical body to enhance Qì circulation and condition the physical body, it is classified as Muscle/Tendon Changing Qìgōng. However, if Qì is led inward to the bone marrow to nourish and cleanse marrow, it is considered as Marrow Washing Qìgōng. If the Qì stored at the Real Lower Dāntián is led upward to nourish the brain cells and further open the Third Eye (Tiānmù/Tiānyǎn, 天目／天眼), it is classified as Brain Washing Qìgōng.

2. **Dual Cultivation Grand Circulation.** 雙修大周天 (Shuāngxiū Dàzhōutiān). As I mentioned in Chapter 1, Dual Cultivation (Shuāngxiū, 雙修) is called "Herb Picking Outside of the Dào" (Dàowài Cǎiyào, 道外採藥) in Daoist society. In this practice, you exchange Qì with your partner(s) and help each other's Qì circulation either for Muscle/Tendon Changing or Marrow/Brain Washing. It is most common for two persons, but in some cases, Qì exchange for multiple partners are also practiced.

3. **Nature-Human Qì Exchange Grand Circulation.** 自然與人交氣大周天 (Zìrán Yǔ Rén Jiāoqì Dàzhōutiān). In this practice, you exchange Qì or regulate your Qì status with the assistance of natural objects such as the sun, moon, earth, trees, grass, and animals such as dogs, cats, or horses.

4. **Enlightenment Grand Circulation.** 神通大周天 (Shéntōng Dàzhōutiān). In this practice, you exchange your Qì with the spiritual energy in the Yīn space (Yīnjiān, 陰間). This is the practice of reaching Buddhahood (Chéngfó, 成佛) or immortality (Chéngxiān, 成仙).

In the next section of this chapter, I will first review the definitions and purposes of Small and Grand Circulations. In Section 2.3, I will discuss the contents of Muscle/Tendon Changing Grand Circulations. Next, I will summarize the contents of Marrow/Brain Washing Small Circulations (i.e., Two Poles Small Circulation) in Section 2.4. Then, the contents of Marrow/Brain Washing Grand Circulation will be introduced in Section 2.5.

Remember, as I mentioned earlier, since the contents of both Grand Circulations are so abundant and wide, it is impossible for anyone to know and experience them in one lifetime. All I can share here is what I know and have experienced.

2.2 Definitions and Purposes of Small Circulation and Grand Circulation (Xiǎozhōutiān Yǔ Dàzhōutiān Zhī Dìngyì Yǔ Mùdì, 小周天與大周天之定義與目的)

In this section, I will define the Small Circulation and Grand Circulations based on the two main Qìgōng practices, Muscle/Tendon Changing and Marrow/Brain Washing. Once you have understood these definitions, you will have a clear idea of how various applications of Grand Circulation (i.e., branches and flowers) can branch out from these main practices (i.e., trunks).

Muscle/Tendon Changing Small and Grand Circulation 易筋經小／大周天 (Yìjīnjīng Xiǎo/Dà Zhōutiān)

WHAT IS MUSCLE/TENDON CHANGING SMALL CIRCULATION MEDITATION?

From Chinese medicine and Qìgōng practices we know that the Conception and Governing Vessels (Rèn/Dū Mài, 任/督脈) are the Qì reservoirs (Qìbà, 氣壩) which govern and regulate the quantity and quality of Qì circulation in the twelve primary Qì channels or meridians (Shíèrjīng, 十二經). When there is an abundant and smooth Qì circulation in these twelve meridians, your entire physical body, including the twelve internal organs, can be conditioned to a healthier, stronger, and durable state. Due to this reason, Muscle/Tendon Changing Small Circulation has become one of the most frequently studied and important Internal Elixir Qìgōng (Nèidāngōng, 內丹功) practices in Qìgōng society. To the martial arts Qìgōng group, this Small Circulation not only gives them health, but also offers a way to enhance their power.

Marrow/Brain Washing Small Circulation (Xǐsuǐjīng Xiǎozhōutiān, 洗髓經小周天), Muscle/Tendon Changing Small Circulation (Yìjīnjīng Xiǎozhōutiān, 易筋經小周天) is classified as Yáng, while Marrow/Brain Washing Small Circulation is Yīn. This is because Muscle/Tendon Changing Small Circulation is the root of your physical body's conditioning while Marrow/Brain Washing Small Circulation between the two poles of the body is the foundation of spiritual cultivation. We will discuss the Marrow/Brain Washing Small Circulation later.

Though there are many possible routes of Muscle/Tendon Changing Small Circulation in Qìgōng society, the most common two are Fire Path (Huǒlù, 火路) (Yáng-Yáng) and Wind Path (Fēnglù, 風路) (Yáng-Yīn). In the Fire Path, a practitioner will use their mind to lead the built-up Qì, following the natural Qì's Small Circulation orbit, to enhance Qì circulation, thus increasing the fire. In the Wind Path (Fēnglù, 風路), a practitioner will reverse the Fire Path route to lead Qì against the natural Small Circulation path, therefore reducing the Qì's circulation (Figure 2-1).

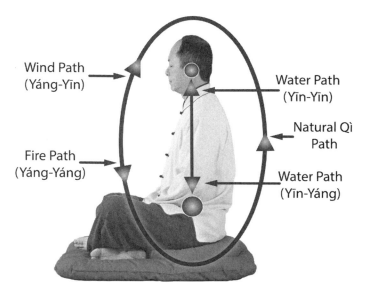

Wind Path (Yáng-Yīn)

Water Path (Yīn-Yīn)

Natural Qì Path

Fire Path (Yáng-Yáng)

Water Path (Yīn-Yáng)

Figure 2-1. Four Small Circulation Paths.

Purposes of Muscle/Tendon Changing Small Circulation Meditation Practice

1. **Increase the Quantity of Qì Storage in both the Conception and the Governing Vessels.** As mentioned, when Qì storage is abundant in these two vessels, there is plenty of Qì to condition the physical body. In order to reach this goal, you must know how to generate more Qì by converting fat stored in your abdominal area into Qì. About two inches below your navel is an area called the Elixir Field (Dāntián, 丹田) or Elixir Furnace (Dānlú, 丹爐) in Qìgōng society. This is because this place (i.e., field) is able to grow or produce Qì (i.e., elixir) like a field. This place is also called Qì Sea (Qìhǎi, Co-6, 氣海) in Chinese medicine since this area is able to provide unlimited Qì like a sea. When Qì is generated to an abundant level, it will be distributed and stored at the Conception and Governing Vessels.

2. **Use the Mind, in Coordination with the Breath, to Circulate the Qì Smoothly in the Conception and Governing Vessels.** It was discovered that when you grow older, the passage for the circulation in these two vessels would narrow down and the Qì's circulation would become more stagnant. Therefore, these two vessels will not be able to regulate the Qì's quantity and circulation smoothly in the twelve primary Qì channels effectively. Consequently, the organs would not receive the proper amount of Qì to maintain their healthy functions, which is the cause of aging and sickness. From past experience, it was realized that there are three areas where the passages are narrow and more dangerous than other places. These three narrow areas are called Three Gates (Sānguān, 三關). This has become the second goal of Small Circulation practice—to widen the passages of three gates (Tōngsānguān, 通三關). Unfortunately, without guidance from a qualified and experienced teacher, this practice can be dangerous and harmful.

Once you are able to produce more Qì and circulate it smoothly in your entire body, you will be able to condition your physical body. Since the content of the theory and training method of Muscle/Tendon Changing Small Circulation is complicated and extensive, I will not be able to cover this topic in this book. If you are interested in knowing more about Muscle/Tendon Changing Small Circulation, please refer to the book: *Qìgōng Meditation—Small Circulation*, by YMAA Publication Center.

What Is Muscle/Tendon Changing Grand Circulation Qìgōng?

Once you have accomplished your Small Circulation, the Qì circulating in the Twelve Primary Channels (Meridians) will be abundant and smooth, and then you can extend the Qì from the meridians outward to the muscles, tendons, ligaments, bones, skin, and beyond. For example, through Grand Circulation you will be able to lead the Qì to the joints to condition and improve the strength and endurance of muscles and tendons. This is the key training of Chinese martial artists. You may also lead the Qì to the Girdle Vessel (or Belt Vessel) (Dàimài, 帶脈) to strengthen your immune system. Naturally, you will also be able to exchange the Qì with your partners or other lives such as animals or plants.

Each person will experience Small Circulation in different ways and each session may be experienced differently each time. I do not want to bind you to one way of thinking. Some may feel a tingling along the vessels, and some may feel a warm wave. Keep your mind open in each practice. Pay attention. Do not preconceive what you may feel.

Theoretically, the higher the level of Small Circulation you have experienced and practiced, the higher accomplishments you will achieve in Grand Circulation. There are many Grand Circulation practices in Qìgōng society. I will list some of the common practices in the next section. Here, I would like to summarize some keys of these practices.

KEYS OF MUSCLE/TENDON CHANGING GRAND CIRCULATION QÌGŌNG

Since there are so many possible Grand Circulations derived from Small Circulation, you must have some important ideas such as what, why, and how. Without knowing these, it will be like driving a car without knowing where to go and why.

1. **Knowing Which Grand Circulation Practice Meets Your Need.** For example, the Grand Circulation for Iron Shirt (Tiěbùshān, 鐵布衫) will be different than others. Not only do you have to know what Iron Shirt is and what results you can expect from training, you must also know what the side effects will be. There are two ways to do Iron Shirt training: from the outside in and from the inside out. The outside-in method commonly used for external martial arts is faster but can also have the side effect of energy dispersion (Sàngōng, 散功). Training Qì exchange with a partner will be different than training with a tree. Different Grand Circulations serve different purposes and have a different theory behind them. Understanding theory is just like knowing how to read a map. Without knowing the theory behind the practice, the training may be shallow and even harmful. Again, since there are so many possible Grand Circulations, it is very difficult to find a qualified teacher who has had all the various experiences. Therefore, knowing the theory behind the training remains the crucial key to safety and success.

2. **Knowing Why You Want to Train a Specific Grand Circulation.** Other than knowing the nature of the Grand Circulation you choose to train and what the theory is behind it, you must also know why you want to know it, why it works, and how it serves your purpose. For example, Iron Sand Palm (Tiěshāzhǎng, 鐵砂掌) is a powerful and destructive training to condition your palms for fighting. However, you must also recognize that the side effect of the training can be harmful for your Qì circulation in the twelve meridians. If you train Iron Sand Palm just to show off your destructive power, then it is not worth the risk to your health. In addition, since guns are more powerful and destructive compared to your palm, it seems this motivation for training is shallow. However, the beginning stage of Iron Sand Palm training, before the harsh conditioning, which teaches you how

to lead the Qì to the palms, can be very beneficial for health. In this case, your training purpose is different. Recognition of why you do want to train is a crucial question before your training.

3. **Knowing How to Train.** This is the final crucial key and the most important one. Without knowing how to train correctly, you may encounter various side effects or negative consequences. Other than knowing the foundational theory, you usually need a qualified and experienced teacher to guide you to the right path. Unfortunately, there are not too many qualified teachers around in today's society. However, if you understand the foundational theory (i.e., map) clearly and proceed cautiously, you may attain a high level of training. For example, once you know the theory clearly, you may practice rooting Grand Circulation Yǒngquán Breathing (Yǒngquán Xí, 湧泉息) without a teacher. This training can be very beneficial for your stability and health. Another example is Grand Circulation of Qì exchange with a partner (i.e., dual cultivation) (Shuāngxiū, 雙修). Once you know the theory, and if you are cautious, usually there is no harm. I remind you, however, that this is serious training.

I will discuss both the theory and practice methods of Muscle/Tendon Changing Grand Circulation in Chapter 3.

MARROW/BRAIN WASHING SMALL AND GRAND CIRCULATION

The same as with Muscle/Tendon Changing practice, Embryonic Breathing Meditation remains the foundation or root of Marrow/Brain Washing Qìgōng practice. Here, I will review the importance of this practice.

1. **Condition the Real Lower Dāntián** (Zhēnxià Dāntián, 真下丹田)—Human Biobattery. If the Qì storage capability of your bio-battery is the same as the standard level, how do you expect to store the Qì at an abundant level? From science we understand that every brain cell consumes approximately twelve times the oxygen as a regular cell. This implies that every brain cell consumes twelve times the amount of Qì compared with a regular cell as well. So in order to activate more brain cells' function and increase the storage of the Qì in the brain, we will need a huge battery. Without the ability to focus the mind and accumulate abundant Qì, the Third Eye or Heaven Eye (Tiānyǎn/Tiānmù, 天眼/天目) will be hard to reopen. Reopening the Third Eye is a step toward spiritual enlightenment. Therefore, conditioning the bio-battery is the first task for enlightenment. If you are interested in bio-battery conditioning, please refer to the book: *Qìgōng, Secret of Youth*, by YMAA.

2. **Wake Up the Subconscious Mind.** The subconscious mind leads you to a focused state, while the conscious mind makes your mind confused, scattered, and disturbed. In order to reach a high level of concentration so the Qì can be focused

like a lens focusing a sunbeam, you need to wake up your subconscious mind and learn how to focus it. Without this, the Qì will be weak and it will be hard to reopen the Third Eye. This training can be done through Embryonic Breathing Meditation. If you are interested to know more about Embryonic Breathing Meditation, please refer to the book: *Qìgōng Meditation—Embryonic Breathing*, by YMAA.

3. **Store the Qì in the Real Lower Dāntián at an Abundant Level.** Naturally, once you know how to generate more Qì, you must also know how to store it in the Real Lower Dāntián. Without abundant Qì storage, even if you are able to lead it up to the brain, it will not be easy to reopen the Third Eye. Again, Embryonic Breathing Meditation is the training that provides this key.

WHAT IS MARROW/BRAIN WASHING SMALL CIRCULATION MEDITATION?

As mentioned earlier, Marrow/Brain Washing Small Circulation (Xǐsuǐjīng Xiǎozhōutiān, 洗髓經小周天) is the Water Path (Yīn Path) (Shuǐlù, 水路) while Muscle/Tendon Changing Small Circulation is the Fire Path (Huǒlù, 火路) (Yáng Path). Marrow/Brain Washing Small Circulation is also called Two Poles Small Circulation (Liǎngyí Xiǎozhōutiān, 兩儀小周天). Again, this Small Circulation can also be divided into two categories, a Yīn-Yáng path (Figure 2-2) and a Yīn-Yīn path (Figure 2-3). The Yīn-Yáng path is to build and store the Qì at the Real Lower Dāntián at an abundant level while the Yīn-Yīn path is to establish a firm foundation for Brain Washing.

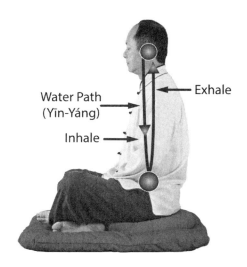

Figure 2-2. Yīn-Yáng Path Two Poles Small Circulation.

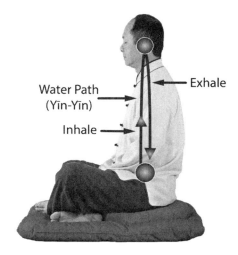

Figure 2-3. Yīn-Yīn Path Two Poles Small Circulation.

This Water Path (Shuǐlù, 水路) has mostly been practiced in monasteries for spiritual enlightenment. The path focuses the cultivation of Qì on the central Qì line connecting the two human poles, the Upper Dāntián (Shàng Dāntián, 上丹田) and Real Lower Dāntián (Zhēn Xiàdāntián, 真下丹田). Once the Qì has been built up to an abundant level, the practitioners would then lead the Qì upward to the Limbic System of the head and then forward, following the space between the two lobes of the brain to reopen the Third Eye or Sky Eye (Tiānmù/Tiānyǎn, 天目/天眼).

Following are some main reasons Marrow/Brain Washing Small Circulation (Xǐsuǐjīng Xiǎozhōutiān, 洗髓經小周天) or Two Poles Small Circulation (Liǎngyí Xiǎozhōutiān, 兩儀小周天) are not commonly practiced in laymen society.

1. If you have already studied and practiced Embryonic Breathing Meditation, you may have discovered that Embryonic Breathing practice is actually very similar with Marrow/Brain Small Circulation. In fact, many monks believed in the past that since they had already built a firm root of Embryonic Breathing Meditation, they didn't really need more Marrow/Brain Small Circulation practice. This is probably why Embryonic Breathing Meditation has become well known, but not Marrow/Brain Washing Small Circulation.

2. Muscle/Tendon Changing has been known and long practiced in laymen society. In addition, since Muscle/Tendon Changing Qìgōng is able to improve martial artists' strength and endurance, it was also commonly practiced in martial arts society.

3. The secret of Muscle/Tendon Changing Qìgōng has been known to laymen society since 550 CE while Marrow/Brain Washing Qìgōng was not revealed to laymen society until the 1980s.

4. Conception/Governing Vessel Small Circulation has an orbit and the cycle is repeated by following the time of day (i.e., following the sun). However, Marrow/Brain Washing Small Circulation follows the Thrusting Vessel alone (i.e., spinal cord) connecting the two poles. To many Qìgōng practitioners, it is not considered an orbital circulation.

5. Except for monks, most people are more concerned about health and longevity. Very few laymen Qìgōng practitioners were interested in spiritual enlightenment or attaining Buddhahood.

6. Compared to Conceptional/Governing Vessel Small Circulation, Marrow/Brain Washing Small Circulation does not have similar obstacles or gates. The passage is wide open (i.e., spinal cord) between the Upper Dāntián and Real Lower Dāntián (i.e., two poles). To laymen Qìgōng practitioners, there is no need to widen the passage as with Muscle/Tendon Changing Small Circulation.

You should understand that even though Marrow/Brain Washing Small Circulation can be trained easily, reaching a profound level of cultivation remains difficult. In order to reopen the Third Eye (Tiānyǎn/Tiānmù, 天眼/天目) for enlightenment, this Small Circulation remains the root of the whole practice.

Keys to Marrow/Brain Washing Small Circulation Meditation Practice

1. If there is no teacher available, the best way of reaching the goal of the practice is to thoroughly comprehend the theory behind the practice. Theory is the map. It offers you a logical direction for your practice. You must understand the body's two poles and the roles they play in health, longevity, and spiritual cultivation. Without a clear picture, it is just like driving without knowing how to drive or where to go. If you understand the theory of Embryonic Breathing Meditation and have practiced it for a while, you have already built up a foundation of practice. This is because Embryonic Breathing practice is the foundation and it shares a theoretic root similar to Marrow/Brain Washing Qìgōng.

2. The best time for practicing Marrow/Brain Washing Small Circulation is from midnight to early morning. This is because when we fall asleep, our Qì begins to condense inward and consequently the body temperature drops and the heartbeat slows down. After a couple hours or so, the Qì will be concentrated in the center Qì line connecting the two poles (Upper Dāntián and Real Lower Dāntián). When this happens, the hormone production from the pineal gland, pituitary gland, and ovaries/testes, all located in the central Qì line, will be enhanced. The body's metabolism will be supported and increased.

   However, after you wake up and you begin to move physically, the Qì from the center line begins to distribute outward to support the body's activities. That means the Qì's circulation in the Conception and Governing Vessels will be enhanced. Naturally, the Qì's circulation in the twelve primary Qì channels will be intensified as well. Finally, the Qì will be spread out to the skin for Guardian Qì's expansion.

   By understanding this natural Qì circulation timing, you can see that the best time for practicing Muscle/Tendon Changing Small Circulation and Grand Circulation is early morning right after waking up. The best time for practicing Marrow/Brain Washing Small and Grand Circulation is from midnight to early morning.

3. You should always remember that the quantity of Qì and quality of Qì manifestation are the crucial keys to success. That means you must have an abundant storage of Qì at the Real Lower Dāntián and also a highly focused subconscious mind. Without these two basic requirements, you will have a hard time achieving your goal.

4. In order to have enough Qì for your training, you must condition your bio-battery (Real Lower Dāntián).

What Is Marrow/Brain Washing Grand Circulation Meditation?

After you have practiced Marrow/Brain Small Circulation (or Two Poles Small Circulation) for a while and have reached a certain level, you can then apply this Small Circulation in Grand Circulation. The applications can be divided into two categories. (Each person should decide for themselves when that level is attained. I do not want to bind you to one way of thinking.)

1. **Pure Marrow/Brain Washing Grand Circulation.** In this form of Grand Circulation, you should keep your Qi development between the two poles (i.e., central Qì line). The common practice is to lead the Qì down to the Huìyīn (Co-1) (會陰) (i.e., perineum) and outward, and then lead it back to the Real Lower Dāntián. This practice is called "Ground Gate Breathing" (Dìhùxí, 地戶息). In this practice, you learn how to exchange Qì with the ground or use the Earth Qì to nourish your Real Lower Dāntián. Naturally, you may do the same for the Upper Dāntián and lead the Qì out and in through the Bǎihuì (Gv-20) (百會) (i.e., crown) for Qì exchange or nourishment. This practice is called "Heaven Gate Breathing" (Tiānmén Xí, 天門息). To monks, the final goal is to lead the Qì upward to reopen the Third Eye (i.e., enlightenment). We will discuss these practices in more detail in Chapter 5.

2. **Mixture of Marrow/Brain Washing and Muscle/Tendon Changing Grand Circulation.** Since the Real Lower Dāntián provides you the required quantity of Qi for all Qìgōng practice, once you have established the root of your two poles and have an abundant Qì storage, you can use this Qì to combine with Muscle/Tendon Changing Grand Circulation. For example, you may apply it in Martial Grand Circulation or rooting training. You may also combine it with Girdle Vessel Breathing training to boost your Guardian Qì (Wèiqì, 衛氣). Not only that, once you are able to cultivate and condition your spirit to a high level, you may apply this higher spirit in all practices. In summary:

A. Marrow/Brain Washing is Yīn training and in comparison Muscle/Tendon Changing is Yáng. Yīn is the origin of Yáng's manifestation, so when the Yīn is strong and deep, the Yáng manifestation will be effective and efficient.

B. The root of Two Poles Small and Grand Circulation is Embryonic Breathing, a singularity. It is called "Embracing Singularity" (Bàoyī, 抱一) in the Dào Dé Jīng, the beginning of life. When this center is strong, all developments from this center will naturally be strong. That's why we can conclude that the root all Qìgōng practice is Embryonic Breathing.

Keys to Marrow/Brain Washing Grand Circulation Meditation

1. **Have a Firm Root of Embryonic Breathing.** You should keep pondering and practicing Embryonic Breathing. The deeper your understanding and experience, the more your chance of success.

2. **Don't Be rushed. Take Your Time.** Since the crucial key to Marrow/Washing Qìgōng is your mind, you cannot be emotional and rush the training. This will only take you farther away from the correct path. It is just like when you try to sleep: the more you try to sleep, the more you push sleep away. Remember, when you practice Qìgōng, you are cultivating your subconscious mind. Too much disturbance from the conscious mind will only hinder your practice. That means you must reach a stage of "regulating of no regulating" (Wútiáo Értiáo, 無調而調) or Wúwéi (無為) state.

2.3 Contents of Muscle/Tendon Changing Grand Circulation (Yìjīnjīng Dàzhōutiān Zhī Nèihán, 易筋經大周天之內涵)

Purposes of Muscle/Tendon Changing Grand Circulations

For laymen:

1. To maintain a healthy physical body (Jiànkāng, 健康)
2. To boost the strength of the immune system (Zēngqiáng Miǎnyìlì, 增強免疫力)
3. To condition the physical body (include internal organs) (Qiángshēn, 強身)
4. To extend the life span (Chángshòu, 長壽)

For martial artists (in addition to the purposes of laymen training):

1. To improve strength and endurance (Lìqì Yǔ Nàilì, 力氣與耐力)
2. To increase power manifestation (Jìnglì, 勁力)
3. To reach a high level of alertness and awareness (Jǐngtìxìng Yǔ Jǐngjuéxìng, 警惕性與警覺性)

For monks (in addition to the purposes of laymen training.):

1. To reach the goal of spiritual enlightenment (Shéntōng, 神通)
2. To reach Buddhahood or Immortality (Chéngfó/Chéngxiān, 成佛/成仙)

The Contents of Muscle/Tendon Changing Grand Circulation

In this section, I will list only the Muscle/Tendon Changing Grand Circulation practices I am familiar with and also have had some experience with. Once you have comprehended the theory and experienced these practices, you may always apply it to other Grand Circulation practices. For a detailed discussion of these practice, please refer to Chapter 3.

1. Girdle (Belt) Vessel Breathing—Enhance immune system

    (Dàimài Xī—Zēngqiáng Miǎnyìlì, 帶脈息－增強免疫力) (Section 3.2)

2. Turtle Shell Breathing—Iron Shirt

    (Guīké Xī—Tiěbùshān, 龜殼息－鐵布衫) (Section 3.3)

3. Twelve Meridian Grand Circulation—Regulate Qì for health

    (Shíèrjīng Dàzhōutiān—Tiáoqì, 十二經大周天－調氣) (Section 3.4)

4. Four Gates Breathing—Balance

    (Sìxīn Xī—Pínghéng, 四心息－平衡) (Section 3.5)

5. Martial Grand Circulation—Power and endurance

    (Wǔxué Dàzhōutiān—Jìnglì, Nàilì, 武學大周天－勁力、耐力) (Section 3.6)

6. Joint Breathing—Loosen and relax the body

    (Guānjié Xí—Sōngshēn, 關節息－鬆身) (Section 3.7)

7. Skin/Marrow Breathing (Body Breathing)—Enhance immune system

    (Fūsuǐ Xī (Tǐxī)—Zēngqiáng Miǎnyìlì, 膚髓息（體息）－增強免疫力) (Section 3.8)

8. Internal Organs Breathing—Foundation of life

    (Qìguān Xī—Shēngmìng Zhújī, 器官息－生命築基) (Section 3.9)

9. Other Dual Circulation (with Human)

    (Qítā Shuāngxiū Dàzhōutiān (Yǔbàn), 其他雙修大周天（與伴）) (Section 3.10)

10. Qì Exchange with Nature

    (Yǔ Dàzìrán Huànqìfǎ, 與大自然換氣法) (Section 3.11)

2.4 Contents of Marrow/Brain Washing Small Circulation (Xǐsuǐjīng Xiǎozhōutiān Zhī Nèihán, 洗髓經小周天之內涵)

As mentioned earlier, Marrow/Brain Washing Small Circulation (Xǐsuǐjīng Xiǎozhōutiān, 洗髓經小周天) can also be called Two Poles Small Circulation (Liǎngyí Xiǎozhōutiān, 兩儀小周天). This is because this Small Circulation is completed between the two poles in a human (human polarity).

Two Poles Small Circulation

(Liǎngyí Xiǎozhōutiān, 兩儀小周天) (Water Path) (Chōngmài, 衝脈)—Foundation (Zhújī, 築基)

As also mentioned earlier, there are two routes for Two Poles Small Circulation. One is considered a Yīn-Yáng path and the other is a Yīn-Yīn path.

Yáng Longevity Path (Yīn-Yáng Path) (Yángshòulù, 陽壽路)

In this Yīn-Yáng path, you are leading the Qì down from the upper pole to the lower pole with an inhalation first and then upward to the upper pole with an exhalation. This will enhance the storage of Qi and hence the physical body can be conditioned and longevity can be achieved. This practice is commonly called "Sink the Qì to Dāntián" (Qìchén Dāntián, 氣沉丹田) or "Lead the Qì to Its Origin" (Yǐnqì Guīyuán, 引氣歸元) (Figure 2-2).

Yīn Spiritual Path (Yīn-Yīn Path) (Yīnshénlù, 陰神路)

In this Yīn-Yīn path, you are leading the Qì up from the lower pole to the upper pole with an inhalation first, and then down to the lower pole with an exhalation. This will enhance the storage of Qi in the brain and raise the spirit. This practice is commonly called "Refine Qì to Sublimate" (Liànqì Shēnghuá, 煉氣昇華)" or "Return Essence to Nourish the Brain" (Háijīng Bǔnǎo, 還精補腦) (Figure 2-3).

2.5 Contents of Marrow/Brain Washing Grand Circulation (Xǐsuǐjīng Dàzhōutiān Zhī Nèihán, 洗髓經大周天之內涵)

As mentioned in Chapter 1, Xǐsuǐjīng Qìgōng includes both marrow and brain washing. You should know that Marrow Washing can be done through either external elixir (i.e., physical stimulation) or internal elixir (i.e., mind leading with coordination of breath). Relatively speaking, physical stimulation through Muscle/Tendon Changing for Marrow Washing is easier than internal marrow breathing with the mind, but we cannot deny that the internal way is more effective and efficient than the external way.

Marrow Washing Grand Circulation (Gǔsuǐ Díxǐ Dàzhōutiān, 骨髓滌洗大周天)

In this practice, you use the mind to lead the Qi from the Yáng pole (lower pole) to the marrow for nourishment. I will explain this practice in more detail in Section 5.2.

Brain Washing Grand Circulation (Nǎosuǐ Díxǐ Dàzhōutiān, 腦髓滌洗大周天) Ground Gate Breathing Grand Circulation (Dìhù Díxǐ Dàzhōutiān, 地戶息大周天) (Section 6.3)

1. Ground Gate Breathing (Huìyīn Breathing Grand Circulation)
   地戶息（會陰息大周天）(Dìhù Xí, Huìyīn Xí Dàzhōutiān)
2. Exchange Qì with Earth Qì 地人氣交 (Dìrén Qìjiāo)
3. Releasing Qì 洩氣 (Xièqì)
4. Pick Up Earth Qì 採地氣 (Cǎidìqì)

Heaven Gate Breathing Grand Circulation (Tiānmén Xí Dàzhōutiān, 天門息大周天) (Section 6.4)

1. Heaven Gate Breathing (Bǎihuì Breathing Grand Circulation)
   天門息（百會息大周天）(Tiānmén Xī, Bǎihuì Xī Dàzhōutiān)
2. Exchange Qì with Heaven 天人氣交 (Tiānrén Qìjiāo)
3. Pick Up Heaven Qì 採天氣 (Cǎitiānqì)
4. Raise Up Spirit 提神 (Tíshén)

Heaven/Ground Gates Grand Circulation (Tiānmén/ Dìhù Xí Dàzhōutiān, 天門／地戶息大周天) (Section 6.5)

1. Heaven/Ground Gates Two Poles Breathing—Foundation
   (天門／地戶兩儀息大周天)—築基
   (Tiānmén/ Dìhù Liǎngyí Xí Dàzhōutiān—Zhújī)
2. Heaven/Ground Gates Cleansing Body Breathing—Yáng
   (天門／地戶淨身息)—陽 (Tiānmén/ Dìhù Jìngshēn Xí—Yáng)
3. Heaven/Ground Gates Raise Up Spirit Breathing—Yīn
   (天門／地戶提神息)—陰 (Tiānmén/ Dìhù Tíshén Xí—Yīn)
4. Heaven/Ground Gates Nourishing Qì Breathing—Yáng
   (天門／地戶充氣息)—陽 (Tiānmén/ Dìhù Chōngqì Xí—Yáng)
5. Heaven/Ground Gates Nourishing Brain Breathing—Yīn
   (天門／地戶補腦息)—陰 (Tiānmén/ Dìhù Bǔnǎo Xí—Yīn)

Buddhahood Grand Circulation (Spiritual Immortality) (Chéngfó Dàzhōutiān— Chéng Xiān, 成佛大周天（成仙）) (Section 6.6)

The final stage of Grand Circulation for Buddhist and Daoist monks is Buddhahood (Chéngfó, 成佛) or Immortality (Chéngxiān, 成仙) as it known to Daoists. Since becoming a Buddha or celestial being would have set them free from human emotional bondage, those who had achieved enlightenment would not bother to write down anything they had experienced after they were enlightened. However, from my personal understanding, in order to become a Buddha or celestial being, you must first reopen your Third Eye. This stage is called "spiritual enlightenment" or "spiritual communication" (Shéntōng, 神通). Those who have reached this stage of spiritual communication will be able to access all the knowledge recorded in the spiritual dimension or world. This knowledge is the accumulation of experiences and discoveries of all intelligent beings evolving in this universe. Once you have opened your Third Eye, you will be able to access this tremendous amount of knowledge and learn from it. It was said that once you have reached this level, you have no need for a physical teacher.

The Third Eye is called "Sky Eye" or "Heaven Eye" (Tiānmù/Tiānyǎn, 天目/天眼) in Buddhist and Daoist societies. When this eye is reopened, you will resume your ability to telepathically communicate with people or animals and you will also be able to see the change in energy of natural phenomena before it happens. Awakened people were often called prophets in the Western world.

There are very few documents in Buddhist and Daoist societies about enlightenment or attaining Buddhahood. However, the Muscle/Tendon Changing and Marrow/Brain Washing Qìgōng documents give some information. These documents tell of the Four Stages (Sìjiē, 四階) or Refinements (Sìhuà, 四化) to become a Buddha or a celestial being. I will list these procedures and briefly discuss the practice in this section. If you would like to know more, you may read Section 5.6 of this book. To learn even more about this practice than is introduced in this book, you may refer to *Qìgōng, The Secret of Youth*, from YMAA Publication Center.

1. Refine the Essence and Convert It into Qì 練精化氣 (Liànjīng Huàqì)
   —One Hundred Days of Building the Foundation 百日築基 (Bǎirì Zhújī)
2. Purify Qì and Convert It into Shén 練氣化神 (Liànqì Huàshén)
   —Ten Months of Pregnancy 十月懷胎 (Shíyuè Huáitāi)
3. Refine Shén and Return It to Nothingness 練神返虛 (Liànshén Fǎnxū)
   —Three Years of Nursing 三年哺乳 (Sānnián Bǔrǔ)
4. Crushing the Nothingness 粉碎虛空 (Fěnsuì Xūkōng)
   —Nine Years of Facing the Wall 九年面壁 (Jiǔnián Miànbì)

2.6 RECOVERY FROM THE MEDITATIVE STATE (JÌNGZUÒHÒU ZHĪ HUĪFÙ, 靜坐後之恢復)

The correct way to recover from meditation is very important. If you don't do it correctly, you may experience a headache (mental imbalance) or some physical tightness, especially in the spine. Correct recovery methods remove Qì stagnation caused by meditation.

The methods of recovering from meditation are both mental and physical. The trick is to reverse the normal regulating process of meditation. First regulate your mind, then your breathing, and finally your body. I will summarize the recovery methods that I have been using in my life for your reference. Naturally, you may compile or create your own ways. However, it does not matter what you choose since the basic theories and principles remain the same. I will explain these recovery methods in more detail in Section 6.7.

Regulate the Mind, Qì, and Breathing

1. Wake up from the semi-sleeping and subconscious state.
2. Use your mind to lead the Qì down to the Real Lower Dāntián. This is called "lead the Qì and return to its origin" (Yǐnqì Guīyuán, 引氣歸元).
3. Take a few breaths to regulate your breathing.

Regulate the Body

1. **Upward Torso Stretching.** Stretching the torso upward is always the first step in regulating the body. When the torso is tensed continuously, you will not be able to relax. This stretch will also awaken the cells from their semi-sleeping state.
2. **Sideways Torso Twist.** After the upward stretch, continue to stretch upward and at the same time twist your torso side to side a few times. Finally, tilt your torso sideways, to both sides, to stretch the sides of your torso. This will loosen up the fasciae and remove Qi stagnation around the torso (i.e., Triple Burners) (Sānjiāo, 三焦).
3. **Spine Waving.** After you have stretched your torso, then wave your spine, vertebra by vertebra. This will loosen up the tendons and ligaments of your spine.
4. **Loosening the Shoulders.** Shoulders are the junctions of the torso and upper limbs. If the shoulders are tensed, the Qì circulating to your arms will be stagnant. Furthermore, loosening up the shoulders will help you relax your neck and upper back and improve the Qì and blood circulation.
5. **Turning the Head.** The neck is the junction of the torso and the head. A tense neck and stagnant Qì and blood circulation in the head may trigger a headache and lead to abnormal brain function.
6. **Massage the Head.** Massaging and stimulating the skin in the head area will lead the Qì trapped under the skeleton to the surface of the skin and release it. Stagnant Qì trapped in the head will cause various problems.
7. **Massage the Three Yīn Channels on the Legs—Spleen, Liver, And Kidneys.** Stretch the legs and massage them, especially the soles of feet. This will loosen up the legs and allow the Qì and blood circulation to resume its normal state after meditation. It is also very important to stimulate and massage the cavity of the junction point of three Yīn meridians (Sānyīnjiāo, 三陰交). The three Yīn organs are the spleen, liver, and kidneys.
8. **Chanting.** The three sound chant (see Section 6.7) will help you to calm down your mind and settle your Qì down following the central Qì line to the Real Lower Dāntián. This is a very effective and powerful technique to return the Qì to its origin (Yǐnqì Guīyuán, 引氣歸元).
9. **If Necessary, Walk for a Few Minutes.** If you find that your legs are still numb or uncomfortable from sitting a long time, you may just walk for a few minutes to enliven the Qì and blood circulation.

PART II

Muscle/Tendon Changing Grand Circulation

CHAPTER 3

Muscle/Tendon Changing Grand Circulation

3.1 INTRODUCTION (JIÈSHÀO, 介紹)

As mentioned earlier, the foundation of Grand Circulation (Dàzhōutiān, 大周天) is built upon Embryonic Breathing (Tāixī, 胎息) and Small Circulation (Xiǎozhōutiān, 小周天) practices. Therefore, if an Internal Elixir Qìgōng (Nèidān Qìgōng, 內丹氣功) practitioner wishes to reach a profound level of Grand Circulation practice, usually he needs to practice Embryonic Breathing and Small Circulation first.

Embryonic Breathing Meditation builds two crucial foundations of internal elixir practice: improving the efficiency of Qì manifestation and conserving the Qì to store it to an abundant level. That means that through Embryonic Breathing Meditation practice, you will learn how to wake up your subconscious mind and feeling and use them to efficiently manifest the Qì at a high level. You will also learn how to generate more Qì and store it in your Real Lower Dāntián (Zhēn Xiàdāntián, 真下丹田) at an abundant level.

Small Circulation Meditation teaches you how to lead the Qì stored at the Real Lower Dāntián to the Conception and Governing Vessels (Rènmài, Dūmài, 任脈、督脈) (i.e., Qì reservoirs) to fill them robustly. In addition, you also learn how to use your mind to lead the Qì to circulate in these two vessels evenly and amply. If this is done, the Qì circulating in the Twelve Meridians (Shíèrjīng, 十二經) (i.e., Twelve Qì Rivers) will be fluent and strong. Consequently, your entire body (including the twelve internal organs) will be conditioned. From this you can see that Small Circulation Meditation is the root of Muscle/Tendon Changing Grand Circulation Meditation.

In the next ten sections, I will introduce ten common Muscle/Tendon Changing Grand Circulation practices for your reference. Once you are familiar with these practices, you will have a good idea of how it works and know to create different Grand Circulations to meet your needs.

1. Girdle (Belt) Vessel Breathing—Strengthen Immune System
   (Dàimài Xī—Zēngqiáng Miǎnyìlì, 帶脈息－增強免疫力) (Section 3.2)
2. Turtle Shell Breathing—Iron Shirt
   (Guīké Xī—Tiěbùshān, 龜殼息－鐵布衫) (Section 3.3)
3. Twelve Meridian Grand Circulation—Regulate Qì
   (Shíèrjīng Dàzhōutiān—Tiáoqì, 十二經大周天－調氣) (Section 3.4)
4. Four Gates Breathing—Balance
   (Sìxīn Xī—Pínghéng, 四心息－平衡) (Section 3.5)
5. Martial Grand Circulation—Power and Endurance
   (Wǔxué Dàzhōutiān—Jìnglì, Nàilì, 武學大周天－勁力、耐力) (Section 3.6)
6. Joint Breathing—Loosen and Relax the Body
   (Guānjié Xí—Sōngshēn, 關節息－鬆身) (Section 3.7)
7. Skin/Marrow Breathing (Body Breathing)—Strengthen Immune System
   (Fūsuǐ Xī (Tǐxī)—Zēngqiáng Miǎnyìlì, 膚髓息（體息）－增強免疫力) (Section 3.8)
8. Internal Organs Breathing—Foundation of Life
   (Qìguān Xī—Shēngmìng Zhújī, 器官息－生命築基) (Section 3.9)
9. Other Dual Circulation (with Human)
   (Qítā Shuāngxiū Dàzhōutiān (Yǔbàn), 其他雙修大周天（與伴）) (Section 3.10)
10. Qì Exchange with Nature
    (Yǔ Dàzìrán Huànqìfǎ, 與大自然換氣法) (Section 3.11)

3.2 Girdle (Belt) Vessel Breathing—Enhance Immune System (Dàimài Xī—Zēngqiáng Miǎnyìlì, 帶脈息－增強免疫力)

As mentioned in Section 1.4, the Girdle or Belt Vessel (Dàimài, 帶脈) around the waist area is the most Yáng vessel among the eight extraordinary vessels. As is well known, this is the only vessel from which the Qì can be led inward and outward horizontally in the body (Figure 3-1). Thus, this vessel is responsible for the body's balance. When the Qì in the Girdle Vessel is expanded outward, the entire body's Guardian Qì (Wèiqì, 衛氣) (i.e., aura energy) can be enlarged and strengthened. This is a crucial key in Skin Breathing (Fūxī, 膚息) or Body Breathing (Tǐxī, 體息) in Qìgōng practice. Through this breathing, the body's immune system can be boosted.

Theoretically, through correct breathing, the Qì from the Real Lower Dāntián can be led out from the Yīnjiāo (Co-7) (陰交) and Mìngmén (Gv-4) (命門) cavities and then distributed to the Girdle Vessel. Yīnjiāo means "Yīn junction" since it is the junction of two Yīn vessels, the Thrusting (Chōngmài, 衝脈) and Conception Vessels (Rènmài, 任脈).

Mìngmén belongs to the Governing Vessel (Dūmài, 督脈) and means "life door" since it is the door connecting to the root of life, the Lower Dāntián or bio-battery.

Practice (Solo):

You may practice Girdle Vessel Breathing sitting or standing as long as the waist area is relaxed. First, use your mind to regulate your breathing and bring the Qì to the center of the Real Lower Dāntián (i.e., bio-battery). Once they are regulated, inhale deeply and pay attention to your center of gravity (i.e., physical and Qì center). Next, use your mind in coordination with your breathing, exhaling to lead the Qì out from the Real Lower Dāntián through the Yīnjiāo (Co-7, 陰交) and Mìngmén (Gv-4) (命門) cavities evenly to the outside of the waist area (Figure 3-2). In order to open your Mìngmén so the Qì can be led out, you need to gently push your lower back backward (i.e., L2 and L3). Naturally, you should use Reverse Abnormal Breathing since you are leading the Qì outward intentionally. When you exhale, you should also gently push out your Huìyīn (Co-1) (會陰) (perineum or anus) to open the Qì gate. Your exhalation should be slow, smooth, slender, and longer than the inhalation. Keep your mind outside of your body around the waist area like a ring expanding from the center. While you are doing so, you may or may not make a Hā (哈) sound. If you make the sound, the expansion will be more aggressive and stronger. However, many practitioners practice this without making sound so the Qì can be expanded softer and farther. Once you are near the end of the exhalation, hold your breath for five seconds to allow the Qì to expand continuously.

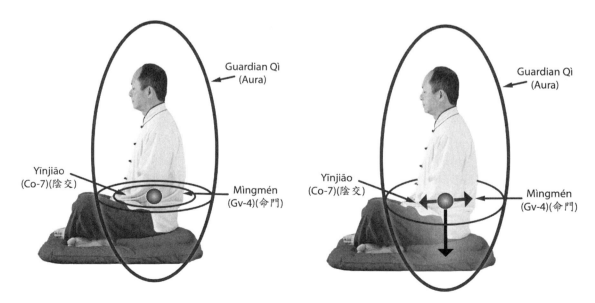

Figure 3-1. Girdle Vessel Qì and Guardian Qì (Wèiqì, 衛氣).

Figure 3-2. Expand Girdle Vessel Qì with Exhalation.

Next, inhale naturally to allow the Qì ring to retreat by itself. Then you may repeat the same process. You may practice till you feel warmer, an indication that your Guardian Qì (Wèiqì, 衛氣) is strengthened.

If you wish to enhance the expansion of Qì (i.e., strengthen your immune system), you may create resistance on your waist area. This will make your mind stronger and the Qì can be led more efficiently and aggressively. To create resistance you may simply tie up your waist area with a belt and repeat the same training process (Figure 3-3). You may also push a staff against the wall with your False Lower Dāntián.

This training will not only boost your immune system; it also raises your Spirit of Vitality. If you are catching a cold, this practice is very effective to prevent it from getting worse. It can also be used to raise your spirit when you are depressed.

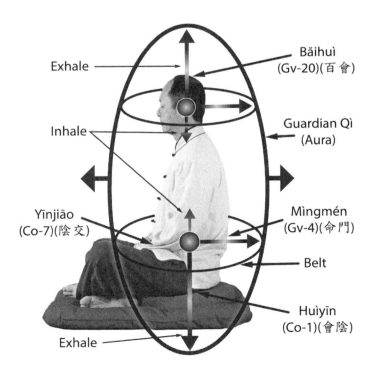

Figure 3-3. Using Belt to Boost Guardian Qì.

Practice (Dual):

When you practice with a partner, both of you should sit facing the same direction. In this practice, the one who has more abundant Qì should sit in front while the one with weaker Qì sits behind (Figure 3-4). The rear person should overlap both palms with the Láogōng (P-8) (勞宮) cavities aligned and placed gently touching their partner's Yīnjiāo (Co-7) (陰交) cavity. The front person should also overlap their palms with the Láogōng cavities aligned and placed on the top of their partner's hands. The person in front is the Qì supplier while the rear one is the leader. When the rear person initiates the practice, the front just follows. Use the same practice process as in the solo practice. After a few minutes, both should feel the Qì expanding from the waist area, combined and acting as one. You may practice as long as you wish till the leader decides to stop. After you have practiced for some time, you may switch positions. It may be only five minutes at the beginning, but once both have mastered the practice, the session can be longer.

3.3 TURTLE SHELL BREATHING—IRON SHIRT (GUĪKÉ XĪ—TIĚBÙSHĀN, 龜殼息—鐵布衫)

Turtle Shell Breathing is another crucial training for leading the Qì out of the skin. This practice is commonly used for martial arts Iron Shirt (Tiěbùshān/Jīnzhōngzhào, 鐵布衫/金鐘罩) conditioning. As a matter of fact, both this practice and the Girdle Vessel Breathing (Dàimài Xī, 帶脈息) practice are considered to be foundational for Muscle/Tendon Changing (Yìjīnjīng, 易筋經) training. This is because when the Qì is expanding from the center to the skin, the muscle/tendon can be energized and conditioned efficiently.

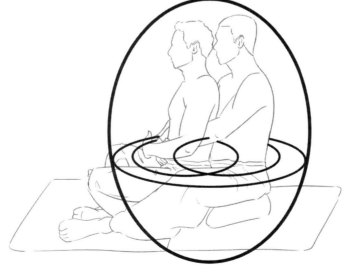

Figure 3-4. Guardian Qì Dual Cultivation.

In the past, this practice was usually done by those who were competent in Muscle/ Tendon Changing Small Circulation (Yìjīnjīng Xiǎozhōutiān, 易筋經小周天) training. Naturally, these practitioners were able to smoothly lead the Qì in the Governing Vessel (on the back) more efficiently and abundantly. From this vessel, the Qì is then led sideways and along the rib cage to expand to the entire back. When this is done, the Qì can be spread over the entire back, forming a strong shield like a turtle shell. Thus the term iron shirt, which is an external layer of protection for the internal organs. Since there is not much danger involved in this practice, many Qìgōng beginners have also practiced it.

Practice (Solo):

In this practice, you may sit or stand as long as your torso is relaxed. Bring your mind and Qì to the Real Lower Dāntián to gather your Qì. After you have calmed down physically and your mind is clear and peaceful, you inhale deeply to firm the Qì at the center of your Real Lower Dāntián. When you are doing so, you also gently lift up your Huìyīn (Co-1) (會陰) (perineum or anus). Next, you exhale deeply and use your mind to lead the Qì to the Huìyīn while gently pushing it out (Figure 3-5). Then, you inhale deeply again and use your mind to lead the Qì following the Governing Vessel (Dūmài, 督脈) (i.e., spine) upward to the Dàzhuī (Gv-14) (大椎) on your upper back. Finally, exhale deeply and use your mind to lead the Qì from the Governing Vessel following the rib cage outward horizontally and spread the Qì to your entire back. In order to charge the cells to a higher energized level, once you reach the end of the exhalation, simply hold your breath for five to ten seconds. Again, if you wish to enhance the spreading of the Qì, you may make a Hā (哈) sound while you are exhaling. The sound should be slow, gradual, and

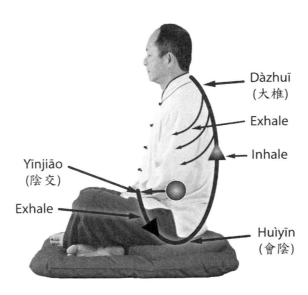

Figure 3-5. Turtle Shell Breathing.

soft. Since the peripheral nervous system branches out from the central nervous system along the rib cage, you will feel a strong sensation of Qì expansion following the rib cage.

Then, you may just relax and allow the breathing to return to its normal state. Naturally, in this practice, you are spending your Qì for manifestation. You may repeat the same process as many times as you wish if you feel comfortable. This practice can boost your immune system very fast. However, you should be aware that both Girdle Vessel Breathing and Turtle Shell Breathing are the training that would boost your Guardian Qì so the body would be more Yáng. If you have high blood pressure, you should be cautious. Naturally, these practices are good for depression and those who have low blood pressure.

Those who have mastered the Martial Grand Circulation (Wǔxué Dàzhōutiān, 武學 大周天) will be able to combine Martial Grand Circulation with Turtle Shell Breathing. This combination will increase the expansion of Qì significantly. We will discuss this combination practice in Section 3.6.

Practice (Dual):

In dual practice with a partner, both of you should sit facing the same direction as you did in Girdle Vessel Breathing. Your hands are in the same position as they were in dual practice Girdle Vessel Breathing (Figure 3-6). The one who has stronger Qì should sit in front while the experienced practitioner should sit behind. The person in the rear position initiates the Qì movements, and the front person will just follow and coordinate his breathing. After you practice for a while, you may switch positions, or not, depending on the agreement of you and your partner.

After you both have reached a deep level of coordination, the Qì circulation of both of you will combine into one. You may practice as long as you feel comfortable.

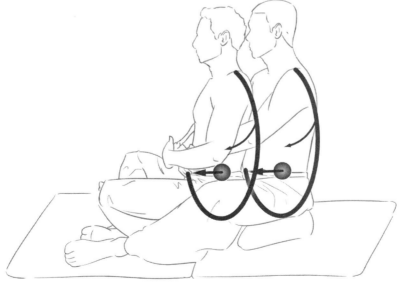

Figure 3-6. Dual Cultivation of Turtle Shell Breathing.

3.4 TWELVE MERIDIAN GRAND CIRCULATION—REGULATE QÌ (SHÍÈRJĪNG DÀZHŌUTIĀN—DIÀOQÌ, 十二經大周天－調氣)

Meridian Grand Circulation is also called Primary Channels Grand Circulation. In this practice, a practitioner uses his mind, massage, or Qì induction to manipulate the Qì circulation by either following with or against the flow of the meridians. If the Qì is led following the torso to the tips of the limbs, it is considered to be "releasing" (Xiè, 洩) (Figure 3-7). However, if the Qì is led from the tips of the limbs to the torso, the Qì in the channels will accumulate at a higher level. This is considered to be "nourishing" (Bǔ, 補) (Figure 3-8). The techniques applied depend on the condition of the corresponding organs. From these basic rules, Tuīná (推拿) (i.e., push and grab), Diǎnxué (點穴) (i.e., cavity press or acupressure), and Qì massage (Qì Ànmó/Wàiqì Liáofǎ, 氣按摩/外氣療法) were developed. Since these Grand Circulations are used to correct the meridians' Qì status, they are commonly used for health maintenance or treatments.

You may also lead the Qì following the natural meridian Qì flow. If you do so, you are enhancing the Qì's circulation and thus nourishing the organs. However, if you lead Qì against the natural meridian Qì flow, then you are slowing down or weakening the Qì's circulation to the organs, thus reducing the fire (i.e., Qì's flow) to the organs and cooling them down.

This information may be confusing at first. However, after you read through this section, you will have a better understanding. However, in order to practice, you must first

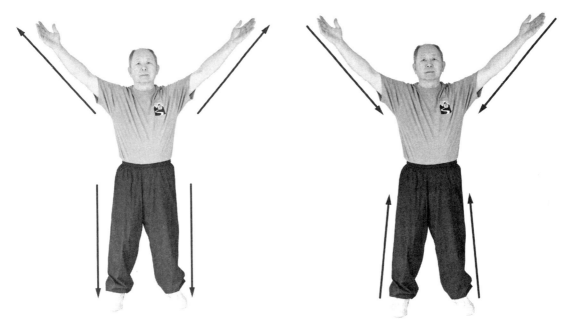

Figure 3-7. Releasing Qì from Torso.   Figure 3-8. Nourishing Qì to Torso.

know the order of the Qì's flow in the meridians. There are a few rules of meridian Qì flow that you should understand and remember.

1. If you raise your arms, the Qi of the Yīn meridians flow from low to high and the Qi flow of the Yáng meridians flow from high to low (Table 3-1) (Figure 3-9).

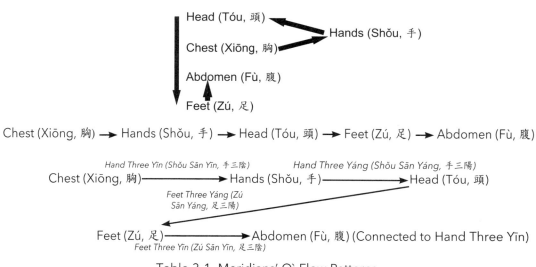

Chest (Xiōng, 胸) → Hands (Shǒu, 手) → Head (Tóu, 頭) → Feet (Zú, 足) → Abdomen (Fù, 腹)

Table 3-1. Meridians' Qì Flow Patterns.

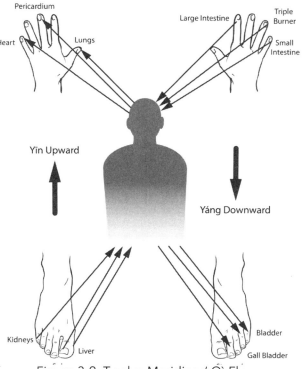

Figure 3-9. Twelve Meridians' Qì Flow.

2. You need to know how Qì circulates from one meridian to the next one following the time of day. From Chinese medicine, we know that major Qì flow switches from one meridian to the next every two hours (Table 3-2). It is called "Zǐ (midnight) Wǔ (midday) Major Qì Flow" (Zǐwǔ Liúzhù, 子午流注). When you practice, you should know these patterns so you are able to adopt the natural major Qì flow into your practice. The order to Qì circulation is:

3. To practice Grand Circulation effectively and successfully, you also need to know the relationship of the five elements (Wǔxíng, 五行): Metal (Jīn, 金), Wood (Mù, 木), Water (Shuǐ, 水), Fire (Huǒ, 火), and Earth (Tǔ, 土) (Figure 3-10) (Table 3-3).

From	To	Meridian	Name	Time
Top of Chest	Outside of Thumb	Hand Tàiyīn	Lungs	3-5 am
Tip of Index Finger	Side of Nose	Hand Yángmíng	L. Intestine	5-7 am
Under the Eye	Second Toe	Foot Yángmíng	Stomach	7-9 am
Big Toe	Top of Chest	Foot Tàiyīn	Spleen	9-11 am
Armpit	Little Finger	Hand Shàoyīn	Heart	11 am-1 pm
Little Finger	Front of Ear	Hand Tàiyáng	S. Intestine	1-3 pm
Inner Corner of Eye	Little Toe	Foot Tàiyáng	Bladder	3-5 pm
Little Toe	Collarbone	Foot Shàoyīn	Kidneys	5-7 pm
Chest	Middle Finger	Hand Juéyīn	Pericardium	7-9 pm
Ring Finger	Outside of Eyebrow	Hand Shàoyáng	Triple Burner	9-11 pm
Outside Corner of Eye	Fourth Toe	Foot Shàoyáng	Gall Bladder	11 pm-1 am
Outside of Big Toe	Side of Nipple	Foot Juéyīn	Liver	1-3 am

Note: Tàiyīn (太陰): Greater Yīn; Shàoyīn (少陰): Lesser Yīn; Juéyīn (厥陰): Absolute Yīn; Tàiyáng (太陽): Greater Yáng; Shàoyáng (少陽): Lesser Yáng; Yángmíng (陽明): Absolute Yáng.

Table 3-2. Twelve Meridians' Major Qì Flow Following the Time.

	Metal	Water	Wood	Fire	Earth	Mutual Fire
Yáng Channel	Hand	Foot	Foot	Hand	Foot	Hand
(External)	Yángmíng	Tàiyáng	Shàoyáng	Tàiyáng	Yángmíng	Shàoyáng
Bowels	Large Intestine	Bladder	Gall Bladder	Small Intestine	Stomach	Triple Burner
Yīn Channel	Hand	Foot	Foot	Hand	Foot	Hand
(Internal)	Tàiyīn	Shàoyīn	Juéyīn	Shàoyīn	Tàiyīn	Juéyīn
Viscera	Lungs	Kidneys	Liver	Heart	Spleen	Pericardium

Table 3-3. Relationship of Meridians and Five Elements.

Practice #1: Following or Against the Limbs (Shùnzhī Huò Nìzhī, 順肢或逆肢)

There are two common Grand Circulation exercises in this practice; one is for releasing and the other is for nourishing. Releasing is used when you have excess and stagnant Qì accumulated in the body; for example, fatigue and lack of sleep. It can also be used to relax the mind and body so the Qì can circulate smoothly. This is the common path used by a Chinese Qìgōng masseur to release patients' trapped energy and make them relax. Nourishing is used when you need to prevent Qì from being lost; for example, right after sickness such as diarrhea. This practice can also keep you warm in wintertime.

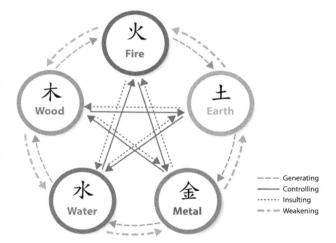

Figure 3-10. Five Elements (Wǔ Xíng, 五行).

In this practice, the mind is not on the meridians but on the path of the arms and legs. Allow the Qì to flow by itself. As mentioned earlier, there is a simple rule: when the Qì is led away from central body (i.e., torso), it is releasing, and when the Qì is led toward the central body, it is nourishing (Figures 3-7 and 3-8). This can be understood easily. If there is a channel along which the Qì flows from torso to the tip of the limb and you lead the Qì by following this path, you are enhancing the Qì's circulation from the torso or internal organs to the tips and thus removing the stagnant Qì in the torso and internal organs. However, if the Qì's natural flow in a channel is from the tips of the limbs toward the torso and you lead Qi against the path, you are weakening the Qì's flow from tip to torso and internal organs, thus reducing the torso and organ's Qì intake. The rules are simple and logical.

Releasing (Xiè, 洩):

Find a comfortable place and position that allows your body to relax. Lying down on a bed or leaning back on a sofa or couch are good choices. Standing is not a good position since your legs will be tensed.

First, bring your mind to the Real Lower Dāntián (i.e., Qì center) and take several deep breaths. Since you are leading the Qì following the limbs outward, it is more effective if you use Normal Abdominal Breathing (Zhèng Fùhūxī, 正腹呼吸). Normal Abdominal Breathing is commonly used for relaxing the body. The mind and the body should be as relaxed and calm as possible. First, inhale deeply and bring your mind to the Qì center while gently pushing out your abdomen and Huìyīn (Co-1) (會陰) (or anus). Next, exhale slowly, softly, and slenderly while using your mind to lead the Qì from the Real Lower Dāntián to the shoulder and hip joints, then to the finger tips and toes while gently withdrawing your abdomen and Huìyīn (or anus) (Figure 3-11). Naturally, you should pay more attention to your exhalation. The exhalation should be as long as possible. You may repeat as many times as you have the time and inclination.

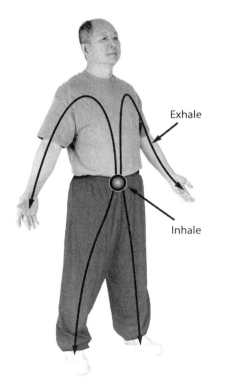

Figure 3-11. Releasing Qì (Method 1).

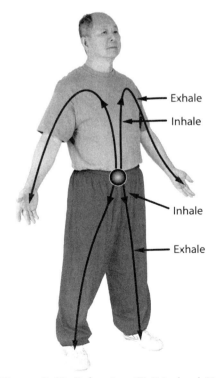

Figure 3-12. Releasing Qì (Method 2).

You may also use an alternative way of leading the Qi. When you inhale, lead the Qì to your shoulder and hip joints, and when you exhale, lead the Qì to the finger tips and toes (Figure 3-12). You should coordinate your breathing with your abdomen and Huìyīn as well.

This practice is commonly used when there is excess Qì trapped in your muscles, especially in the torso. When Qì is trapped in the muscles, the internal organs will receive excess Qì and cause them to be on fire. Once the excess Qì is released following the limbs, you may prevent the Qì from affecting the normal function of the organs. Consequently, you are relaxed. This practice is very effective for releasing excess Qi right after heavy physical exercises.

For those who have mastered the skills of Reverse Abdominal Breathing, their mind can be focused to a high level and the abdominal muscles can be controlled efficiently. Such practitioners often prefer using Reverse Abdominal Breathing (Nì Fùhūxī, 逆腹呼吸) instead of Normal Abdominal Breathing.

Nourishing (Bǔ, 補):

In this practice, the direction for leading Qì is exactly opposite from that of releasing. For nourishing you need to lead Qì inward toward your body center. It would be more effective if you know how to use Reverse Abdominal Breathing (Nì Fùhūxī, 逆腹呼吸) since your mind is very important for leading Qì in this practice. However, if you feel uncomfortable or are not familiar with Reverse Abdominal Breathing, you may also use Normal Abdominal Breathing.

First, lie supine in a comfortable position so your body is relaxed. Remember, when your body is relaxed, the Qi's circulation will be smoother. Next, inhale deeply and use your mind to lead the Qi from your fingers tips and toes toward your shoulders and hips and finally to the Qì center. While you are doing so, withdraw your abdomen and gently lift your Huìyīn (or anus). You should pay more attention to your inhalation and make the breathing as slow, slender, and soft as possible. Once the Qi is led to the

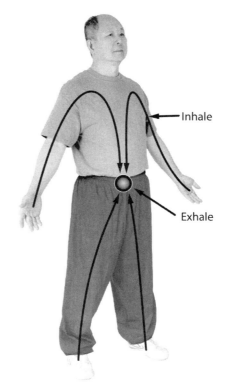

Figure 3-13. Nourishing Qì (Method 1).

center, just exhale and allow the air to flow out naturally and smoothly. Also relax your abdomen and Huìyīn (or anus) (Figure 3-13).

An alternative method is when you inhale, you lead the Qì from finger tips and toes to your central Qì line and when you exhale, you lead the Qì down to the Real Lower Dāntián (i.e., Qì center) (Figure 3-14).

Practice #2: Follow or Move Against the Natural Meridian Qì Flow

Again, this practice can be divided into releasing and nourishing. Depending on the internal organ, the direction in which you lead the Qì can be different. If you look at Tables 3-1 and 3-2, you can see the direction of the meridian's Qì flow. But the simple rule is when the Qì led toward the organ is enhanced, it is nourishing. However, when the Qì led away from the organs is intensified, then it is releasing. For example, the natural Qì flow of the heart channel is from armpit to pinky. That means that if you lead the Qì from armpit to pinky, you are leading the Qì away from the heart, and then it is releasing. However, if you reverse the direction, you are nourishing the heart (Figure 3-15). But when you take a look at the liver channel, it is very different. The natural Qì flow of the liver channel is from outside of the big toe to the side of the nipple. That means if you lead

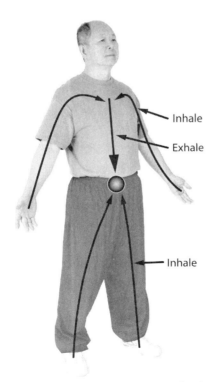

Figure 3-14. Nourishing Qì (Method 2).

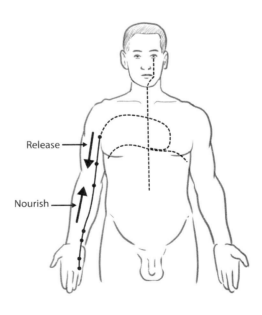

Figure 3-15. Nourish and Release of Heart.

the Qì following the natural Liver Qì flow direction, you are leading the Qì toward the center and the liver, and then it is nourishing. However, if you use your mind to lead the Qì in the reverse direction of the natural liver Qì flow, from the side of the nipple to the big toe, then you are preventing excess Qì from flowing to the body center and liver, and thus it is releasing (Figure 3-16).

From here, you can see that when you practice Grand Qì Circulation in the meridians, you must know and be very careful about the natural Qì flow of the organs or else the purpose can be completely reversed. The simple rule is *when you lead the Qì toward the torso, you are nourishing the organs; when you lead the Qì away from the torso, you are releasing Qi from the organs.*

Some people would practice all twelve meridians' Qì to enhance its circulation. Again, there are two ways of doing so: releasing and nourishing. The theory is very simple in this practice. If you use your mind to lead the Qì following the natural Qì flow, then you are enhancing the Qì's circulation. Naturally, all organs will receive more Qì than normal. This is nourishing. However, if you reverse the Qì flow, then you are reducing the Qì's circulation from entering the internal organs, thus releasing.

Example #1: Lead Qì Away from the Central Body—Releasing

We will use the lung meridian as an example. The natural Qì circulation in the lung meridian is from the top of the chest to the outside tip of the thumb (Table 3-2). When you practice, you may use either Normal Abdominal Breathing or Reverse Abdominal

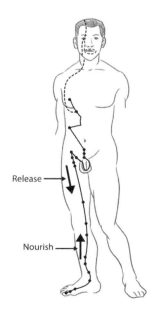

Figure 3-16. Nourish and
Release of Liver.

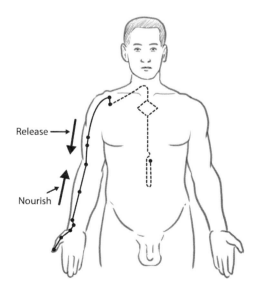

Figure 3-17. Nourish and Release of Lungs.

Breathing. If you are not familiar with Reverse Abdominal Breathing, you may use Normal Abdominal Breathing. You simply let a relaxed body and a firm mind leading do the job. Inhale deeply and place your mind on your upper chest. When you exhale use your mind to lead the Qì following the lung meridian and down to the thumb (Figure 3-17). This will enhance the Qì circulation from your upper chest to the thumbs and release it. However, if you wish to nourish the lungs, then you may just reverse the direction and lead Qì from the thumbs to the upper chest. Naturally, coordination with your Huìyīn (Co-1, 會陰) (or anus) and breathing are crucial keys to making this practice successful.

If you are familiar with Reverse Abdominal Breathing and use it to achieve the goal, the leading can be more effective and efficient. However, you should keep your body as relaxed as possible.

Example #2: Lead Qì Toward the Central Body—Nourishing

Here we use the kidney meridian as an example. The natural Qì circulation of the kidneys is from the little toe to the collarbone. Use the same breathing method as in example #1. If you lead the Qì from the little toe to the collarbone (i.e., toward the central body), you will enhance the Qì circulation in the kidney meridians (Figure 3-18). This is nourishing. However, if you lead the Qì from the collarbone to the little toe, that goes against the natural Qì flow and thus will weaken the Qì flowing into the kidneys, thus reducing the kidneys' excess fire.

Example #3: Twelve Meridian Grand Circulation

You may use the mind to lead the Qì to either follow (i.e., nourishing) or go against (i.e., reducing) the natural Qì flow patterns of all twelve meridians. That means, for nourishing, you would enhance the Qì circulation. Thus you follow the natural Qì circulation path and begin from the lungs, next the large intestine, then the stomach, and so on until the liver and return to the lungs again to repeat the practice (Table 3-2). Whenever the Qì is led from the central body to the limbs, exhale, and when Qi is led toward the central body, inhale. This practice will expedite the Qì circulation in the meridians and thus enhance the Qì's nourishment in the organs.

However, if you lead Qi against the natural meridian Qì circulation path, you

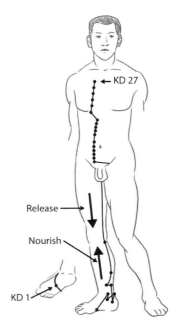

Figure 3-18. Nourish and Release of Kidneys.

are slowing down or cooling down the Qì in the organs. So leading Qì in this way is for reducing. You begin with the liver meridian, from the side of the nipples to outside of the big toes, then move to the gall bladder meridian, from the fourth toe to the outside corner of the eyes, and so on, until you reach the lungs, and then repeat (Table 3-2). Again, you will exhale when the Qì is led outward to the limbs and inhale when it is led toward the central body.

You need to be aware that this twelve meridian Qì manipulation has not commonly been practiced, especially by beginning Qìgōng practitioners. There are three reasons: first, if you are not an expert in Chinese medicine and know exactly the paths of the meridians, you may lead the Qì to the wrong place; second, unless you really know your body's Qì status, especially the internal organs, if your mind is not clear to practice this, you may also trigger abnormal Qì circulation in the meridians; third, you must already have abundant experience in leading the Qì, otherwise, normal Qì circulation can be disrupted.

The examples #1 and #2 were chosen because they are safer, simpler, and effective if you are not yet an expert in leading the Qì.

Example #4: Meridian Grand Circulation with Applications of Five Elements

If you are skillful in using your mind to lead the Qì and if you know how to apply the theory of Five Elements (Wǔxíng, 五行), you will be able to effectively manipulate the circulation of Qi in your practice. If you take a look at Figure 3-10 and Table 3-3, you will see that the natural Qì production pattern is:

Kidneys (Water) –> Liver (Wood)–> Heart (Fire) –> Spleen (Earth) –> Lungs (Metal)

This means the Qì flow in the kidneys will influence the liver's Qì, the liver's Qì will influence the Qi of the heart, the Qì in the heart will affect the Qì circulation in the spleen and, finally, the spleen's Qì will impact the Qì circulation in the lungs. If you circulate your Qì following this order, it will be productive and the Qì flow will be enhanced.

However, if you reverse the order, then it is conquest and will thus reduce the Qì's flow. Again, if you are not familiar with Chinese medicine and the theory of Five Elements, you must be very careful in this practice.

3.5 FOUR GATES BREATHING—BALANCE (SÌXĪN XÍ—PÍNGHÉNG, 四心息－平衡)

Four Gates Breathing Qìgōng is a common practice in martial arts society. In this practice, a practitioner will normally first learn how to lead the Qì to the Láogōng (P-8) (勞宮) cavity at the center of palms. This is because the hands are used to strike, grab, and carry weapons. Through this practice, the sensitivity of the hands can be increased, and strength and endurance will be enhanced. Strong hands mean greater endurance and fighting capability in martial arts.

Next, practitioners will learn how to lead Qì to the Yǒngquán (K-1) (湧泉) cavity at bottom of the feet to improve the feeling of the soles. This will promote better balance and centering, thus helping to establish a firm root.

Only after practitioners are able to lead the Qì to the palms or feet efficiently and smoothly should they combine these two practices, which then becomes Four Gates Breathing. This will offer practitioners an upward and downward balanced feeling.

Láogōng Breathing—Enhance Hands' Sensitivity (Láogōng Xī—Zēngyì Shǒugǎn, 勞宮息－增益手感)

In this practice, a practitioner will use his mind, with some specific physical movements, to lead the Qì to the Láogōng (P-8, 勞宮) cavity and allow the Qì to be distributed to the entire hand (Figure 3-19). This practice has also been commonly used to improve

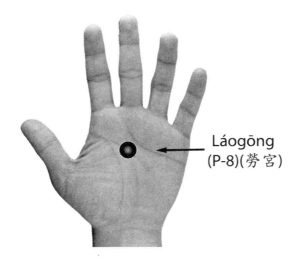

Figure 3-19. The Láogōng (P-8) Cavity.

the Qì circulation in the six Qì channels, circulating to the tip of the fingers. These six channels are the: Heart, Lungs, Pericardium, Small Intestine, Large Intestine, and Triple Burners.

Practice (Solo):

When you practice, you may sit or stand. Here, we use standing as an example. Stand comfortably with palms facing downward. First, inhale deeply and gather all the Qì at the Real Lower Dāntián. Use Reverse Abdominal Breathing and gently withdraw your abdomen and Huìyīn (Figure 3-20).

Next, exhale and imagine you are pushing your palm down against some object (Figure 3-21). While you are doing so, firmly but gently push out your abdomen and Huìyīn. You should not pay attention to the meridian; just allow the Qì to flow naturally and smoothly by itself. All you need is a strong and focused mind to lead the Qì using the image of pushing an object. Remember, it is your mind that leads the Qì. The more focused the mind, the stronger the Qì will be led. In this position, your arms are more relaxed and Qì will flow easily. Once you have mastered the skill, you should gradually raise your arms and finally

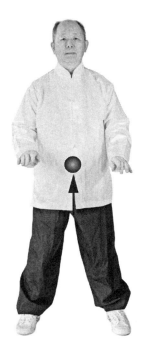

Figure 3-20. Gather Qì at Real Lower Dāntián.

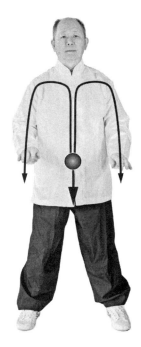

Figure 3-21. Lead Qì to Láogōng.

push forward. Naturally, because your arms are raised, they will be more tensed and the Qì flow will be more difficult.

Next, inhale deeply again and lead the Qì back to the Real Lower Dāntián. Repeat the training for as long as you have the time and inclination. If you wish to keep leading the Qì out and extending your Qì beyond your palms farther and farther, when you have reached the end of exhalation, simply hold your breath for five to ten seconds. This will allow the continuous expansion of your Qì. Then when you inhale, simply relax your abdomen and Huìyīn and allow the breathing to return to its normal state. Naturally, the more repetition, the farther the Qì will reach.

Once you are able to lead the Qì to the Láogōng at the center of your palms easily and smoothly, you may practice extending the Qì to the tips of your five fingers (Figure 3-22). This will allow your Qì to circulate more abundantly in the six meridians in the arms for health. These six meridians are the Lungs, Pericardium, Heart, Large Intestine, Triple Burner, and Small Intestine. This practice is commonly called Finger Tip Qì Releasing Practice (Zhǐjiān Fàngqì Liànxí, 指尖放氣練習).

Later, once you know the Martial Grand Circulation (Wǔxué Dàzhōutiān, 武學大周天) in Section 3.6, you may apply Martial Grand Circulation in this practice. This will enhance the Qì circulation significantly.

Practice (Dual):

This dual cultivation practice is commonly called Láogōng Dual Cultivation (Láogōng Shuāngxiū, 勞宮雙修) or Láogōng Qì Exchange Practice (Láogōng Huanqì Liànxí, 勞宮換氣練習). This dual cultivation is the most basic and safest Dual Cultivation training for beginners. It is also the most basic training for Qì masseurs and Qì healers. In this practice, you and your partner mutually exchange the Qì through the Láogōng cavity and lead it to

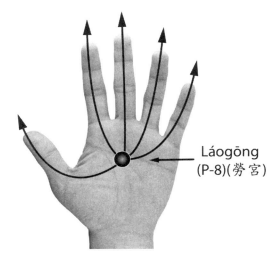

Láogōng
(P-8)(勞宮)

Figure 3-22. Extend Qì to Finger Tips.

different areas of your partner's body. For example, by using your mind in coordination with your breathing, you may first lead the Qì to the partner's wrist and your partner will do the same. After both of you can smoothly lead and govern the Qì through this exchange, you can then extend the exchange to areas further away from the wrist, to the elbows or shoulders. The final goal of this Qì exchange is to reach each other's Real Lower Dāntián. Naturally, the farther your Qì enters your partner's body, the more difficult it will be.

When you practice, you and your partner sit and face each other. The person who has more experience will be the leader while the other is the follower. The follower places their palms on their partner's knees with palms facing up. The leader will place their palm on the top of follower's palms facing down with Láogōng lined up with each other.

First, you both regulate the mind and breathing for a few minutes until you are calm and natural. Next, the leader will exhale and use their mind to lead the Qì from the Real Lower Dāntián to their palms and beyond till the Qì reaches the follower's wrists (Figure 3-23). When they initiate this action, they should gently push the follower's palm physically with a very slight movement. From this movement, the follower will feel the leader's action and can coordinate with it. Once the follower feels the action, they should inhale and lead the Qì from the palms to their wrists. Next, the leader will lead the Qì back to their wrists with an inhalation while the follower will coordinate and lead the Qì to the

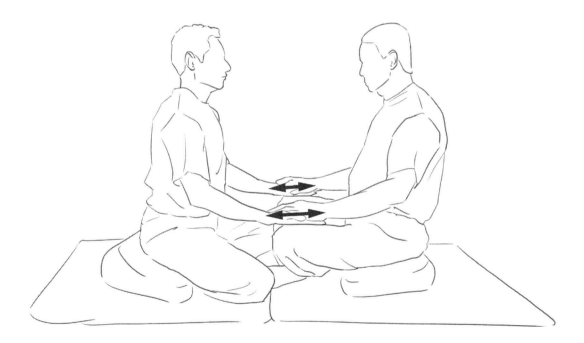

Figure 3-23. Qì's Exchange to the Wrists.

leader's wrists. Naturally, both should use Reverse Abdominal Breathing since both have the intention to lead the Qì.

After you have mastered this Qì exchange, advance to the elbows, then the shoulders, and finally to each other's Real Lower Dāntián.

If you have practiced with palms touching, you may then enter into the more advanced practice of Dual Cultivation without touching. That means the leader will place his palms above the follower so their palms are a couple inches apart (Figure 3-24). After practicing until you can both strongly feel the Qi exchange, you may increase the distance between your palms.

Again, once you have learned Martial Grand Circulation in Section 3.6, you may then apply it to this practice and make the Qì exchange stronger.

Yǒngquán Breathing—Rooting (Yǒngquán Xí—Zāgēn, 湧泉息－紮根)

Martial artists have commonly practiced this Grand Circulation for rooting—a crucial key to winning in a battle. In this practice, the Qì is led by the mind to the Yǒngquán (K-1) (湧泉) cavity and distributed to the entire sole (Figure 3-25). This will increase the sensitivity of the nerves, thus promoting better balance and centering, and in turn allowing a firm root to be established. The Yǒngquán breathing technique can also be used to condition the soles of the feet of the elderly and increase their sensitivity to help them walk with more balance. Through this practice, the Qì circulating in the legs will be

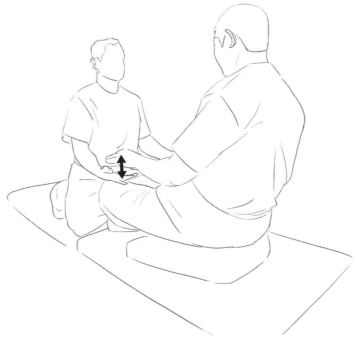

Figure 3-24. Qì Exchange without Touching.

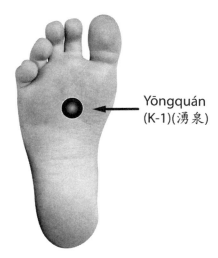

Figure 3-25. The Yǒngquán (K-1) Cavity.

smoother and more abundant; consequently, the strength and endurance of the legs can be improved. This practice has commonly been used to improve the Qì circulation in the six Qì meridians circulating to the tip of toes, which is beneficial for health maintenance. These six channels are: Liver, Kidneys, Spleen, Gall Bladder, Bladder, and Stomach.

In practice, since all channels to the feet are wide open, it will be much easier to lead the Qì with the mind. These meridians are wide open because our legs (with body's weight) are constantly used to walk and have evolved since the beginning of human history for this purpose. Our legs have evolved to be much bigger and stronger than our arms. Naturally, in order to supply plenty of Qì for leg function, the Qì circulation is more abundant.

Practices (Solo):

Practice #1:

The best position for Yǒngquán Breathing is lying supine. This is because when you lie down, your legs are more relaxed, thus allowing the Qì to be more easily led. Lie down comfortably with your arms next to your torso. First, calm down your mind and gather your Qì at the Real Lower Dāntián. Next, inhale deeply and gather your Qì at your Real Lower Dāntián in coordination with the abdomen and Huìyīn. Since you are using your mind to lead the Qì, it is better if you use Reverse Abdomen Breathing. Next, exhale and

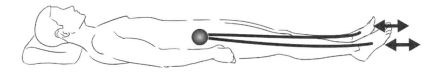

Figure 3-26. Yǒngquán Breathing Practice.

lead the Qì to the bottom of your feet while pushing out your abdomen and Huìyīn (or anus) (Figure 3-26). Then inhale and lead the Qì back to your Real Lower Dāntián while withdrawing your abdomen and Huìyīn. You may repeat the practice for as long as you have the time and inclination.

If you wish to use Yǒngquán Breathing to train your rooting, then it is better to do the practice standing. When you exhale, squat down slightly and use your mind to lead the Qì to the soles of your feet and beyond. At the end of the exhalation, hold your breath for five to ten seconds (Figure 3-27). After that, return to the neutral standing position and simply relax your mind and allow the inhalation to occur naturally. Practice daily for approximately five minutes. Naturally, the more you practice, the deeper the root you can develop.

After you have developed a sense of the soles of your feet from practicing while standing on the ground, if you wish to extend your Qì farther beneath your soles, then practice while standing on bricks and repeat the same process (Figure 3-28). When you stand on bricks, you must place your mind on the bottom of the bricks to prevent you from falling. With this training, the root will grow deeper. Once you have mastered the practice standing on a single brick under each leg, then you may increase the number of bricks to two or

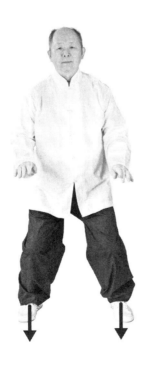

Figure 3-27. Rooting Training.

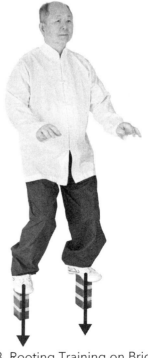

Figure 3-28. Rooting Training on Bricks.

three. Of course, the more bricks you are able to manage, the deeper the root will be. Be careful when standing on bricks. The instability creates more potential for falling. If you want more information about training refer to *Tai Chi Theory & Martial Power*, available from YMAA Publication Center.

Practice (Dual):

Yǒngquán Dual Cultivation (Yǒngquán Shuāngxiū, 湧泉雙修) is also called Yǒngquán Qì Exchange Practice (Yǒngquán Huanqì Lianxi, 湧泉換氣練習). Similar to Láogōng Dual Cultivation, you are exchanging the Qì with your partner through the Yǒngquán in this practice. And like Láogōng Breathing, you develop the exchange slowly. Begin the Qì exchange to each other's ankles, then progress to the knees, then hips, and finally to the Real Lower Dāntián.

When you practice this dual cultivation, you and your partner may lie down or sit with each other's soles touching gently (Figures 3-29 and 3-30). Reverse Abdominal Breathing should be used since you have an intention to lead the Qì. As in all practices, to begin you and your partner should calm your minds and regulate the breathing to a smooth and relaxed state. After that, the leader will exhale and lead the Qì from his Real Lower Dāntián to his Yǒngquán, then lead the Qi to enter the partner's Yǒngquán, and then to the partner's ankles. When the leader is doing so, the follower should inhale and allow the leader's Qì to enter their soles and then to their ankles. In order to synchronize with each other, when the leader exhales, they should gently push the toes forward to hint at their action. Again, coordination with the abdomen and Huìyīn is very important.

Next, the follower exhales and leads the Qì out from their Real Lower Dāntián to the leader's ankles. After practicing for a while and when both are familiar with the practice, they can extend the Qì's exchange to the knees, hips, and finally the Real Lower Dāntián.

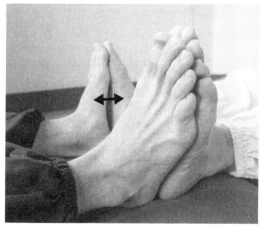

Figure 3-29. Yǒngquán Qì Exchange with Lying-Down Position.

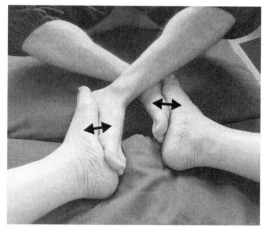

Figure 3-30. Yǒngquán Qì Exchange with Sitting Position.

Four Gates Breathing—Balancing (Sìxīn Xí—Pínghéng, 四心息－平衡)

Once you have mastered both the Láogōng and Yǒngquán Breathing, then you are ready for the Four Gate Breathing practice. This is a very important training for a martial artist since they need a firm root whenever they strike. Without a firm root, the power emitted will be shallow. It is just like when you push a heavy object: if you are not rooted, the power generated will not be as strong since there is no balance to support the push.

In this practice, start in the standing posture with the palms facing downward. First, regulate your breathing and gather your Qì at the Real Lower Dāntián. After you have regulated to a comfortable stage, then exhale and use your mind to lead the Qì to the palms by imagining you are pushing something downward. At the same time, slightly squat downward and lead the Qì to the soles by imagining you are pushing your feet downward (Figure 3-31). Next, inhale and lead the Qì back to the Real Lower Dāntián. Naturally, you should use Reverse Abdominal Breathing since you have an intention to lead the Qì strongly. You may repeat the training for as long as you have the time or inclination.

If you intend to extend your Qì farther from the palms and soles, then once you have reached the end of your exhalation, hold your breath for five to ten seconds. This will allow the Qì to expand farther. If you wish to continuously enhance the Qì's expansion, then when you inhale, simply relax and allow the inhalation to happen naturally. Then, repeat the same process. The more you practice, the further the Qì will expand. It is like taking three steps forward and two steps backward. In no time you will have advanced beyond your original position. You may practice the Four Gates Breathing while standing on bricks.

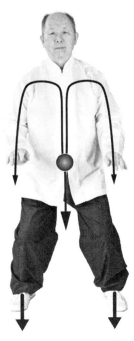

Figure 3-31. Four Gates Breathing Practice.

The Fifth Gate Breathing—Raise the Spirit of Vitality (Dìwǔxīn Xí—Tíshén, 第五心息—提神)

One of the most important keys to emitting power with a firmed root is your spirit. When your spirit is high, your mind and actions are effective and manifest powerfully. The fifth gate is on the top of your crown, Bǎihuì (Gv-20) (百會) cavity. Since the Fifth Gate Breathing belongs to Marrow/Brain Washing Qìgōng, we will discuss this practice later in Chapter 6-4.

3.6 Martial Grand Circulation—Power and Endurance (Wǔxué Dàzhōutiān—Jìnglì, Nàilì, 武學大周天—勁力、耐力)

In Martial Grand Circulation Breathing, a martial artist learns how to open an additional door, the Mìngmén (Gv-4) (命門), which is on the lower back between the L2 and L3 vertebrae, to enhance the Qì supply for manifestation (Figure 3-32). Mìngmén is a Chinese medical term and means "life-door" since it is the gate to access the Real Lower Dāntián (i.e., human bio-battery), the life source. When this door is opened and the Qì is led correctly, more Qì can flow into the Small Circulation orbit to increase the quantity of the Qì in circulation. As a result, the power manifested by the physical body can be enhanced significantly. Your endurance can also be improved because of the abundant Qì circulation that allows muscles to be used more efficiently.

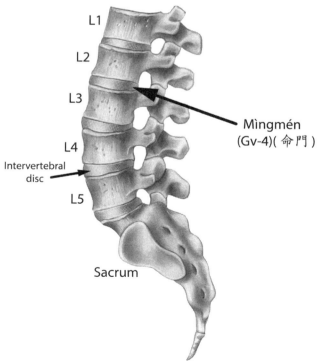

Figure 3-32. Mìngmén (Gv-4) (命門).
(Illustration by Shutterstock)

However, in Daoist society, Mìngmén is called "closed gate" (Bìhù, 閉戶) since it was closed long ago in human history. According to their understanding, originally there were two gates in our body to access the Real Lower Dāntián, the Qì residence or storage place. However, it is believed that when we were still not yet evolved to stand and walk upright, we were like chimpanzees and our back was curved forward so that the Mìngmén gate was opened. Later, we learned how to stand and walk upright due to the contraction of the back muscles, so we shut down the Mìngmén cavity gradually. Now, we have only one gate called Yīnjiāo (Co-7) (陰交), one inch below the navel, opened to supply the Qì to the entire body from the Qì center. Today, Daoists call the Yīnjiāo cavity the "life door" (Shéngmén, 生門). Actually, many Daoists also considered the navel to be the "life door" since it is where an embryo received life nourishment from the mother (Figure 3-33).

If you understand this, you understand the importance of this cavity. You need to learn how to push the vertebrae of the lower back backward so you can open the Mìngmén cavity again. Consequently, you will have another door to connect to the Real Lower Dāntián (Figure 3-34).

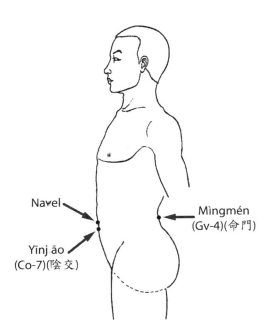

Figure 3-33. Yīnjiāo (Co-7), Mìngmén (Gv-4), and Navel.

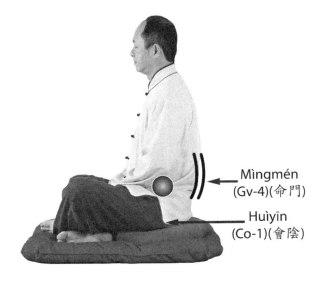

Figure 3-34. Open Mìngmén by Pushing Lower Back Backward Gently.

Practices (Solo):

There are two ways of leading the Qì with the mind in Martial Grand Circulation practice. One is for beginners who have not had much experience in leading the Qì with the mind. For this group, two methods of respiration are commonly used to lead the Qì. The other method is for those who are able to lead the Qì efficiently and wish to apply the Martial Grand Circulation in martial power manifestation.

For experienced martial artists, after they have mastered their Grand Circulation to a stage where they can feel their Qi flow smoothly in the Grand Circulation path, they will learn how to apply this Grand Circulation in their techniques. They have to practice till they are able to subconsciously lead the Qì with martial Grand Circulation into the techniques. That is because when they are in a combat situation, they will not have time to use their conscious mind to lead the Qì. Everything has to happen subconsciously.

If you are a beginner, it is better and easier to use two respiration cycles. First, place your mind at the Real Lower Dāntián and gather your Qì there till you feel comfortable. Once you are ready, inhale deeply while still keeping your mind at the Real Lower Dāntián to firm the gathered Qì. Then you exhale and use your mind to lead the Qì out through the Yīnjiāo to the Huìyīn, following the Conceptional Vessel (Rènmài) (任脈) (Figure 3-35). You should use Reverse Abdominal Breathing since you are leading with strong intention. Next, inhale and lead the Qì upward following the Governing Vessel (Dūmài, 督脈) to the Dàzhuī (Gv-14) (大椎) cavity. While you are leading the Qi and when the Qì is passing the Mìngmén cavity, gently push your lower back backward to open the joint between the L2 and L3 vertebrae. This will open the Mìngmén gate and allow the Qì to exit from the Real Lower Dāntián. In this case, an additional Qì flow will join the one going up from the Huìyīn and thus will enhance the Qì flow. Once you have led the Qì to the Dàzhuī, then you exhale and lead the Qì to the palms for manifestation. To repeat, inhale again and bring your mind back to the Real Lower Dāntián and repeat the process.

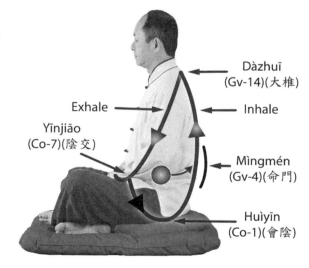

Figure 3-35. Two Respirations Grand Circulation.

If you are able to comfortably lead the Qì following two breathing cycles, you should practice this circulation with one breathing cycle. When you apply Martial Grand Circulation in a battle, you will not have time for two. You would need to lead the Qì out as soon as possible for manifestation. In this practice, again gather your Qì at the Real Lower Dāntián. Next, inhale and use your mind to lead the Qì out of Yīnjiāo, through the Huìyīn, and then upward to Dàzhuī. When the Qì is passing Mìngmén, you gently push your lower back backward to open it to allow additional Qì to join the flow (Figure 3-36). Once the Qì has reached the Dàzhuī, exhale and lead the Qì out to the palms for manifestation. You may apply this Grand Circulation to enhance the power of martial techniques. You may also use this additional Qì flow to condition your muscles and tendons. As a matter of fact, this is the crucial key to Muscle/Tendon Changing practice.

A common concern of practitioners is if they practice this Martial Grand Circulation too much, they will exhaust their Qì storage. However, you should remember one thing: your body is alive and it will always find ways to adjust to your demands. Therefore, the more you train, the more Qì will be generated and stored in the Real Lower Dāntián. It is one of the ways to condition the production of Qì.

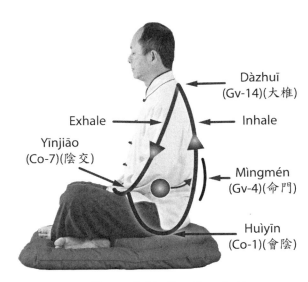

Figure 3-36. One Respiration
Grand Circulation.

Remember, in Martial Grand Circulation training you are consuming your Qì for manifestation. If you wish to cultivate and build the Qì in the circulation to an abundant level without losing your Qì, then you must build a route that allows your Qì to return to the Real Lower Dāntián. In this case, you may sit or stand while placing both hands over the Yīnjiāo cavity with the Láogōng lined up. This will prevent the Qì from flowing out of the palms and will return Qi back to the Real Lower Dāntián or into the Conceptional Vessel. To practice, when you have led the Qì to the palms with an exhalation, simply inhale to lead the Qì from the palms into the Real Lower Dāntián through the Yīnjiāo cavity. At the same time, you are again leading the Qì from the Real Lower Dāntián to the Huìyīn and upward to Dàzhuī (Figure 3-37). Remember, when the Qì is passing the Mìngmén, you must gently push your lower back backward to open the Mìngmén again. You may practice this Qì cultivation for a long time without problems. The more you practice, the stronger and the smoother the Qì will be built up.

Practice (Dual):

To practice Dual Martial Grand Circulation (Wǔxué Dàzhōutiān Shuāngxiū) (武學 大周天雙修), if you are a beginner, it is better to have an experienced partner. This will expedite the learning process but also allow the Qì to circulate more abundantly.

In this practice, the leader should sit behind the beginner. Both persons' palms should overlap each other with the Láogōng lined up. It does not matter whose palms are on the bottom or top. What is most important is the coordination of the breathing and mind.

First, both should regulate the mind and gather the Qì at the Real Lower Dāntián. After both are regulated, the leader will inhale and lead the Qì out of the Yīnjiāo to the Huìyīn and upward to the Dàzhuī. When the Qì is passing the Mìngmén cavity, gently push the lower back backward to allow additional Qì from the Real Lower Dāntián to

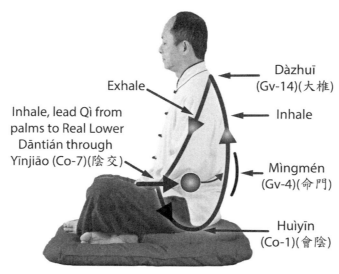

Figure 3-37. Routed Grand Circulation.

join the upward Qì flow. When the leader is doing this, the follower should synchronize the breathing and the leading of Qi with the leader. Next, both will exhale and lead the Qì from the Dàzhuī to the palms (Figure 3-38). Once the Qì has reached the palms, then inhale and lead the Qì inward to join the new cycle. Practice until you are able to coordinate with each other. Be patient as this may take a long time. When you are ready for the next step, you inhale from the palms and lead the Qì so that it passes through both the Real Lower Dāntián and exits from the leader's Mìngmén to join the Qì flow from Huìyīn. Once you have reached a high level, you will feel that the two Qì routes have been combined into one.

3.7 Joint Breathing—Loosen and Relax the Body (Guānjié Xí—Sōng-shēn, 關節息－鬆身)

Joint Breathing Grand Circulation is the foundation of Muscle/Tendon Changing practice. It is probably one of the most common forms of Qìgōng training in Qìgōng society. That is because this practice gives a practitioner a healthy body and also a calm and relaxed mind. There are a few purposes for this Grand Circulation.

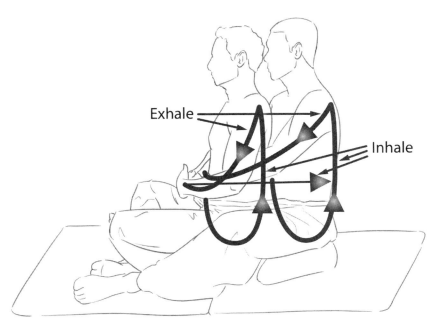

Figure 3-38. Dual Martial Grand Circulation.

Purposes:

1. **Loosening and Relaxing the Body.** One of the main goals in this practice is to relax the joints using the mind in coordination with your breathing. When the joints are relaxed, the ligaments and tendons will be loosened. When ligaments and tendons are loosened, the muscles will be relaxed. When muscles are relaxed, the body is relaxed. Consequently, the Qì circulation in the body, especially the internal organs, will be natural and smooth. Since this practice is able to provide a high level of relaxation, it has commonly been used for recovery from fatigue. As a matter of fact, this practice is especially important for those who often engage in heavy physical training or work.

2. **Conditioning the Joints.** Another important goal of this training, especially for a martial artist, is to use the enhanced Qì circulation to condition the joints and make them stronger and develop more endurance. Strength and endurance are always crucial keys to surviving in battle. Joint Breathing Grand Circulation will provide the foundation for this training.

3. **For Healing.** Since this practice is able to enhance the Qì circulation at the joints, it is also commonly used for self-healing for injury or arthritis.

4. **For Bone Marrow Washing.** When joints are loosened and the Qì's circulation is enhanced at the joints, a person will be able to lead the Qì to the center of the bones for Marrow Washing (i.e., bone marrow nourishment). Therefore, Joint Breathing Grand Circulation is also considered as the foundation of Marrow Washing Qìgōng practice.

Orders of Joints Grand Circulation Practice:

1. **Spine.** The torso is the most important place for relaxing the body. This is because almost all the internal organs are wrapped within the torso. When the torso is tensed, the body is tight and the Qì circulation, especially to the internal organs, will be stagnant. In addition, when the torso is relaxed, the mind is relaxed and peaceful. The key to relaxing the torso's muscles and tendons is relaxing the spine, especially the lower back and neck area. The Qì's circulation at the lower back, where the Girdle Vessel (Dàimài, 帶脈) is located, is the crucial area for affecting your immune system. When the lower back is loosened and relaxed, the Guardian Qì (Wèiqì, 衛氣) can strongly expand from the Girdle Vessel and thus boost the immune system.

In addition, relaxing the neck joints is also very important. This is because the neck is the junction of the Qì and blood circulation to the brain. In order to have a healthy, functioning brain, you must keep this junction opened.

2. **Shoulder and Hip Joints.** The joints at the shoulders and hips are the junctions for Qì and blood exchange between the torso and limbs. In order to have strong Qì and blood circulation to the limbs, these joints must be loose and relaxed.

3. **Elbow and Knee Joints.** Once you are relaxed at the shoulder and hip joints, you can extend the training to the elbows and knees. These are the midpoints of the arms and legs. When these midpoints are relaxed, the Qì and blood can smoothly circulate to the fingertips and toes.

4. **Wrist and Ankle Joints.** Next, relax and loosen the wrists and ankles. Usually, these are the first places for physical conditioning in the martial arts. This is because when the wrists are strong, the weapons carried can be heavier and the power manifested can be stronger. When ankle joints are conditioned, the root can be firmer and more rooted.

5. **Hands and Feet.** Finally, pay attention to the hands and feet. The hands' sensitivity is very important since we use them for touching and carrying things. The feet's sensitivity is also important since it provides us with a firm root and balance. From the Chinese medical point of view, the hands and feet are the extremities of Qì and blood circulation. If Qì and blood cannot circulate smoothly to reach these extremities, it implies the initiation of sickness. As matter of fact, the fingers and toes have commonly been used for diagnosis. Therefore, to keep the joints of the hands and feet loosened and relaxed is a crucial key to Qì and blood circulation.

6. **Entire Body's Joints.** After you have completed and mastered different Joint Breathing exercises, the final practice is to loosen the joints of the entire body all at the same time. Since you have already built up a sensitive feeling of the joints, you may relax them at the same time using the coordination of mind and breathing.

To make your practice successful, there are a few crucial keys. Without these keys the effectiveness will be shallow.

Crucial keys of practice:

1. **Feel the Joints.** Feeling the joints is the most important key. Just think: if you cannot feel your joints clearly, how will you be able to lead the Qì to the joints and manipulate their condition? Since the joints are essential to the many different ways we can move, by placing your mind there, you will feel how each joint is constructed and how they function. Once you are able to feel the joints deeply, you may also use the movements to stretch the ligaments and tendons. In order to relax the joints, you usually must open them through stretching.

2. **Lead the Qì to the Joints.** Next, you must also know how to lead Qì to the joints from the Real Lower Dāntián. This will enhance the Qì's quantity and circulation at the joints. If you don't do so, the Qì circulating at the joints will be local and the quantity will not be increased significantly. Learning how to manipulate the Qì circulation has always been a crucial key to successful Qìgōng practice.

3. **Know How to Use the Qì Pump—Huìyīn.** The Huìyīn (or anus) is the pump that controls the in-and-out movement of Qi from and to the Real Lower Dāntián. When the Huìyīn (or anus) is pushed out gently, the Qì is led outward from Real Lower Dāntián and when the Huìyīn (or anus) is lifted upward gently, the Qì is led into the Real Lower Dāntián. In order to lead the Qì effectively, Reverse Abdominal Breathing is recommended.

4. **Breathe the Joints.** Once you have led the Dāntián Qì to the joints, then through breathing you lead the Qì to the center of the joints and out to the skin surface of the joints. This is the exercise of Joint Breathing. Once you know how to do so, you may apply it for healing, Marrow Washing, or conditioning of the joints.

5. **Apply Martial Grand Circulation to the Practice.** If you are familiar with Martial Grand Circulation and know how to open the Mìngmén to lead additional Qì from the Real Lower Dāntián, you should do so. This will increase the quantity of Qi circulating to the joints.

When you practice, first regulate your mind and breathing, and gather Qì at the Real Lower Dāntián. Next, inhale deeply and then exhale to lead the Qì from the Real Lower Dāntián to the joint. Once the Qì arrives, inhale to lead the Qì into the midpoints of the joints (Figure 3-39). Next, exhale and lead the Qì out from the joints. Practice leading Qi in and out a few times. If you wish to increase the Qì at the joint, exhale again and lead the Qì from the Real Dāntián to the joint. You may repeat the same process till the joint is warm.

If you are familiar with Martial Grand Circulation, add it to this exercise. This will enhance the Qì's buildup and the circulation at the joint.

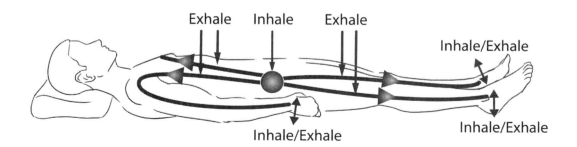

Figure 3-39. Joints Breathing.

3.8 Skin/Marrow Breathing (Body Breathing)—Enhance the Immune System (Fūsuǐ Xí (Tǐxí)- Zēngqiáng Miǎnyìlì, 膚髓息（體息）－ 增強 免疫力）

Skin Breathing is considered Yáng since the Qì is led outward to the skin surface to enhance the Guardian Qì (Wèiqì, 衛氣). When the Guardian Qì is enhanced, the body feels warm and the immune system is strengthened. Marrow Breathing is considered Yīn since the Qì is led inward to the marrow for nourishing. Marrow is considered to be like electric plasma or liquid metal. That means the electric conductivity in marrow is extremely high. Therefore, marrow, like the brain, is able to absorb a high quantity of bioelectricity. When Qì is led to the marrow for nourishing, the body feels cold. Naturally, when you lead Qì to the marrow, the Guardian Qì shrinks and the immune system is weakened. This is important to know when you practice these two breathing methods.

1. **Skin Breathing.** Begin to practice at mid-autumn when the weather is getting cold and your Guardian Qì is shrinking and weakening. If you are able to lead more Qì to the skin surface to maintain or even strengthen your Guardian Qì, you will be able to keep your immune system strong. Other than knowing how to keep yourself warm, if you can practice Skin Breathing consistently and frequently, you will be able to keep your immune system at a high level of defense against sickness when winter arrives.

2. **Marrow Breathing.** Practice should begin at the mid-spring when the weather is getting warm and you don't need as much Qì to support your Guardian Qì as you do in wintertime. When the season enters summer, that is the best time for Marrow Washing since the demand for Guardian Qì is at the minimum.

3. **Skin/Marrow Breathing (Body Breathing).** Skin/Marrow Breathing is also called Body Breathing. In this practice, you lead Qì to the marrow to nourish it and also to the skin to enhance the Guardian Qì. To make this successful, you must know how to generate and store the Qì to an abundant level. If you don't have plenty of Qì to serve these two practices, you will find your Qì is deficient. Learning how to generate more quantity and store it at the Real Lower Dāntián is the crucial key to practice. However, if you don't have plenty of Qì to be used, you can still practice during spring and autumn when the weather is comfortable.

Once you are skillful, you may use the Yīn and Yáng condition of the day to fit into your practice. For example, the early afternoon, when the temperature is warmest, is a good time for Marrow Washing practice. However, if the temperature is getting cold, you should practice Skin Breathing.

To practice these breathing techniques, you must know three keys to make the practice successful. Though we have mentioned them earlier, here is a brief summary.

1. To lead the Qì inward.

    A. Inhalation is longer than exhalation.

    B. Make a Hēng (哼) sound.

    C. Hold the breath for five to ten seconds at the end of the inhalation.

2. To lead the Qì outward.

    A. Exhalation is longer than inhalation.

    B. Make a Hà (哈) sound.

    C. Hold the breath for five to ten seconds at the end of the exhalation.

3. To keep Qì's inward and outward balance.

    A. Exhalation and inhalation are the same length.

    B. Make a Hēng (哼) sound for inhalation and Hā (哈) sound for exhalation. You may also practice without making sounds.

    C. Hold the breath at the end of the inhalation and the exhalation.

Practice (Solo):

1. Skin Breathing

First, regulate your mind and breathing, and gather your Qì at the Real Lower Dāntián. Once you have regulated them to a comfortable and stable stage, inhale and draw in your abdomen and Huìyīn. Since you are leading the Qì horizontally to the skin, it is more effective if you use Reverse Abdominal Breathing. Next, exhale slenderly, softly, and gently and use your mind to lead the Qì to the surface of the skin and beyond. Once you have reached the end of the exhalation, hold your breath for five to ten seconds (Figure 3-40). If you want to quickly enhance the expansion of Qì, you may add the Hā (哈) sound while you are exhaling. However, you should understand that if you use the Hā sound, though the Qì circulation is stronger, it does not expand as far as if you keep your body relaxed and quiet. You may repeat the process as many times as you need. This breathing can help you raise your spirit and ease depression. This breathing is also very effective against catching a cold, especially at the beginning stages of the disease.

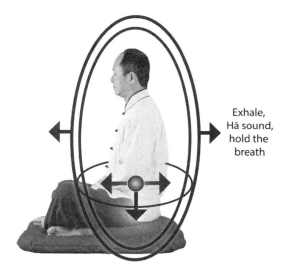

Exhale, Hā sound, hold the breath

Figure 3-40. Skin Breathing.

2. Marrow Breathing

After you have regulated your mind and breathing and gathered your Qì at the Real Lower Dāntián, exhale and allow the air to go out naturally, then inhale deeply, slowly, gradually, and slenderly and use your mind to lead the Qì inward toward the center of your bones. After you have reached the end of your inhalation, hold your breath for five to ten seconds to allow the Qì to be absorbed into the marrow (Figure 3-41). If you intend to lead the Qì in quickly, you may add the sound Hēng (哼). If you are familiar with Joint Breathing, you may feel a big portion of Qì entering the bone marrow through the joints. This will enhance the Qì you are leading to the marrow for nourishment.

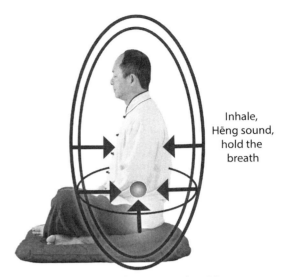

Inhale, Hēng sound, hold the breath

Figure 3-41. Lead Qì Inward to Marrow.

Once you have mastered Joint Breathing and Skin Breathing, you may combine both breathing methods and make the Qì circulation to the marrow more efficient. If you analyze the electric structure of a section of the bone, you will see that the tendon is a fibrous tissue that connects muscle to bone. It is known that the electric conductivity of tendons is higher than that of the muscles, thus in comparison the tendons belong to Yīn and the muscles belong to Yáng (Figure 3-42). In addition, if you analyze the structure of the bones, you can see that the density at the center is higher than the joint area. The middle of a section of bone is stronger and more compact and thus is considered to be Yáng while the end is Yīn. From this, you may conclude that the joint area of a piece of bone is Yīn while the middle section is Yáng. This relationship forms a Yīn and Yáng Qì's natural circulation route. The joints are where the Qì enters while the middle section is where the Qì exits (Figure 3-43).

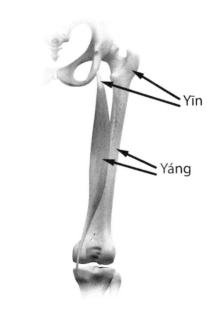

Yīn

Yáng

Figure 3-42. Yīn and Yáng Status of Bone and Muscles/Tendons.
(Photo by Shutterstock)

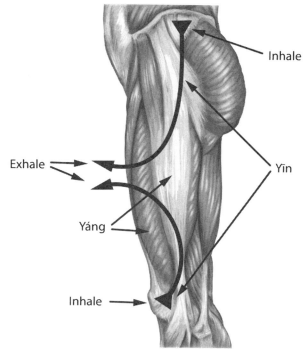

Figure 3-43. Qì's Circulation
in a Section of a Limb.
(Illustration by Shutterstock)

When you know this theory, you can easily apply it to your practice. When you inhale, you lead the Qì from the joints into the center of the marrow and while you are exhaling, you lead the Qì from the marrow out of the skin. This is to enhance the natural bone breathing and thus is able to nourish and clean the marrow. This is the Muscle/Tendon Grand Circulation of bone washing.

3. Skin/Marrow Breathing

If you do Skin and Marrow Breathing at the same time, your body will remain neutral. This practice will maintain the Qì circulation horizontally, smoothly, and healthfully. As mentioned earlier, this should be practiced during spring and autumn when the weather is not too hot or cold.

You may follow the above training principles to keep your inhalation and exhalation the same length. Naturally, your mind remains the crucial key to leading the Qì. When you inhale, use your mind to lead the Qì inward to the marrow and then hold your breath for five to ten seconds. Next, exhale and use the mind to lead the Qì out to the surface of the skin and beyond. When you reach the end of the exhalation, again hold your breath for five to ten seconds. If you intend to quickly enhance the results, you may add the Hēng and Hā sounds.

3.9 Internal Organs Breathing—Foundation of Life (Qìguān Xī— Shēngmìng Zhújī, 器官息－生命築基)

When a Qìgōng practitioner has developed to a high level of feeling and sensitivity, he will be able to feel or sense the Qì status of the five important internal Yīn organs. These five internal organs are the heart, lungs, spleen, liver, and kidneys. Usually, the lungs and the heart are the organs that can be felt more easily than the liver, kidneys, or spleen. Some advanced Qìgōng practitioners are able to sense the colors of these organs. As we noted earlier, the heart is red (Hóng, 紅), liver is green or blue (Lǜ/Qīng, 綠/青), spleen is yellow (Huáng, 黃), lungs are white (Bái, 白), and kidneys are black (Hēi, 黑). Once you are able to feel or sense the organs, then through correct breathing and mind-body communication (i.e., feeling), a practitioner will be able to lead the Qì toward or away from the organs. In addition, if you are familiar with the Five Elements (Wǔxíng, 五行) theory, you may also apply that theory for nourishing or releasing (Figure 3-44) to the practice. For example, the kidneys (water) (Shuǐ, 水) produce wood that enhances the Qì of the liver (wood) (Mù, 木), and the liver (wood, 木) (Mù, 木) generates the fire of the heart (Huǒ, 火). If you follow this order, you are nourishing the organs. Another example: the heart is fire (Huǒ, 火) and the lungs are metal (Jīn, 金). If you enhance the lungs' Qì, the heart's fire will be reduced. For example, when your heart is beating quickly, a few deep breaths will reduce the heart fire and slow down the speed of the heartbeat.

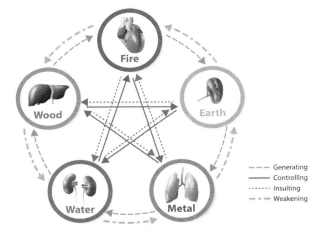

Figure 3-44. Relationship of Five Elements.
(Illustrations by Shutterstock)

To practice, you use the same breathing strategies. If you wish to lead the Qì to a specific organ for nourishing, inhale deeply and use your mind to lead the Qì to that organ. When you have reached the end of the inhalation, hold your breath for five to ten seconds. Then, just relax and allow the air to go out naturally. This will continue to build up the Qì in that organ. For example, if your kidneys' Qì is deficient, you may inhale to lead the Qì to the kidneys and then hold the breath for five to ten seconds. Then, simply relax and allow the breathing to return to its normal state. You may repeat the process till you feel the kidneys are warm.

However, if the organ is too Yáng and you wish to release the excess Qì, then place your mind at the organ and inhale naturally first. After that, exhale and lead the Qì out of the organ and to the limbs. If the organs are the heart and lungs, lead the Qì to the hands, and if the organs are liver, kidneys, and spleen, then lead the Qì to the feet. Again, when you reach the end of exhalation, you should hold your breath for five to ten seconds to enhance the releasing process. Remember, you may direct your mind to all organs except the heart. When you put your mind at the heart, you will lead Qì to the heart and make the heart more Yáng. In most cases, you will lead excess Qì in the heart away to reduce the heart fire.

When you regulate the Qì status of a specific organ, you may also use the organ's corresponding healing sound to enhance the regulating process. There are six sounds that correspond to the six internal organs. Heart corresponds to the sound "Hē" (呵), Spleen to "Hū" (呼), Lungs to "Sī" (四), Triple Burner to "Xī" (嘻), Liver to "Xū" (嘘), and Kidneys to "Chuī" (吹). When you exhale to release the excess Qì in the organ, simply make a very light and long vocalization of the sound corresponding with the organ. This will vibrate and relax the organs so the Qì can be released more easily.

3.10 Other Dual Circulation (with Human) (Qítā Shuāngxiū Dàzhōutiān (Yǔbàn), 其他雙修大周天（與伴）)

There are many other possible methods of dual cultivation in Qìgōng practice. In the past, Qì exchange practices often involved more than two persons. This multiple-person Qì exchange was one of the common practices in monasteries and Chinese martial arts society. Historically, Buddhists or Daoists might practice Qì exchange with six (hexagon) or eight practitioners (i.e., eight trigrams) simultaneously, sitting in a circle. In this multiple-person training, synchronization is the key to success. If anyone in the ring does not coordinate their breathing and mind with the group, the result will be poor. Today, it is extremely difficult to find many people who have reached similar levels and are both committed and available to train this exercise.

In the past, another common Qì exchange group meditation practice in monasteries was done in the early morning, without touching. The group faced to the east to absorb the Qi of the rising morning sun. If the practice was done in the evening, they faced to the south to absorb the earth's Qì. Usually, the chiming of a bell was used to synchronize the breathing and Qì expansion and withdrawing. From this kind of group-synchronized meditation, the Qì in the whole group could be harmonized and strengthened and the mind could be more oriented and focused.

Here, we will discuss a few examples of dual cultivation with a single partner. Once you know the theory and acquire abundant experience, you may create many ways of practicing Qì exchange. As mentioned earlier, your partner does not have to be of the same sex as you. However, there are a few keys that make this practice successful, especially those Qì exchange practices in which you touch each other. These few keys are:

1. You and your partner must know what, why, and how to practice. Otherwise, the mind will be scattered and the Qì led will be chaotic.

2. To reach a high efficiency of dual cultivation, the practitioner who has experience in leading the Qì (i.e., quality of Qì's manifestation) should be the leader. The other person with less experience, usually younger, and who has more abundant Qì (i.e., quantity of Qì), is the follower.

3. Due to having your skin touching, you and your partner must feel comfortable with each other. If any one of you has an uncomfortable feeling, this person will not open their paths for Qì exchange. They will shut them down subconsciously. Therefore, finding a suitable partner is not as easy as most people think.

4. If any one of the practitioners loses their patience, confidence, and willingness, the achievement will be shallow.

Real Lower Dāntián Mutual Nourishment Dual Cultivation

This practice is also called Embryonic Breathing Dual Cultivation (Tāixí Shāngxiū, 胎息雙修). Usually, this practice is used for an experienced Embryonic Breathing Meditation practitioner to teach a Qìgōng beginner to grasp the key to Embryonic Breathing. In this practice, through mind and breathing synchronization, you and your partner help each other to increase the Qì storage at the Real Lower Dāntián to an abundant level.

When you practice, you and your partner sit facing the same direction and align the Real Lower Dāntián in a straight line (Figure 3-45). The leader should be sitting behind

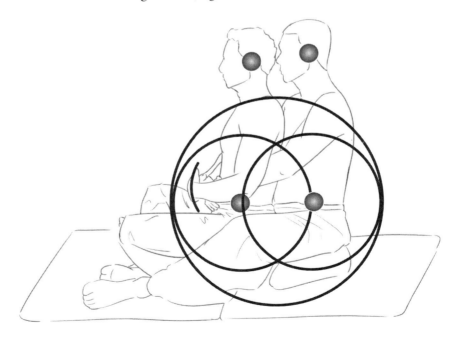

Figure 3-45. Embryonic Breathing Dual Cultivation.

and the follower sits in front. Both your palms should overlap; you then align the Láogōng and place your overlapped hands on the follower's Yīnjiāo cavity. It does not matter if the leader or follower's hands are on top or bottom. You may use Normal or Reverse Abdominal Breathing. After both of you have regulated your mind and breathing to a calm and peaceful state, the leader will give a signal to the follower to begin. In this practice, the synchronization is not difficult since you can hear and feel each other's breathing. Once both of you have reached the final stage of Embryonic Breathing and the spirit (i.e., son) and the Qì (i.e., mother) are united at the Real Lower Dāntián (i.e., unification of mother and son) (Mǔzǐ Xiànghé, 母子相合) through the Yīnjiāo (Co-7) (陰交) and Mìngmén (Gv-4) (命門) cavities, your Qì will unite.

Chest/Back Qì Dual Cultivation

According to Chinese medicine, the front of the torso is considered Yīn while the back is Yáng. It is also known that through the skin, the Qì can be exchanged outside of the body. If done correctly, this practice can be very beneficial and effective. The best part is that if you and your partner are healthy, there is not much danger involved.

1. Chest-to-Chest Dual Cultivation (i.e., Hugging)

Chest-to-Chest Dual Cultivation can often be seen in our society. We call it hugging. Whenever a close friend or relative is sad or depressed, we hug them. Through hugging, they feel comforted from the Qì they receive through your hugging.

Of course, Qìgōng practice goes further than just hugging. It is a Qì exchange with intention and coordination of breathing. In this practice, you may stand, sit, or even lie down as long as your chest feels comfortable. The practice is more effective without barriers on your chest area such as a shirt. Gently hug each other with arms behind each other's back. Next, one person inhales while the other exhales. You may use either Normal or Reverse Abdominal Breathing. If Normal Abdominal Breathing is used, you will be more relaxed. If Reverse Abdominal Breathing is used, the intention is stronger and naturally the Qì exchange will be enhanced.

2. Chest-to-Back Dual Cultivation (i.e., Hugging)

If you wish to have Qì exchange between the back and chest, then both of you face the same direction and the one behind gently hugs the one in front. Again, you may stand, sit, or lie down. There are two ways of doing this dual cultivation. In the first method the person sitting behind exhales, the person in front inhales, and vice versa. Again, you may use either Normal or Reverse Abdominal Breathing. In this practice, the one who exhales expands the Qì while the one inhaling will absorb the Qì.

The other method is that both of you inhale and exhale at the same time. After practicing a while, your Qì will unite with each other.

3. Back-to-Back Dual Cultivation

Though this practice is not common, it can be used to boost Qì expansion for a person who is weak. In this practice, the Qì circulation in the Governing Vessel (Dūmài, 督脈) can be enhanced and thus you help each to build up Yáng. Therefore, it can be used for healing.

In this practice, you and your partner sit back against back. If you both know how to apply Martial Grand Circulation to this dual cultivation practice, it will make this practice more effective. Through the lower back's movement, the follower should be able to feel the leader's intention and coordinate with the leader's movement and synchronize the breathing.

After both you and your partner have regulated your mind and breathing and have gathered the Qì at the Real Lower Dāntián, the leader will exhale to lead Qì to the Huìyīn and then inhale and lead the Qì to the Dàzhuī (Gv-14) (大椎). When the Qì passes the Mìngmén, gently push the lower back out to open Mìngmén (Gv-4) (命門) and allow the additional Qì to exit from the Real Lower Dāntián. Naturally, the follower should follow and synchronize with the leader. Once the Qì has been led to the Dàzhuī, the leader can decide to either lead the Qì out to the arms (i.e., Martial Grand Circulation) or spread it out following the rib cage (i.e., Turtle Shell Breathing). You may repeat the practice as long as you feel comfortable. In order to boost the energy, both of you should cover the body to keep warm during practice.

Small Circulation Dual Cultivation

Small Circulation Dual Cultivation was probably one of the most common Qìgōng Dual Cultivations in traditional Chinese martial arts society. This was because Small Circulation was the foundation of Muscle/Tendon Changing, and a beginner, with an experienced partner as a leader, would be able to build their Qì to an abundant level in a short time. From this dual cultivation, they could also grasp the key to leading the Qì quickly. Those who do not know Small Circulation should first read the book, *Qìgōng Meditation—Small Circulation*, by YMAA Publication Center.

1. Chest-to-Back

To be safe, the leader should first lead the follower into Small-Small Circulation. With this as a foundation, they should advance and complete the circulation.

In this training, the experienced leader will sit behind the follower. The same as with many dual cultivations, it is better that both of you wear nothing on the upper body so the skin can touch.

Both you and your partner should overlap the palms and place them in front of the follower's abdominal area. Both of you should place the tip of your tongue lightly on the palate of your mouth. Next, regulate your breathing and mind, and gather your Qì at the Real Lower Dāntián. Once both of you have regulated, the leader exhales and leads the Qì from the Real Lower Dāntián to the Huìyīn and then inhales to lead it up to the Mìngmén to enter the Real Lower Dāntián. When Qì is entering the Mìngmén, the lower back should be gently pushed back. Naturally, the follower should follow the leader along this cycle. This is a Small-Small Circulation (Figure 3-46).

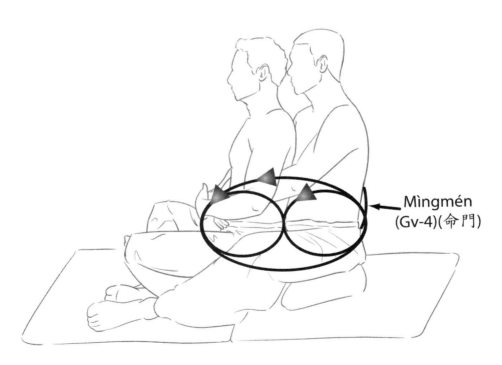

Mìngmén
(Gv-4)(命門)

Figure 3-46. Small-Small Circulation Dual Practice.

After both of you are able synchronize with each other harmoniously, then instead of re-entering the Real Lower Dāntián, the leader should lead the Qì from the Huìyīn upward following the Governing Vessel to the Bǎihuì (Gv-20) (百會) and down to the mouth area. Then, exhale to lead the Qì down to the Huìyīn. While the Qì passes to the Yīnjiāo (Co-7) (陰交) cavity, another additional flow of Qì will join the flow to enhance the Qì quantity (Figure 3-47). You may practice as long as you decide is appropriate.

Once both of you have achieved a high level of synchronization with abundant Qì circulation in the Governing and Conceptional Vessels, the leader will add additional Qì to the orbit by opening the Mìngmén (Gv-4) (命門) each time the Qì passes it (Figure 3-48). Naturally, this will enhance the Qì buildup in the orbit.

When both of you have decided to stop, you should lead the Qì back to settle in the Real Lower Dāntián.

2. Back to Back

If you wish, you may also practice with your partner back against back. Just follow the above training procedures for this practice.

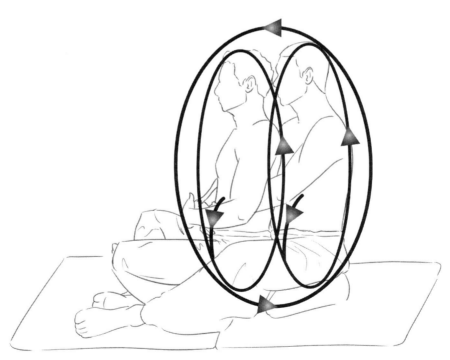

Figure 3-47. Small Circulation Dual Practice.

External Qì Exchange Treatments (Wàiqì Liáofǎ, 外氣療法)

External Qì Exchange Treatments for injuries or illnesses are commonly used in Chinese hospitals. Naturally, the doctor needs to be an experienced Qì healer and practitioner. The doctor commonly leads the Qì to their Láogōng (P-8) (勞宮) and emits their Qì to manipulate the Qì of the patient. There are two options for this Qì manipulation: with touch and without touch. If using touch, the Qì (i.e., bioelectricity) will be conducted and exchanged between doctor and patient directly. However, doctors often do not like to touch patients unless the patients are close relatives or friends. This is because when the doctor and patient touch each other, the abnormal Qì of the patient will flow into the doctor's body directly and affect the Qì circulation. Therefore, Qì healers need to know how to get rid of or balance negative Qì invading their body after treatment. That's why the most common Qì treatments in hospitals use the method of Qì induction without touching. This is the same theory as when a charged object is near an uncharged object: the uncharged object will be ionized and the opposite charges will be gathered near the charged object. Through this Qì correspondence, a doctor will be able to manipulate the Qì.

There are many ways to manipulate Qì. Here, we will give a few examples for your reference.

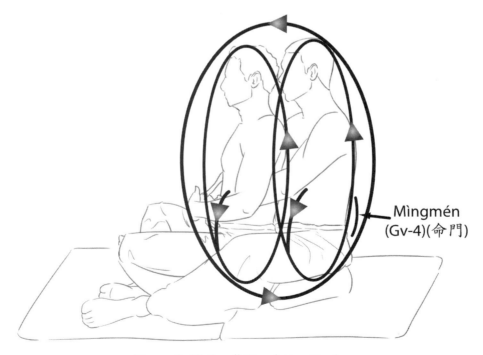

Mìngmén
(Gv-4)(命門)

Figure 3-48. Small Circulation Dual
Practice with Mìngmén Opened.

1. **Releasing the Excess Qì in the Body.** This can be used for those who have hypertension (high blood pressure), fatigue, nervousness, and stress. This technique can help to release excess Qì trapped in the body and thus create relaxation both mentally and physically.

As mentioned earlier, the four limbs are just like four big Qì passageways that regulate the status of Qì in the body. In each of these passageways, there are six rivers (i.e., meridians) that are used to regulate the Qì status of internal organs. If you lead the Qì away from the torso, you are releasing the excess or trapped Qì in the body and if you lead the Qì toward the torso, you are nourishing the organs.

In this practice, a doctor will first build up the Qì correspondence from the shoulders or hips joints. The doctor will place their palms a couple inches from the joints with the Láogōng (P-8) (勞宮) cavity aimed toward the joints' center. After a few deep breaths, the doctor will inhale to lead the patient's Qì to the patient's elbows or knees (Figure 3-49). Next, the doctor will exhale to lead the Qì out to the patient's fingertips or toes. Often, if patients are able to coordinate with the doctor's breathing and follow the doctor's lead, they can make the treatment more effective.

In this case, when the doctor is exhaling to induce Qì correspondence, at the beginning the patient should be inhaling. This will build up the connection very quickly. After a few breaths to build the connection, when the doctor exhales to lead the Qì to the patient's fingers and toes, the patient should exhale to open all of the joints or limbs to allow the doctor to lead the Qì out of the fingertips or toes.

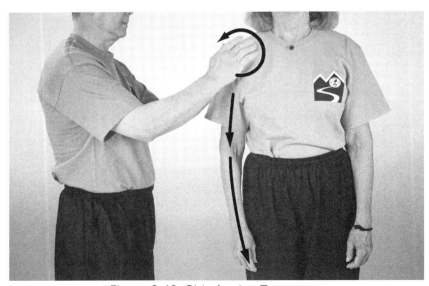

Figure 3-49. Qì Induction Treatment.

If a doctor reverses the path from hands or feet to shoulders and hips, then it is a nourishing treatment. For example, use this reverse path treatment right after the patient has experienced diarrhea or sickness and needs to be nourished.

This is just a brief explanation. We will leave this practice for you to ponder. Remember one thing: everyone has healing power. The difference between you and a doctor is that the doctor has more experience and practice. If you practice and study, you can become an expert as well.

2. **Treating Injuries.** External Qì treatment has also been commonly used for injuries, especially in martial arts society. This occurred because martial artists often got injured during practice. Since many martial artists lived in remote mountain areas where there was no doctor available, they had to find ways of self-healing or mutual healing.

For example, if the injury is at your shoulder area, your partner will first build up the Qì connection with your shoulder through Qì induction. Once the connection or Qì communication is established, your partner will circle their hand around the injured area to loosen it up and initiate Qì circulation (Figure 3-50). Next, the partner will exhale to lead the Qì away from the injured area. If both you and your partner are able to coordinate your breathing and your mind, the treatment will be more effective.

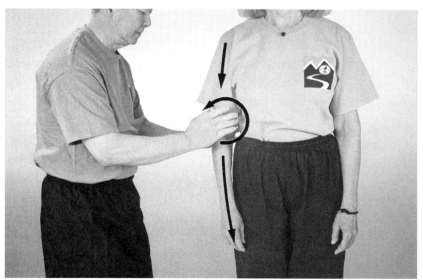

Figure 3-50. Shoulder Injury Treatment through Qì Induction.

3. Treating Mental Instability.
External Qì treatment has also been used for helping mental patients to feel their center. Usually the Bǎihuì (Gv-20) (百會), Shéntíng (Gv-24) (神庭), and Yìntáng (M-NH-3) (印堂) cavities are used (Figure 3-51). Unfortunately, in this situation, it is harder to receive cooperation from a patient. Having an experienced Qì healer is important for this treatment. We will not discuss this subject further.

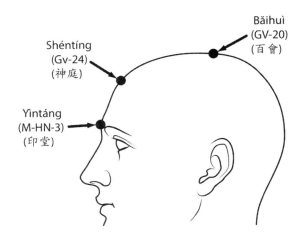

Figure 3-51. Cavities for Mental Treatment.

3.11 Qì Exchange with Nature (Yǔ Dàzìrán Huànqìfǎ, 與大自然換氣法)

Qì exchange with nature is probably the most common, natural, and safe practice in Qì exchange Grand Circulation. This is because we are part of nature and cannot therefore separate ourselves from it. We already have an automatic and subconscious Qì exchange with nature. However, if you know the theory clearly and are able to apply it into your practice, then you can expedite and enhance your Qì exchange with nature. In Chinese Qigong society this is called "feeding the Qì technique" (Shíqìfǎ, 食氣法).

The strongest and the most abundant Qì natural resource is the sun, then the moon, earth, trees, grass, and other animals. As matter of fact, almost everything in nature is able to exchange Qì with you. This exchange can be done through Muscle/Tendon Change Grand Circulation or Marrow/Brain Washing Grand Circulation. We will discuss Muscle/Tendon Change Grand Circulation with nature in this section and discuss the other exchanges in Chapter 6.

Qi Exchange with the Sun (Shí Tàiyáng Qì, 食太陽氣)

As we know, without the sun's energy, all life on the earth would die. It is from this sun Qì that all life derives and exists. Therefore, if we know the theory and how to adopt sun Qì into our practice, we will make this Qì exchange more efficient and effective.

The early morning sun is mild, comfortable, and nourishing. This is the best time to absorb the sun's Qì for our body. The sun's energy at noontime and early afternoon is often too strong and if we expose ourselves to it, the body will reject this strong input and it could also cause damage to our bodies. The energy of the setting sun is weakening and the Qì is also reducing. That is why when you expose yourself to the sun in the morning, you feel comfortable and delightful, around noontime you feel hot and uncomfortable, and at dusk you feel relaxed since your body, like other natural lives, is releasing Qì with the setting sun.

Therefore, the best time to absorb the sun's Qì is early morning right after sunrise. There is another advantage to the early morning. As we know, plants absorb oxygen and release carbon dioxide at night. However, under strong sunshine, plants release the excess oxygen produced during photosynthesis. During this transmitting period, the chemical reaction occurring packs the atmosphere with ions. If you practice Qìgōng at this time, you will be able to join in the natural chemical reaction/cycle and cleanse your body.

You should avoid prolonged exposure to the sun during the midday hours. This is the time to relax. If you have too much Qì trapped in your body, you may release your excess Qì by watching the sun set and practice releasing Qìgōng at that time.

Based on this brief theory, we can summarize a few keys of practice.

Practices (Sunrise):

This is the time for nourishing your Qì. Face the sun in the early morning. Since your front is Yīn while the back is Yáng, if you face the sun, you will be able to absorb the sun's Qì. The process of absorbing is very simple. Once you feel comfortable, inhale deeply and receive the Qì from the sun and then exhale to lead all the Qì absorbed to the Real Lower Dāntián. Once the Qì is led to the Real Lower Dāntián, simply hold your breath for five to ten seconds and allow the Qì to settle and be stored (Figure 3-52). Naturally, if you are experienced in leading your Qì, you may just inhale and lead the Qì directly to the Real Lower Dāntián. Hold your breath for five to ten seconds, then exhale naturally so the Qì absorbed can be distributed to the entire Dāntián. You may practice till the sun begins to feel too warm. Remember, once you feel uncomfortable, you will subconsciously begin to repel the sun's Qì. In this

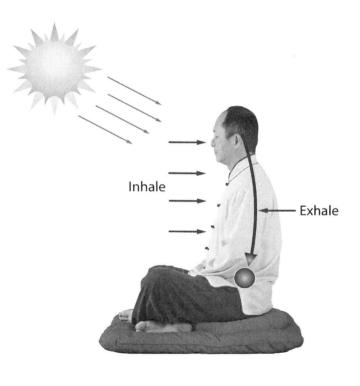

Inhale

Exhale

Figure 3-52. Absorb Sun's Qì Early Morning.

practice, you may use Normal Abdominal Breathing or Reverse Abdominal Breathing. If you use Reverse Abdominal Breathing, your intention to lead the Qì will be stronger.

Practice (Sunset):

This is the best time to release your excess Qì and help you to cool down both mentally and physically. In this practice, you may face toward the setting sun to release excess Qi in the six Yīn organs.

If you face the sunset, you should pay attention to your exhalation. The exhalation should be longer than the inhalation. First, inhale naturally and then exhale slowly, gradually, softly, and slenderly and lead the excess Qì out of the body to join the Qì led by the sun. If you wish to enhance the releasing, you may just add a gentle and soft sound of Hā (哈) while relaxing your body. This practice is good for lowering blood pressure.

Qi Exchange with the Moon (Shí Yuèqì, 食月氣)

From past experience, it is said that three days before the full moon till the day of full moon is the best time to receive the moon's Qì. After that is not a good period for absorbing the moon's Qì. As we know, the moon's energy is very powerful, as evidenced by the gravitational force that causes the tide of oceans and also the amount of radiation that falls upon us that can affect our emotions and the growth of plants. If you know how to pick up the moon's Qì and store it at the Real Lower Dāntián, then you may enhance the storage of Qì.

Practices:

When you adopt the moon's Qì, use the same method you used to absorb the sun's Qì. Face toward the moon and regulate your mind and breathing to a profound state. Next, look at the moon, inhale deeply, and absorb the moon's Qì from the front side of your body toward the center and then exhale to lead the Qì down to the Real Lower Dāntián. Once you reach the end of the exhalation, hold the breath for five to ten seconds to allow the Qì to settle down. Remember, your inhalation should be longer than your exhalation since you are taking and leading the Qì inward to your body.

As when receiving the sun's Qì, you may just inhale to absorb Qì and lead it directly to the Real Lower Dāntián. Once the Qì is led to the Real Lower Dāntián, hold the breath to enhance the gathering of Qì. Next, exhale and allow the air out naturally but keep your mind at the Real Lower Dāntián. Your inhalation should be longer than your exhalation. This will help the Qì absorbed become stored at the Real Lower Dāntián.

Qi Exchange with Plants (Yǔ Zhíwù Qìjiāo, 與植物氣交)

The most common plants used for Qì nourishment and cleansing are trees and grass. Here we will use these two plants as examples. Once you know the theory and methods, you may apply them to other plants.

TREES

Before we talk about this practice, let's analyze a tree's energy. There are a few basic guidelines that will help you to grasp the keys of this practice.

1. Trees with strong and long-lasting wood such as oak or redwood usually carry good Qì for nourishing, releasing, and enhancing Qì circulation.

2. When the sun rises, the tree's Qì circulates upward from the root to the leaves, and the flowers open their petals. As the sun sets, the tree's Qì goes downward from the leaves to the roots and the flowers' petals close (Figure 3-53). From this you can see that if you wish to nourish your Qì, it is better to hug the tree during sunrise. However, if you wish to reduce your excess Qì, then it is better to hug the tree as the sun sets.

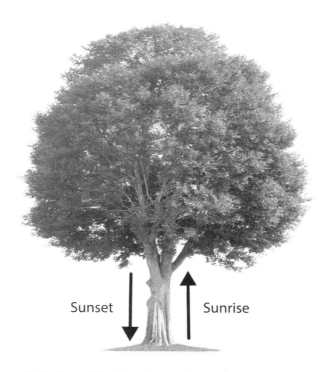

Figure 3-53. Tree Qì's Circulation during Sunrise and Sunset.
(Photo by Shutterstock)

3. Once the sun is up and becomes strong, the side of a tree facing the sun is Yáng while the other side is Yīn (Figure 3-54). In this case, the tree's Qì is flowing from the Yáng to the Yīn side. If you hug the tree on the Yīn side, you will receive the tree's Qì, and if you hug the tree on the Yáng side, you will release your Qì.

4. If you wish to clean your body's evil Qì (Xiéqì, 邪氣), you should stand and hug the tree between the tree's Yīn and Yáng (Figure 3-55) sides. In this case, the circulation of the tree energy from the Yáng side to the Yīn side will help you remove evil Qì. After you practice for approximately five minutes, if you wish to balance your body's Qì, stand on the other side and hug the tree for the same period of time.

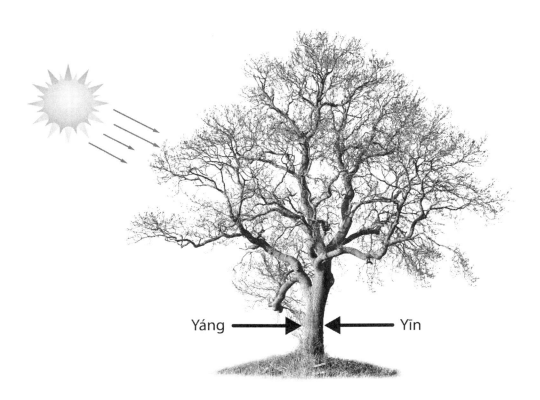

Figure 3-54. Yīn and Yáng of a Tree Under the Sun.
(Photo by Shutterstock)

5. If there is no sun and you are in northern hemisphere, the side of a tree facing north is more Yáng. This is because in order to resist the cold wind in winter, this side of tree is more compact and its density is higher. Correspondingly, the side facing south is more Yīn (Figure 3-56). Using this information, you can find a way to fit it into what your practice needs.

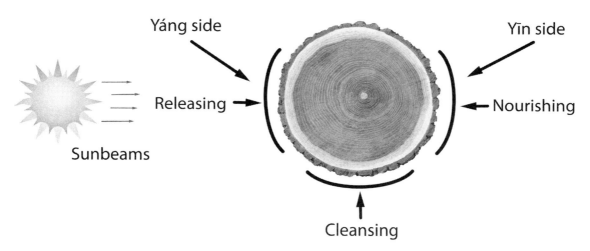

Figure 3-55. Nourishing, Releasing, and Cleansing with Tree Qì.
(Illustration by Shutterstock)

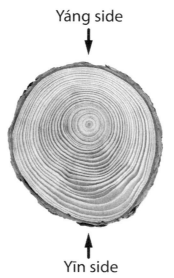

Figure 3-56. Tree Qì's Yīn and Yáng without the Sun.
(Illustration by Shutterstock)

6. In all of these Qì-exchange practices, you should use Reverse Abdominal Breathing since you have an intention to regulate the body's Qì. If you use Normal Abdominal Breathing, though you are more relaxed, the Qì led will not be as strong.

Practices:

1. **Nourishing.** If you wish to absorb tree Qì for nourishing yourself, hug the tree in the early morning when the tree's Qì is flowing upward to the leaves and outward from the trunk's center. If the tree is exposed to the sun, if you hug the trunk from the shadow side (i.e., Yīn side), you make use of the tree's circulation. Once you hug the tree, first regulate your mind and breathing until you feel comfortable and natural. Next, inhale deeply and absorb the tree Qì into your body to your centerline. Then exhale and lead the Qì down to the Real Lower Dāntián (Figure 3-57). Once the Qì is led there, hold your breath for five to ten seconds to let the Qì settle. You may repeat the absorbing process as long as you wish. Remember, your inhalation should be longer than your exhalation since you are absorbing the Qì inward.

   You may also use another method. Inhale and lead the Qì inward and then downward to the Real Lower Dāntián. Hold your breath for five to ten seconds and then exhale naturally to let the Qì dissipate into the biobattery (Figure 3-58). You may try both ways and see which one works better for you.

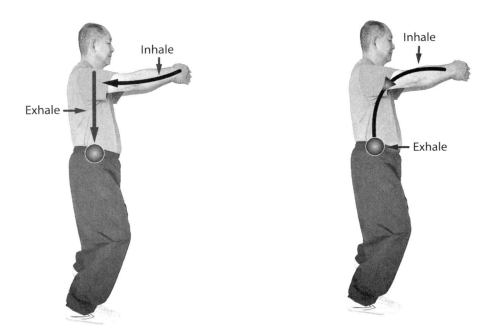

Figure 3-57. Absorbing Qì from Tree–1.   Figure 3-58. Absorbing Qì from Tree–2.

2. **Releasing.** If you wish to release excess Qì from your body, you should hug the tree when the sun is setting, when the tree's Qì is returning to its root. Again, regulate your mind and breathing first until they are calm and natural. Next, inhale naturally. Then exhale and lead the Qì out of your front side to enter the tree (Figure 3-59). Your exhalation should be longer than your inhalation. Once you have reached the end of your exhalation, you may hold your breath for five to ten seconds to enhance the releasing.

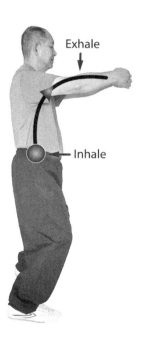

Figure 3-59. Releasing Qì to Tree.

3. **Cleansing.** There are two ways to use the tree's Qì to cleanse your body's evil Qì. The first way is to hug the tree on the shadow side. Absorb the tree's Qì inward toward the center of your body, then exhale to lead it down through the bottom of your feet to enter the ground (Figure 3-60). The second way is to hug the tree on the side between the bright and shadow sides. For example, place your right hand on the bright side and your left hand on the shadow side and hug the tree. Next, inhale and absorb the tree's Qì from the left-hand side of your body and then exhale to release from the right-hand side of your body back into the tree (Figure 3-61).

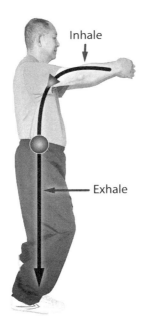

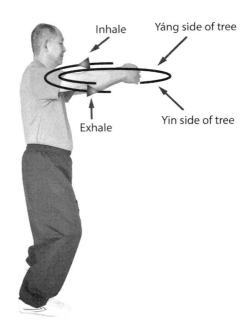

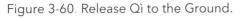

Figure 3-60. Release Qì to the Ground.   Figure 3-61. Cleansing Qì with Tree.

Grass/Ground

Since grass grows close to the ground and the ground is able to absorb unlimited Qì, the grass or ground is commonly used to release or cleanse Qì. In this practice, you may use either Normal or Reverse Abdominal Breathing. Many experienced Qìgōng practitioners are able to absorb the Earth Qì from the Yǒngquán (K-1) (湧泉) and lead it upward to Real Lower Dāntián for storage. If you have an intention to do so, you may use Reverse Abdominal Breathing.

Practice:

1. **Nourishing.** If you wish to adopt Earth Qì or grass Qì for nourishing, you should touch your bare feet to the ground. Sitting is usually better than standing since it is a more relaxing posture and you can more effectively lead the Qì led upward to the Real Lower Dāntián. You may also sit on a comfortable chair with your bare feet touching the grass or ground. Again, first regulate your mind and breathing till they are comfortably regulated. Next, inhale and absorb the grass or Earth Qì through the Yǒngquán and lead it upward to the Real Lower Dāntián. Once the Qì reaches the Real Lower Dāntián, hold your breath for five to ten seconds. Next, exhale naturally and allow the Qì to distribute to the entire Dāntián. You may repeat the same process till you decide to stop. When you practice this nourishing cycle, you must do so in warm weather. If the ground is too cold, the Qì will be led downward automatically and naturally. You would then be losing or reducing your Qì.

2. **Releasing/Cleansing.** It is much easier and more effective to release your excess Qì into the ground (or stream). You may stand or sit, but sitting is more relaxing. First, regulate your mind and breathing until they are comfortably regulated. Next, inhale and gather the Qì at the Real Lower Dāntián and then exhale and lead the Qì downward into the ground or grass through the bottom of your feet (or Yǒngquán). Once you reach the end of your exhalation, hold your breath for five to ten seconds. You may repeat the same process until you decide to stop. In this practice, do not worry that the ground or grass will take too much of your Qì and make you weak. We have evolved touching the ground and it is a part of our nature. Once the Qì is harmonized and balanced between your body and the ground, the releasing will stop. When the weather is comfortable, the ground or grass Qì is grounded (i.e., neutral).

Animals (Cat or Dog)

You may also exchange Qì with animals. The most commonly used animals are cats, dogs, and horses. As long as you are kind to them, they will willingly exchange Qì with you. In the past, it was recognized that the cat's Qì is the strongest among these three. From statistical data, seniors who own pets are usually healthier and live longer.

When people exchange Qì with animals, they often adopt the animals' Qì for nourishment. In this practice, if you hug a pet and inhale longer than exhale, you will take the Qì from them. You should not worry that they will run out of energy. This is because animals still have a strong capability to readjust their Qì supplies. We humans have isolated ourselves from nature for so long that we have lost our capability to regain the balance as quickly as animals.

Others

You may also exchange Qì with natural objects such as rocks, water, crystals, or jade. Actually, many Qì healers, after doing a treatment, use a crystal or jade to neutralize their Qì so they are able to regain their harmonious state quickly. Running water is also commonly used for releasing the evil Qì received from patients.

You may use the same principles involved in Qì exchange with animals and trees and apply them to these objects. The more you practice, the more you are able to feel and use them naturally, the more you are able to use them to benefit yourself. Experience generates profound feeling and feeling is the key to regulating the Qì.

There is another strong and powerful Qì that humans have been exchanging Qi with since ancient times. That is the cosmic Qì falling upon us from the sky. If you know how to adopt this cosmic energy into your body, then you have found the grail of longevity. Since this practice is related to Brain Washing Qìgōng, we will discuss it in Chapter 6.

PART III

Marrow/Brain Washing
Small and Grand Circulations

CHAPTER 4

Scientific Foundation of Brain Washing Qìgōng

4.1 REVIEW OF ANCIENT CHINESE QÌGŌNG UNDERSTANDING (XǏSUǏJĪNG DE KĒXUÉ GĒNJĪ, 洗髓經的科學根基)

Before we enter into the scientific explanation of Brain Washing Qìgōng (Xǐsuǐjīng, 洗髓經), it is good to review what is known from the ancient Chinese Qìgōng practices. Without a clear understanding of these ancient foundations, it will be difficult to link them with today's science.

1. The Body's Polarity

It was recognized long ago that there are two specific points in the human body that are two poles of a very important polarity. They were considered of the utmost importance for health and well-being. One was determined to be the center of the head, and it was named "Mud Pill Palace" (Níwán Gōng, 泥丸宮) or "Upper Dāntián" (Shàng Dāntián, 上丹田). The other was identified as the center of gravity (i.e., your physical center) and named "Real Lower Dāntián" (Zhēn Xià Dāntián, 真下丹田).

While the Upper Dāntián was believed to be the residence of the spirit (Shénshì, 神室), the Real Lower Dāntián was believed to be the dwelling of Qì (Qìshè, 氣舍). The spirit manages the manifestation of Qì in the upper center, and the quantity of Qì is supplied from the lower one. This polarity and relationship was first mentioned in Chapter 16 of the *Dào Dé Jīng* (道德經), a book by Lǎozi (老子), which was written in the sixth century BCE, about 2,600 years ago.

2. Relation of the Two Poles

The Upper Dāntián and Real Lower Dāntián are connected by the Thrusting Vessel (Chōngmài, 衝脈), which is basically an energy reservoir that follows the path of the spinal cord. As the word "thrust" implies, the Chinese believed that Qì moved swiftly and without resistance in this vessel. Therefore, these two poles were understood to function as a single entity, synchronizing with each other simultaneously.

This system is the basis of any human's or animal's central Qì system, a vital and necessary component of life. When an embryo forms, this polarity is constructed first.

The communication between the Upper Dāntián and Real Lower Dāntián must remain smooth and undisturbed, so spinal health is an absolute requisite to living well and living longer (Figures 4-1 and 4-2).

3. Guardian Qì (Wèiqì, 衛氣)

An aura is defined as a type of energy surrounding the body. This concept has sometimes been portrayed across different cultures as halos, which are found in both Eastern and Western cultures—including both Christianity and Buddhism. While scientific research has been unable to confirm the existence of a person's aura, the Chinese understood it to be an elliptical shield-like energy surrounding the body that was directly related to the body's central polarity.

The stronger the Qì is in your center, the stronger your Guardian Qì (Wèiqì, 衛氣)—or aura—can be. Your Guardian Qì is strongly related to your immune system, your ability to fend off diseases and recover. If you are able to build and maintain a strong central Qì core, then your Guardian Qì will be stronger and it will strengthen your spirit and inner purpose.

4. The Body's Energy Pumps

The Chinese discovered that the abdomen and perineum (i.e., anus) could be used to more efficiently move Qì around the body. These pumps are a natural part of the human body's design. For example, when a baby is growing in the womb, it must use these pumps to receive nutrients, water, and oxygen through the umbilical cord. The idea of having

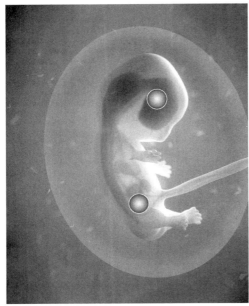

Figure 4-1. Polarity in Embryo–Human.
(Illustration by Shutterstock)

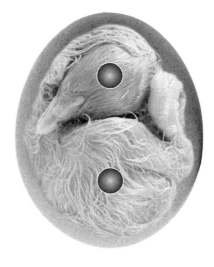

Figure 4-2. Polarity in Embryo–Chicken.
(Illustration by Shutterstock)

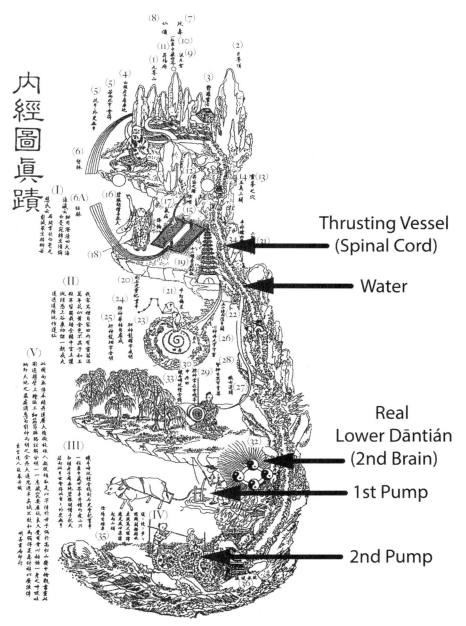

内經圖真蹟

**Thrusting Vessel
(Spinal Cord)**

Water

**Real
Lower Dāntián
(2nd Brain)**

1st Pump

2nd Pump

Figure 4-3. Táng Dynasty Inner Meridian Chart.

such pumps to move water in the body is illustrated in an ancient chart of the human body, the Táng Dynasty Inner Meridian Chart (Tángdài Nèijīng Tú, 唐代內經圖, circa 859 CE) (Figure 4-3). As represented in the chart, water is moved by: 1) a man tilling the field, and 2) children working a water wheel. The man is in the abdominal area, and the children are in the perineal area. The part representing the spinal cord has a path where water flows. Modern science has confirmed that there is a fluid present in the spinal cord. It is actually cerebrospinal fluid, as opposed to water.

I believe these pumps physically move your entire central Qì system up and down, specifically affecting the limbic system. The limbic system oscillations massage, stimulate, and enhance various parts of the body to produce hormones and create conditions for a higher quantity and quality of Qì in the body. This is probably why the ancient Chinese concluded that these areas were pumps for ultimately manipulating Qì flow.

4.2 SCIENTIFIC FOUNDATIONS AND INTERPRETATIONS (KĒXUÉ GĒNJĪ YǓ JIĚSHÌ, 科學根基與解釋)

Focal Points (i.e., Resonance Centers)

A line is defined as having two endpoints. For an ellipse, two focal points exist. The rounder an ellipse is, the closer these focal points are. If the ellipse is a circle, the focal points overlap and become one. The below diagrams illustrate this concept (Figure 4-4). Remember to also consider the three-dimensional cases (an ovoid and a sphere).

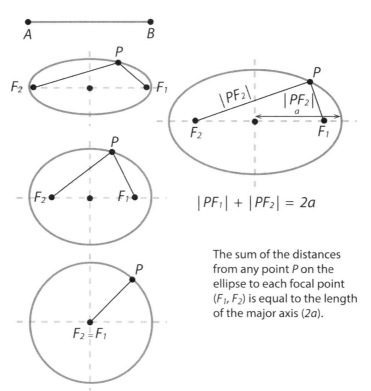

$$|PF_1| + |PF_2| = 2a$$

The sum of the distances from any point *P* on the ellipse to each focal point (*F₁*, *F₂*) is equal to the length of the major axis (*2a*).

Figure 4-4. Focal Points (i.e., Resonance Centers).

If we consider the Upper Dāntián and Real Lower Dāntián as focal points, then an ovoid space would surround the body. Within this space, the Upper Dāntián and Real Lower Dāntián share a synchronized relation to each other, as shown in the illustrations with *PF₁* and *PF₂*. These points are energetic, so I will refer to them as "resonance centers." They are actually what scientists now refer to as the body's two brains. The first brain is the one in our head, and the second brain is our gut (i.e., enteric nervous system). Scientists classified these two entities as brains because they each have the capability to function independently. This undoubtedly highlights their importance and significance.

The spinal cord connects a path between them, attaching directly to the brainstem and going down to the lumbar area of the back. Because the spinal cord is made up of highly electrically conductive nervous tissue, the two brains can synchronize with each other instantaneously and function as a single circuit. The two-brain theory coincides precisely with the Chinese explanation of the Upper Dāntián, Real Lower Dāntián, and Thrusting Vessel.

Resonance Center Origin Points

While it is easy to locate our upper and lower brains, it is worth trying to explore and ponder where the origin point of each resonance center is.

The head's Qì field is spherical, so logically its resonance center should be at the center of the head. The limbic system is at the center of the head and is believed to heavily influence the unconscious mind and may also store genetic memory. I believe it affects the subconscious mind as well. "Unconscious" implies a state where consciousness is entirely not present. Many aspects of Qigong practice, particularly meditation, involve the conscious mind still being at least partially present in a semi-sleeping state. The subconscious mind can provide you with intuition, emotion, and action. In the book *The Second Brain*, the author refers to the lower brain as the source of gut instinct, but I actually believe it has to do more with the second brain being connected to the limbic system. I believe it is accurate to say that the subconscious mind resides in the limbic system and acts as the spiritual center of your life. There is a reference to the "center of doing nothing" in the *Dào Dé Jīng*. It means the "doing of no doing" and the "thinking of no thinking" (Wúwéi, 無為). Essentially, it talks about the center where everything is natural and automatic, without conscious interference or disturbance. I

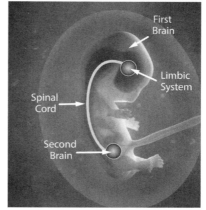

Figure 4-5. Resonance Center Origin Points.
(Illustration by Shutterstock)

believe this passage is further substantiating the limbic system as the true origin of the upper resonance center (Figure 4-5).

The lower resonance center should be the body's physical center of gravity—when standing in a neutral position. Essentially, it is your gut (i.e., the Real Lower Dāntián). The center of gravity is the point on the body where mass seems the most concentrated, and the point around which gravity acts. This location would make the most practical sense for being a resonating energy center because it provides the most equilibrium in terms of body balance, symmetry, and stability—both physically and mentally. It is my belief that this is the location of the very first cell that is formed when an embryo develops and thus should remain the core root of manipulating and controlling all aspects of your life.

Qì Movement in the Body

In addition to the Qì fields produced by the two brains (Figure 4-6), there is another strong, round Qì field (i.e., magnetic field) produced by the heart. Similar to electricity, a potential difference is required in order to circulate Qì. Since the location of the heart is closer to the front and left side of the torso, the resulting energy imbalance creates a major motive force behind Qì spiraling around the body (Figure 4-7). The same effect happens with the spinal cord, which is offset toward the back of the body. Qì circulates from the back of the body to the front because of this energy imbalance. In Turtle Shell Qìgòng, exercises were developed in line with this flow, following the nerves around the ribcage from back to front.

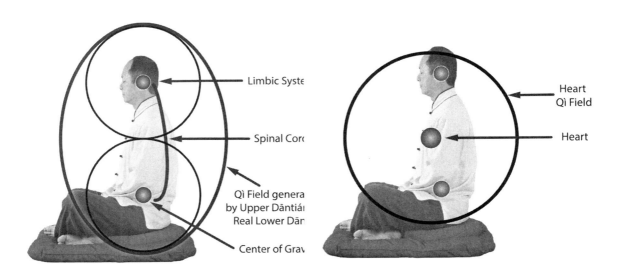

Figure 4-6. Qì Field
Produced by Two Poles.

Figure 4-7. Qì Field
Produced by the Heart.

Unfortunately, science has not been able to provide a detailed map of exactly how these magnetic fields (Qì) flow and change around the body. Through my own Qìgōng practice, I have observed and become aware of general patterns, however. The fields drawn in the diagrams below have been simplified for readability and to present the general concept (Figure 4-8).

Combined Effect of All Qì Fields

When the field formed by the two brains and the field formed by the heart are added together, the resulting Qì field is stronger and denser on the rear side (Figure 4-9). The front side is less compact, so we would classify the front side as Yīn and the rear side as Yáng. Qì extends farther in front of the body than in the back.

Profound results can be achieved by being cognizant of all the different energy fields at play and incorporating this recognition into your daily practice. Something as seemingly small as a heartbeat can produce a subtle but significant change in your body's Qì, influencing both your mind and body. Heart rate variability and amplitude have been shown to correlate with emotional well-being. My theory is that with each heartbeat, your overall body's Qì field changes shape, from being more elongated to more round. Thus, the two resonance centers should also

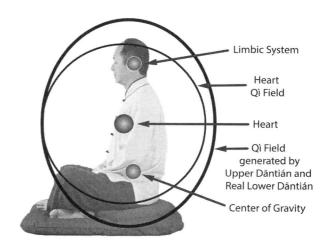

Figure 4-8. Co-Existence of Two Poles Qì Field and Heart Qì Field.

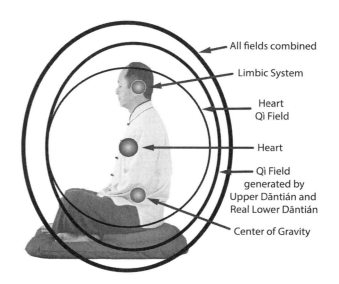

Figure 4-9. All Fields Combined.

oscillate closer and farther away from each other energy-wise, not just physically. The whole process should help contribute to the movement and stimulation of the limbic system, and consequently also hormone production.

Pineal and Pituitary Glands

I am confident that the "pill" of the ancient Chinese name "Mud Pill Palace" was in reference to the pineal and pituitary glands, both of which are located in the limbic system (Figure 4-10). The pineal gland is related to spiritual development, and the pituitary gland is related to physical growth. These two glands oversee most, if not

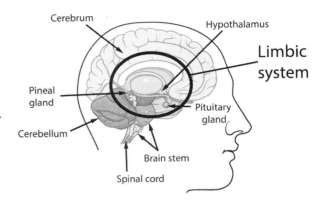

Figure 4-10. Pineal and Pituitary Glands in Limbic System.

all, of the body's spiritual and physical health. The name "palace" implies an echo-like effect, meaning that these glands can be stimulated and vibrated, for example, through the practice of Qìgōng.

Western cultures call the pineal gland our "Third Eye." It produces melatonin, which is commonly related to good sleep, a healthy immune system, and well-being. The effects of higher melatonin production have often been associated with deep meditation, as well as calming, regulatory effects on the body and emotions. Some of our most profound discoveries and epiphanies come in these meditative moments. Consequently, I believe melatonin production plays a major role in our spiritual development.

The pituitary gland is sometimes referred to as the "master gland" of the endocrine system, because it is responsible for the control and function of several other glands that help to maintain the body's physical health. Among those hormones is HGH (human growth hormone), which regulates the physical body's growth, cell production, and tissue repair. Maintaining the operation of this gland helps to prevent physical aging and reduce recovery times.

Circulation/Movement of Cerebrospinal Fluid

Within the brain and spinal cord is a clear fluid known as cerebrospinal fluid (CSF). When we are sleeping and breathing deeply, this fluid helps to remove any accumulated metabolic waste, and it actually moves in a rhythmic, wave-like manner (Figure 4-11). The key to keeping the brain healthy and functioning normally is to keep pumping the CSF and keep it circulating smoothly throughout the brain.

Enhancing the flow of Qì through Qìgōng practice should complement the natural CSF circulation process. To further enhance the cleaning process, you may want to try lying down with your head lower than your torso. It would be worthwhile to explore how this practice may benefit patients with brain disorders, such as tumors or Alzheimer's. I strongly believe that training Qìgōng is a safe and effective practice that can be used to self-clean the brain for better clarity.

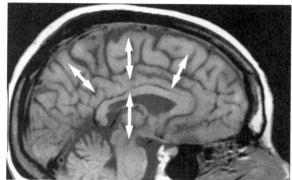

Figure 4-11. Cerebrospinal Fluid Circulates throughout the Brain in a Pulsing, Wave-Like Motion.
(Illustration by Shutterstock)

Limbic System Oscillations

It has been shown that limbic system oscillations (up-down motions) can be enhanced by breathing, particularly from the nose, or influenced by your heartbeat. The pulsing of the heart contributes to the movement of cerebrospinal fluid in and out of the brain (Figure 4-12). According to these findings, it may be surmised that exercising more (i.e., conditioning your heart and breathing) can help to regulate or even increase the levels of hormone production in the limbic system, specifically in the pineal and pituitary glands.

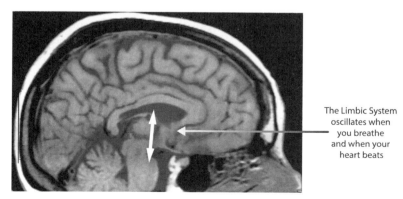

The Limbic System oscillates when you breathe and when your heart beats

Figure 4-12. The Limbic System Oscillates with Breathing and Heartbeats.
(Illustration by Shutterstock)

4.3 Ancient Practice and Guidelines for Practicing Today (Gŭdài De Shíjiàn Yŭ Zhŭnzé Yòngzài Jīnrì De Liànxí, 古代的實踐與準則用在今日的練習)

Abdominal Breathing (Fùshì Hūxī, 腹式呼吸)

Daoists and some Buddhist Qìgōng practitioners emphasized the practice of abdominal breathing. Abdominal breathing is also called "back to childhood breathing" (Fǎntóng Hūxī, 返童呼吸). Through this type of breathing, the limbic system is continuously massaged. As a result, hormone production from the pineal and pituitary glands can be increased.

In order to produce more Qì (i.e., elixir), you need to convert the fat stored in your abdominal area into Qì. This can be achieved through abdominal exercises. In order to increase the efficiency of this conversion, you will need to train and condition your abdominal muscles. This process is called "building the foundation of Dāntián" (Dāntián Zhújī, 丹田築基). Deep abdominal breathing will push and pull the spinal cord and limbic system up and down. Deep breathing can increase the expansion of the diaphragm up to two centimeters, which would then also stimulate and massage the adrenal glands on top of the kidneys. Diaphragmatic breathing has been correlated to increased levels of melatonin production, so there is almost certainly a relation to the pineal gland.

Coordination with the Perineum (or Anus)

When Daoists and Buddhist practitioners trained abdominal breathing, they also coordinated it with the movement of the perineum. Specifically, they focused at the center of the perineal area on an acupuncture cavity called the Huìyīn (會陰) (i.e., meeting point of Yīn) that is considered the exact point of this pump. Oftentimes, documents simply referred to this area as the anus, which, although inaccurate, is close enough to the Huìyīn to produce the same results. The Huìyīn pump can help to promote Qì flow in your brain, gut, and spinal cord (Upper Dāntián, Real Lower Dāntián, and Thrusting Vessel) and is a major component in moving Qì into and out of the body. In coordination with deep breathing, this pump can help to more effectively move the limbic system and spinal cord up and down, creating a more optimized and improved process to enhance hormone production. I believe this pump also promotes better cerebrospinal fluid flow.

In order to make this pump efficient, you must condition the muscles of the perineal area in addition to your abdominal muscles. You must regularly condition and exercise the muscles around Huìyīn until you are able to use your mind to fully control and manipulate them.

Keeping the Mind at Dāntián

To Daoist and Buddhist Qìgōng practitioners, another key to successful practice is being able to keep the mind focused on the Upper Dāntián and Real Lower Dāntián (Yìshǒu Dāntián, 意守丹田).

Dāntián literally translates to "elixir field," which implies an area where you can produce (grow) energy. When the mind can stay on these two centers, Qì will stay in your body's centerline and not be led outward or needlessly consumed. During practice, you should always keep your mind focused on these two points to conserve and build energy, and observe their synchronization. Once you have built a subconscious habit of keeping your mind on these two centers, you will then be able to maintain a supply of Qì for enhancing hormone production through the Upper Dāntián (i.e., limbic system).

Girdle Vessel Exercises

The Girdle Vessel (Dàimài, 帶脈), or Belt Vessel, roughly follows the waist line. It is well-recognized in Chinese medicine and Qìgōng that when the Qì in your Girdle Vessel is abundantly expanded, your immune system can be strengthened and boosted (Figure 4-13).

Exercises for the abdominal area commonly target the Girdle Vessel. The center of the Girdle Vessel is now recognized as the second brain: the center of gravity. When the

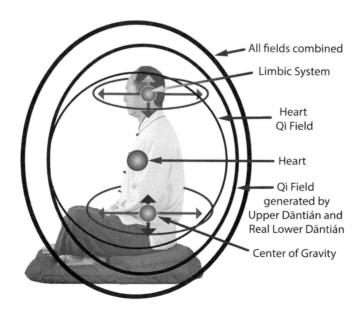

Figure 4-13. All Fields Combined.

Qì in this area (lower resonance center) is strong and expansive, the limbic system (upper resonance center) will also expand, because it will automatically synchronize with its lower counterpart. Chinese martial artists often use cloth belts to enhance the quality of their Qì manifestation and power in their training. When the waist area is restricted by a belt, the resistance pushes the body to expand its energy further. Coordination of breathing and the Huìyīn pump using Reverse Abdominal Breathing will also raise inner vitality and spirit.

Summary of Benefits

1. **Longevity**—This is perhaps the most significant benefit that can be achieved through diligent practice. Due to the stimulation of the pituitary and pineal glands, you will be able to maintain or enhance your body's hormone production, an essential key to extending your life and maintaining your youth.

2. **Stronger Immune System**—Expanding the Qì in the Girdle Vessel and coordinating with the use of your perineum as a pump will enhance your Guardian Qì, strengthening and boosting your overall immunity and internal defense system.

3. **Brain Health**—Focusing Qì on the upper resonance center (upper brain) will help to promote a healthy and consistent flow of cerebrospinal fluid, allowing for regular maintenance and improved function. This may likely contribute to your brain's long-term health, including the prevention of brain disorders.

4. **Raise Your Spirit**—Your Qì's manifestation will be effective and efficient, naturally leading to a higher spirit. Combined with a strong immune system, the meaning of life can become profound and purposeful, making you less prone to depression and passivity.

CHAPTER 5

Marrow/Brain Washing Small Circulation

5.1 INTRODUCTION (JIÈSHÀO, 介紹)

The Third Eye is called "Heaven Eye" (Tiānmù, 天目 or Tiānyǎn, 天眼) in Chinese Qìgōng society. This is because when the Third Eye is opened, you will be able to connect without obstacles to the natural energy and spirit. However, for we humans, our Third Eye have been closed since the beginning of human culture. We have lost direct contact with or feeling for nature. Animals are still able to sense the natural energy's variations but we have lost this capability. Buddhists and Daoists are looking for the way to reopen the Third Eye in order to resume their connections with nature. When the Third Eye is reopened, they will be able to feel or sense natural energy changes and also regain the capability for telepathy. This is the stage of spiritual enlightenment and the necessary step of reaching Buddhahood (Chéngfó, 成佛) or Immortality (Chéngxiān, 成仙).

In order to reopen the Third Eye, we must first understand the reasons why it was shut down in the first place. Only then will we be able to find the way to reopen it. If we don't understand the reasons, then the practice of brain washing will be shallow and meaningless. Here, I would like to list those possible reasons:

1. If we trace back to the beginning of human life as we know it, we were like other animals, hunted and hunter. Animals often hunt at night when visibility is minimized. In order to hunt or escape from being hunted, animals depended on the development of the Third Eye which allowed them to feel and sense danger or to catch prey. However, once humans began to build safe places for protection and learned how to raise cattle and plant food, gradually, due to lack of practice, the Third Eye was closed. Since then we have isolated ourselves from the greater nature.

2. When we humans became smarter and more clever, we became cunning. We learned how to play tricks and lie to each other. Our conscious mind developed rapidly and began to create dogmas and doctrines that suppressed the truthful feeling of the subconscious mind. Since then, we have created a human matrix and hidden our true nature behind masks. In order to keep our hidden lies behind the mask, we closed our Third Eye subconsciously.

These are the two main reasons we have lost our direct feeling connection with the greater nature. It stands to reason that in order to reopen the Third Eye, you must be truthful to yourself and others. Without this priori condition, the Third Eye will remain shut. That is why the Daoists called themselves "Zhēnrén" (真人) which means "truthful person" since they must be truthful.

Marrow/Brain Washing Qìgōng is called Xǐsuǐjīng (洗髓經) in Chinese. Xǐ (洗) means to wash or to clean, Suǐ (髓) means bone marrow (Gǔsuǐ, 骨髓) or brain (Nǎosuǐ, 腦髓), and Jīng (經) means classic. The reason that both marrow and brain washing were put together was that the training theory and techniques are very similar, and they both target the two most Yīn places of the body: the marrow and brain. These two places are constructed of highly electric conductive material and are considered to be electric plasma (i.e., liquid metal). That means the resistance in these two places is so low as to be almost nonexistent. Due to their conductivity characteristics, these two places are the most sensitive to any radiation from natural or artificial sources that penetrate our bodies. Since we have evolved within this environment of natural radiations such as from the sun, the earth, the cosmos, and so on from the beginning of human history, it is not a problem for us to adopt them. However, since the 1920s humans have introduced various forms of artificial radiation into this world and our bodies have not had enough time to evolve with them; arguably; various cancers developed from these forms of polluting radiation. This new artificial radioactive environment has affected all life on earth, such as plants, animals, germs, and viruses. However, unlike humans, these lives are not separated from nature and they have more potential to adapt more quickly than us.

According to scientific understanding, every brain cell consumes about twelve times more oxygen than regular cells. Our anatomy has evolved to reflect this. There are four arteries in our neck that circulate blood from our torso to our head. Relatively, our legs are large, and there is only one artery in each one. Since blood cells are carriers of oxygen and Qì, and oxygen consumption is proportional to the production of energy (or of Qì), we can reasonably assume that each brain cell must also consume twelve times more Qì than regular cells.

The fact is that since we are currently living in a more challenging, polluted environment than in the past, Qìgōng practice has become more important than ever. With routine Qìgōng practice, you will be able continuously bring the abnormal Qì imbalance back to a normal state. This is the way of maintaining health and preventing sickness.

This is also true for Marrow/Brain Washing Qìgōng practice. Through this Qìgōng practice, you will be able to maintain your marrow's healthy function and also keep your brain in its normal operational state. Traditionally, there are two main purposes of Marrow/Brain Washing Grand Circulations:

1. **Longevity.** Marrow washing Qìgōng is effective to maintain healthy marrow cells' function and also to reactivate those aged and degenerated marrow cells. This is to resume blood cell production to its normal and healthy level. Blood cells are carriers of oxygen, water, nutrition, Qì, and any other minerals that are required for cell replacement (i.e., metabolism). It follows that smooth cell replacement is the crucial key to longevity.

2. **Spiritual Enlightenment.** There are two goals of brain washing. One is to activate more brain cells to improve function and increase the capacity for Qì storage. The brain is like a capacitor that is able to store Qì to an abundant level. The other goal is to cleanse the dark side of our genetic thoughts that are passed down to us through genetic memory. If we cannot cleanse these dark thoughts and if we do not stop hiding the truth behind our mask, we will continue to subconsciously shut down our Third Eye. In order to reopen the Third Eye, we must be truthful and have abundant Qì storage in the brain. Then, through Embryonic Breathing, the Qì can be focused into a strong tiny beam like a lens and we can reopen the Third Eye.

The first step of Marrow/Brain Washing is practicing Marrow/Brain Washing Small Circulation (Two Poles Small Circulation or Thrusting Vessel Small Circulation). Then, you may step in with Grand Circulation. You may be curious why this Small Circulation, like Muscle/Tendon Changing Small Circulation (Conception/Governing Vessels Small Circulation or Microcosmic Orbit), though important, is not commonly known and practiced. As we mentioned in earlier chapters, there are two main reasons for this.

1. The secrets of the practice were hidden in monasteries. Since the final main goal of this practice is to reopen the Third Eye for spiritual enlightenment and Buddhahood, usually, only those monks who lived in seclusion were interested and had the right environment for this cultivation. Most laymen were living in a matrix with masks and were more interested in health and longevity, so they were more interested in Muscle/Tendon Changing Small Circulation (Conception/ Governing Vessel Small Circulation or Microcosmic Orbit) that is more related to physical health. Furthermore, Muscle/Tendon Changing Small Circulation was commonly practiced by Shàolín monks for martial arts' power manifestation, and they gradually revealed this practice to the general public.

2. Though this practice is not as difficult and dangerous as that of Muscle/Tendon Changing Small Circulation, the theory of spiritual cultivation behind the practice is harder to comprehend.

Benefits of Marrow/Brain Washing Small Circulation practice:

1. If you wish to reopen your Third Eye, you must first recognize and feel the two poles of your body's Qì central system and know how to manipulate the Qì circulating in this center system. Marrow/Brain Washing Small Circulation will help you build this foundation.

2. Marrow/Brain Washing Small Circulation will help you to firm and strengthen the central Qì system, a crucial requirement for longevity and all Marrow/Brain Washing Grand Circulation.

3. Provide you a firm foundation for Grand Circulation practice.

In the next section, we will first talk about the theory and practice of Two Poles Small Circulation/Thrusting Vessel Small Circulation. Then we will discuss the applications of this Small Circulation practice.

5.2 MARROW/BRAIN WASHING SMALL CIRCULATION AND ITS APPLICATIONS (XǏSUǏJĪNG XIǍOZHŌUTIĀN YǓ YÌNGYÒNG, 洗髓經小周天與應用)

As mentioned, Marrow/Brain Washing Small Circulation is also called Two Poles Small Circulation (Liǎngyí Xiǎozhōutiān, 兩儀小周天). It can also be called Thrusting Vessel Small Circulation (Chōngmài Xiǎozhōutiān, 衝脈小周天). This Circulation is considered to be Yīn (Shuǐlù, 水路) (i.e., Water Path) in relationship to Muscle/Tendon Changing Small Circulation that is considered to be Yáng (Huǒlù, 火路). This Small Circulation establishes a solid ground for enlightenment and Buddhahood spiritual cultivation.

As explained in the first and last chapter, the body's Qì network is built upon two main poles (i.e., human polarity), Upper Dāntián (Shàng Dāntián, 上丹田) (i.e., First Brain) and Real Lower Dāntián (Zhēn Xià Dāntián, 真下丹田) (i.e., Second Brain), which are connected by the Thrusting Vessel (Chōngmài, 衝脈) (i.e., Spinal Cord). This central line is considered the Central Qì System (Qìzhōngshū, 氣中樞) (i.e., Central Nervous System). The Upper Dāntián is considered to be Yīn and the spiritual center (i.e., Spiritual Residence) (Shénshì, 神室) while the Real Lower Dāntián is considered as Yáng and the physical center and Qì dwelling place (Qìshè, 氣舍). While the Upper Dāntián governs the quality of Qì manifestation, the Real Lower Dāntián provides the quantity of the Qì for manifestation. When the Qì is stored abundantly in the Real Lower Dāntián, physical health can be maintained and lifespan can be extended. With abundant storage of Qì, the Qì can also be led upward to nourish the brain and activate more brain cells. When spirit (related to the subconscious mind) residing at the center (i.e., limbic system) of the Upper Dāntián is strong, the Qì manifestation can be efficient and effective. These two centers have form a spiritual triangle for spiritual evolution (Figure 5-1). They also establish a two ellipse Qì field around the body (Figure 5-2).

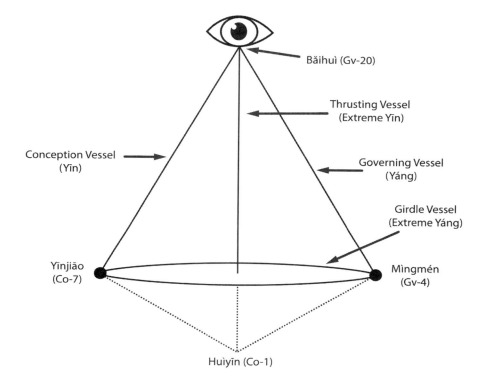

Bǎihuì (Gv-20)

Thrusting Vessel
(Extreme Yīn)

Conception Vessel
(Yīn)

Governing Vessel
(Yáng)

Girdle Vessel
(Extreme Yáng)

Yīnjiāo
(Co-7)

Mìngmén
(Gv-4)

Huìyīn (Co-1)

Figure 5-1. Spiritual Triangle.

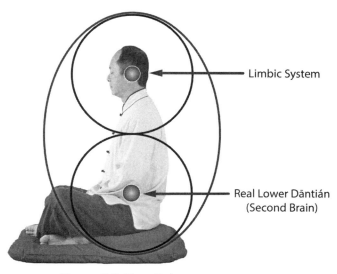

Limbic System

Real Lower Dāntián
(Second Brain)

Figure 5-2. Two Poles
Ellipse Qì Field.

Therefore, the first step of spiritual cultivation is to build up and store abundant Qì at the Real Lower Dāntián through Embryonic Breathing. Then, practice Two Poles Small Circulation to establish a firm foundation for spiritual development.

The next step is that you must develop the feeling of two poles and know how to skillfully manipulate them with your mind. This will help you build a firm foundation of Two Poles Small Circulation. This practice is called Two Poles Synchronization Breathing (兩儀同步息, Liǎngyí Tóngbù Xī). This is a synchronization practice of the two poles, Upper Dāntián (i.e., Limbic System) and Real Lower Dāntián (i.e., Center of Gravity). In this practice, you may use Normal Abdominal Breathing (Zhèng Fùhūxī, 正腹呼吸) or Reverse Abdominal Breathing (Nì Fùhūxī, 逆腹呼吸). Though both techniques serve the same purpose of strengthening the central Qì system, there are still two differences between these two breathing methods.

- The Normal Abdominal Breathing method is more relaxing while Reverse Abdominal Breathing is more tensed and aggressive.
- Normal Abdominal Breathing will enhance the normal up-down circulation of the spinal fluid, while Reverse Abdominal Breathing is more effective in stimulating the pineal and pituitary glands for hormone production.

Two Poles Synchronization Breathing—Foundation

If you practice and use Normal Abdominal Breathing, inhale while moving your abdomen and Huìyīn out. While you are doing so, also use your mind to pull the limbic system and your gut (physical center) downward. When you exhale, simply relax and allow these two poles to return to their original positions (Figure 5-3). This will enhance the up-down movement of your central Qì polarity and improve the circulation of the cerebrospinal fluid. It is a gentle and easy way of conditioning the central Qì line.

If you practice and use Reverse Abdominal Breathing, the up-down motions of your central Qì system will better stimulate the pineal and pituitary glands. Of particular importance is the stimulation of the pituitary gland, which will facilitate hormone production throughout the rest of the body. Remember that hormones are essential to building a stronger foundation for an improved, more robust immune system. In Reverse Abdominal Breathing, when you inhale, you should use your mind to move the limbic system (upper pole) downward while withdrawing your abdomen and lifting the Huìyīn (Figure 5-4). This will actually move your physical center (lower pole) upward. You will feel the distance between these two poles become shorter, and the elliptical Qì field around you should become rounder. When you exhale, gently push your limbic system upward while pushing out your abdomen and Huìyīn.

Two Poles Small Circulation (Liǎngyí Xiǎozhōutiān, 兩儀小周天)

As mentioned earlier, Two Poles Small Circulation is classified as Yīn. Like Conception/Governing Vessels Small Circulation that has a fire path (Huǒlù, 火路) (Yán) and wind path (Fēnglù, 風路) (Yīn) (i.e., reverse Fire Path), there are also two paths for Two Poles Small Circulation, the Yáng longevity path (Yángshòulù, 陽壽路) and Yīn spiritual path (Yīnshénlù, 陰神路).

Before you practice, you should understand one important fact: you need to focus your mind on the central line between the Two Poles connected by the Spinal Cord (i.e., Thrusting Vessel) (Chōngmài, 衝脈). The best result comes from a profound, calm, and focused subconscious mind. Therefore, you should first use Embryonic Breathing to bring your mind to a deep meditative state and gather Qì at the Real Lower Dāntián.

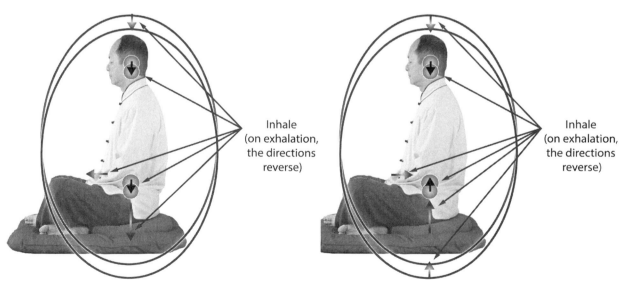

Figure 5-3. Firm the Central Qì Line–Normal Abdominal Breathing (Inhalation Only).

Inhale (on exhalation, the directions reverse)

Figure 5-4. Firm the Central Qì Line–Reverse Abdominal Breathing.

Inhale (on exhalation, the directions reverse)

Yáng Longevity Path (Yángshòulù, 陽壽路)

The purpose of this practice is to learn how to lead the Qì down to the Real Lower Dāntián (i.e., Lower Pole) and then back up to the Upper Dāntián (i.e., Upper Pole) through the Thrusting Vessel (i.e., spinal cord) in coordination with the breathing. In this practice, once you have found and felt the Two Poles, you inhale while leading the Qì down to the Real Lower Dāntián. Since you have an intention to lead the Qì, you should use Reverse Abdominal Breathing (Nì Fùhūxī, 逆腹呼吸). In addition, you should gently hold up your anus (i.e., perineum). Then you exhale and lead the Qì upward to the Upper Dāntián while gently pushing your anus outward (Figure 5-5). *Your inhalation and exhalation should be of equal lengths.*

APPLICATIONS OF THE YÁNG LONGEVITY PATH

A. Qì Sunk to Dāntián (Qì Chén Dāntián, 氣沉丹田)

In this practice, first inhale deeply to lead the Qì down through the Thrusting Vessel to the Real Lower Dāntián and then exhale to allow the Qì back up to the Upper Dāntián by itself naturally. In order to lead more Qì down to the Real Lower Dāntián, you should *inhale longer than you exhale* and gently hold up your anus (Huìyīn, 會陰). When you exhale, just relax the anus and allow some Qì to return to the Upper Dāntián by itself (Figure 5-6). When this happens, the Qì accumulated in the upper body (i.e., above the diaphragm) can be led down to return the Qì to the Real Lower Dāntián. This Grand Circulation practice can be used to lower blood pressure, slow down the heartbeat, and solve the problem of insomnia.

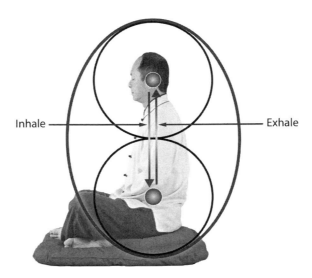

Figure 5-5. Yáng Longevity
Path (Yángshòulù, 陽壽路).

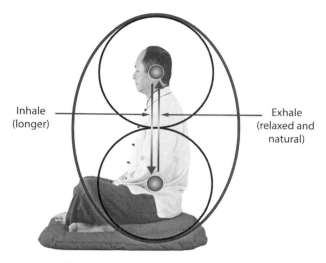

Figure 5-6. Qì Sunken to Dāntián.

Lead Qì to Its Origin (Yǐnqì Guīyuán, 引氣歸原)

This practice allows you to lead Qì down to the Real Lower Dāntián and keep it there for storage. Begin by inhaling deeply and use your mind to lead the Qì down through the Thrusting Vessel to the Real Lower Dāntián while holding your anus (Huìyīn) upward. Next, hold your breath for five seconds and allow the Qì to settle down and then let the air out comfortably, naturally, and smoothly with a relaxed anus (Figure 5-7). This will help you to restore your Qì at the Real Lower Dāntián and conserve it. This practice is commonly used after any type of Qìgōng practice, especially meditation. It can also be used to condition the Real Lower Dāntián for Qì storage.

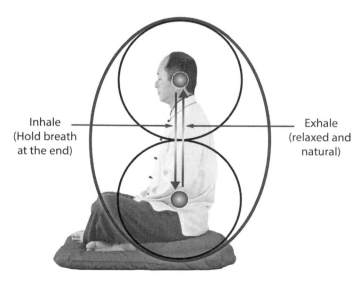

Figure 5-7. Lead Qì to Its Origin.

Yīn Spiritual Path (Yīnshénlù, 陰神路)

The purpose of this practice is to learn how to lead the Qì up and then down the Thrusting Vessel in coordination with your breathing. Find and feel the Two Poles of human polarity, then inhale and lead the Qì upward along the Thrusting Vessel to the Upper Dāntián while gently holding your anus upward. Then exhale and lead the Qì downward to the Real Lower Dāntián while gently pushing your anus outward (Figure 5-8). *Your inhalation and exhalation should be the same length.*

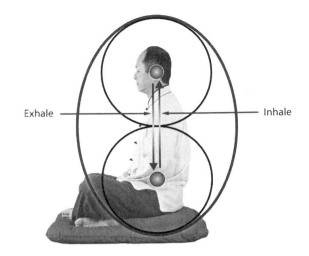

Exhale — Inhale

Figure 5-8. Yīn Spiritual Path.
(Yīnshénlù, 陰神路)

APPLICATIONS OF THE YĪN SPIRITUAL PATH

A. Refining Qì for Sublimation (Liànqì Shénghuá, 煉氣昇華)

In this practice, begin by inhaling deeply and use your mind to lead the Qì upward to the Upper Dāntián following the Thrusting Vessel. When you are doing so, your anus should be gently held upward. Then exhale and allow some Qì to return to the Real Lower Dāntián naturally while gently relaxing your anus (Figure 5-9). In order to lead more Qì up to the upper polarity, you should *inhale longer than you exhale* and gently hold your anus upward. When you are doing so, continue to lead Qì upward to nourish your brain. From this practice, you will be able to lift your spirit to a higher level. Therefore, it can be used for those who have low blood pressure or are mentally depressed.

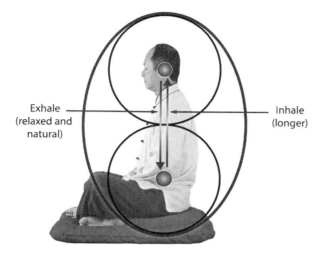

Figure 5-9. Refining Qì for Sublimation.

B. Returning Essence to Nourish the Brain (Huánjīng Bǔnǎo, 還精補腦)

In this practice, begin by inhaling deeply and use your mind to lead the Qì upward to the Upper Dāntián following the Thrusting Vessel. While you are doing so, also gently hold your anus upward. Then hold your breath for five seconds to allow the Qì to reach its maximum. After this, simply relax your anus and let the exhalation happen naturally. This will allow the Qì to be led to and diffused to the brain cells (Figure 5-10). Through this practice, you will be able to activate more brain cells for functioning.

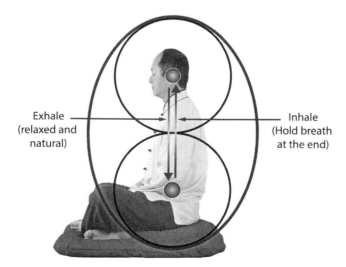

Figure 5-10. Returning Essence to Nourish the Brain.

In monasteries, a technique sometimes used by a few monks and nuns was to hang weights on the testicles (male) or from the vagina (female). It was believed that this would strengthen the upward leading of the Qì by the mind. This technique is called "Diàodāng" (吊襠) and means "hanging groin." However, there were also many practitioners who were able to successfully lead the Qì up with the mind without hanging weight on the groin.

It is not hard to practice Thrusting Vessel Two Poles Small Circulation. However, this practice is of crucial importance since the Central Qì Path is the main Qì path that distributes and dominates the manifestation of Qì in the entire body. When the Qì circulating in this path is smooth and abundant, the Center Nervous System will be strong and function healthily. This is the crucial key to making Muscle/Tendon Changing and Marrow/Brain Washing Qìgōng practices successful.

CHAPTER 6

Marrow/Brain Washing Grand Circulation

6.1 INTRODUCTION (JIÈSHÀO, 介紹)

Spiritual cultivation for Buddhahood or Immortality is probably the highest level of Qìgōng practice one can ever achieve. Chinese Buddhist and Daoist monks practiced it in hope of achieving the final goal of the Unification of the Heaven and Human (Tiān-rén Héyī, 天人合一). If they achieved this final stage, they would be able to acquire the immortality of spiritual eternal life. However, according to existing records, though there were millions of monks who practiced it, the number who had accomplished it were very few.

Though we have felt and experienced the existence of spirit, we still don't have a clear idea of what spirit is. The scientists of our time cannot explain it either. The development of spiritual science is still in its beginning stage. Furthermore, those who had achieved enlightenment and Buddhahood had isolated themselves from the human world to practice and would not write down what they had understood and experienced. All of the available documents passed down to us were written by those who were searching for the final Dào but had not yet acquired it. But these documents are still extremely valuable and can provide us some guidelines to reach the final Dào. As they said, if you wish to get deeper, once you have reopened the Third Eye and reached enlightenment, you would be able to access all the knowledge recorded in the spiritual world that could guide you to the final destination.

I believe and hope that by the end of this century, human science will be able to uncover life's spiritual mysteries and offer answers. If we continue to ignore our spiritual cultivation in this century, human self-destruction will most likely be inevitable.

I will introduce all the available Marrow/Brain Washing Grand Circulation Qìgōng I know. However, please remember that since I am still in the stage of searching for the truth of this spiritual cultivation, you should put a question mark on everything I write in this chapter. My purpose is to offer you inspiration and information for you to ponder and practice. You must keep your mind open and be willing to accept or challenge these concepts. A wise person will borrow knowledge from the past, verify it, experience it, and finally create their own path for the future. This way, you will become a pioneer in this field and be able to offer your experience to following generations.

Before introducing Marrow/Brain Washing Grand Circulation, I would like to review some important points.

1. Both Muscle/Tendon Changing and Marrow/Brain Washing Qìgōng are built upon the same root: Embryonic Breathing (Tāixí, 胎息). This is especially crucial for Marrow/Brain Washing Qìgōng since in that practice, both Embryonic Breathing and Marrow/Brain Washing focus on the same vessel: the Thrusting Vessel (Chōngmài, 衝脈) (i.e., spinal cord).

2. Muscle/Tendon Changing Grand Circulation is considered to be Yáng while Marrow/Brain Washing Grand Circulation is classified as Yīn. This is because Muscle/Tendon Changing trains Qì manifestation in the physical body for health, strength, and longevity while Marrow/Brain Washing focuses on spiritual cultivation.

3. The foundation of Muscle/Tendon Changing Grand Circulation is Conception/Governing Vessel Small Circulation (Rèn/Dūmài Xiǎozhōutiān, 任 / 督脈小周天) while the root of Marrow/Brain Washing Grand Circulation is Two Poles Small Circulation (Liǎngyí Xiǎozhōutiān, 兩儀小周天) or Thrusting Vessel Small Circulation (Chōngmài Xiǎozhōutiān, 衝脈小周天).

4. The reasons that Conception/Governing Vessels Small Circulation was well known while Two Poles Small Circulation was little known were:

   A. Most laymen are concerned about physical health, and longevity while spiritual cultivation was practiced mostly in Buddhist and Daoist monasteries.

   B. Since the fifth century, Muscle/Tendon Changing has been commonly practiced in Chinese martial society for power manifestation and its foundation was Conception/Governing Vessels Small Circulation. The strength of the physical body was the crucial key to executing power effectively and efficiently. It is from martial society that Conception/Governing Vessel Small Circulation was spread to the general public.

   C. The theory of Muscle/Tendon Changing was easier to understand and the practice was relatively simple while the theory of Marrow/Brain Washing was much harder to understand and the practice was difficult.

   D. Marrow/Brain Washing Qìgōng was kept a secret in Buddhist and Daoist monasteries.

E. It is not easy to achieve spiritual enlightenment living in lay society since laymen hide behind masks and it is an untruthful, emotional environment. Those who wished to reopen the Third Eye needed to have a peaceful, calm, and truthful mind so they isolated themselves from lay society by living in monasteries in the mountains.

5. The most common dangers in Internal Elixir Qìgōng (Nèidān Qìgōng, 內丹氣功) practice are the mind and the Qì divergences. When it happens, it is called "walk into the fire and enter to the devil" (Zǒuhuǒ Rùmó, 走火入魔). "Walk into the fire" means the Qì is led into the wrong paths and causes danger or problems, while "enter to the devil" means the mind enters into fantasies. In Two Poles Small Circulation practice, though there is not as much danger in leading the Qì into the wrong path (Zǒuhuǒ, 走火), it happens more often that a practitioner could enter into fantasies (Rùmó, 入魔). One of the hardest challenges of Two Poles Small Circulation practice is achieving a truthful mind. Without a truthful mind, the Third Eye Grand Circulation will not reopen.

6. Suǐ (髓) means "Gǔsuǐ" (骨髓) (i.e., bone marrow) and "Nǎosuǐ" (腦髓) (brain). Spiritual cultivation focuses on the brain instead of the bone marrow.

Brain Washing includes three practices:

A. To cleanse the thoughts generated from the conscious mind and to set ourselves free from emotional bondage.

B. To wash away the evil thoughts in our genetic memory such as conquering, killing, enslaving, raping, and other acts of historical violence. These genetic memories come from repeated instances of past violence and are inherited through our limbic system. These thoughts have hindered our spiritual evolution. To allow our spirit to evolve, we must first cleanse these evil thoughts and promote the good part of our memory such as compassion, love, peace, harmony, righteousness, justice, and fairness.

C. In order to reopen the Third Eye for enlightenment, we must have an abundant quantity of Qì and a high level of ability to focus the mind to lead the Qì to its higher efficient level of manifestation. Only if we have a high level of Qì can we activate more brain cells and increase the brain's capacity to function. The key to increasing the quantity of Qì storage is conditioning the Real Lower Dāntián (Zhēn Xià Dāntián, 真下丹田) (i.e., biobattery) and also knowing how to produce more Qì and to conserve Qì.

7. To achieve the goal of Buddhahood (Chéngfó, 成佛) or Immortality (Chéngxiān, 成仙) after reopening the Third Eye (i.e., enlightenment or the birth of the spiritual baby), you will still need three years of nursing (Sānnián Bǔrǔ, 三年哺乳) Qi, nine years facing the wall (Jiǔnián Miànbì, 九年面壁), and crushing emptiness (Fěnsuì Xūkōng, 粉碎虛空). Crushing Emptiness is the final stage of "unification of human and heaven" (Tiānrén Héyī, 天人合一).

8. Finally, I want to remind you that we are part of nature. Humans used to smoothly exchange Qi with nature. After we learned how to live more comfortably, we gradually isolated ourselves from nature. Thus, we have lost our original capability to smoothly exchange Qì with nature. One of the most powerful Qì resources for us to adopt is natural Qì. If we remember how to communicate with nature, we will have unlimited energy.

Clearly to reach the final goal of spiritual cultivation is a long and difficult path. Though I am able to analyze the theory and have acquired some knowledge from ancient documents, unfortunately, I don't have enough time and the capability to gain enough experience to share the final stages with you. This chapter only offers you some guidelines for you to ponder.

Before we enter the next section, I would like to mention that there are two ways of Marrow Washing. One is from physical training that was commonly practiced in Muscle/Tendon Changing and the other way is by using the mind to lead the Qì though the joints in coordination with the Real Dāntián Breathing (Zhēn Dāntián Xí, 真丹田息)/Cavity Breathing (Xuèwèi Xí, 穴位息). We have already discussed the Marrow Washing practice through Muscle/Tendon Changing. We will discuss the other way in this next section.

Ground Gate and Heaven Gate Breathing Grand Circulation will be discussed in Sections 6.3 and 6.4. Then, the combination practice using both gates will be introduced in Section 6.5. The ultimate goal of reaching Buddhahood or Immortality will be discussed in Section 6.6. Finally, recovery from the meditative state will be briefly summarized in Section 6.7.

6.2 Marrow Washing Grand Circulation (Gǔsuǐ Díxǐ Dàzhōutiān, 骨髓滌洗大周天)

As mentioned earlier, there are two ways to practice Marrow Washing. One is through Muscle/Tendon Changing. (The practice was discussed in Chapter 3.) The other is through Marrow Washing Grand Circulation, which we will discuss in this section.

As explained in Chapter 3, once you have mastered Embryonic Breathing (Tāixí, 胎息) to a profound level, you will be able to apply it to Yáng manifestation practices such as Conception/Governing Vessel Small Circulation (任/督二脈小周天), Girdle Vessel Breathing (Dàimài Xí, 帶脈息), Skin Breathing/Body Breathing (Fūxī/Tǐxī, 膚息/體息), and Turtle Shell Breathing (Guīké Xí, 龜殼息). Naturally, you can also apply it to Yīn practices such as Two Poles Small Circulation (Thrusting Vessel Small Circulation) (Liǎngyí Xiǎozhōutiān/Chōngmài Xiǎozhōutiān, 兩儀小周天/衝脈小周天), Marrow Washing (Gǔsuǐ Xī, 骨髓息), Sexual Qì Exchange (Xìng Shuāngxiū, 性雙修), Heaven Gate Breathing (Tiānmén Xí, 天門息), Ground Gate Breathing (Dìhù Xí, 地戶息), and Third Eye Breathing (Tiānmù Xí, 天目息). In this section, we will introduce Marrow Washing practices.

When you practice Marrow Washing, you must first have reached a profound level of Embryonic Breathing. To begin, inhale deeply while making a light Hēng (哼) sound. When you do this, you should gently hold up your perineum (Huìyīn, 會陰) (anus) and use your mind to lead the Qì from all your joints to the center of your bones such as those of the thighs and pelvis. You also need to use your mind to lead the Qì from all your meridians through the secondary Qì channels (Luò, 絡) to the bone marrow. Once you reach the end of the inhalation, hold your breath for five seconds. After this, simply relax and allow the air to go out *while continuing to gently hold up your perineum (Huìyīn) (anus).* What you are doing is leading the Qì from the skin surface inward to the bone marrow, using the mind to lead the Qì from your joints to the marrow in the center of your bones, and finally allowing the Qì to spread and nourish the marrow (Figure 6-1).

When you practice Bone Marrow Washing, you must remember something very important. Do not practice during autumn and winter. Your need Qì to strengthen your immune system by expanding your Guardian Qì (Wèiqì, 衛氣). If you practice during these two seasons, you may catch a serious cold. The best seasons to practice Marrow Washing are spring and summer.

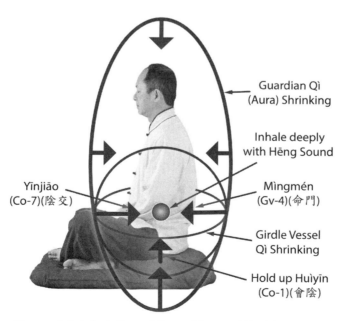

Figure 6-1. Inhalation of Bone Marrow Washing.

6.3 GROUND GATE GRAND CIRCULATION BREATHING (Dìhù Dàzhōutiān Xí, 地戶大周天息)

The Huìyīn (Co-1) (會陰) (perineum) is also called Ground Gate (Dìhù, 地戶) or Sea Bottom (Hǎidǐ, 海底). The Huìyīn has always been considered to be a crucial but tricky gate (Qiàomén, 竅門) in Qìgōng practice because this gate is the junction of four Yīn Vessels: the Conception (Rènmài, 任脈), Thrusting (Chōngmài, 衝脈), Yīn Heel (Yīnqiāomài, 陰蹻脈), and Yīn Linking (Yīnwéimài, 陰維脈) Vessels. This gate is used as a piston or pump of the Qì chamber (i.e., Real Lower Dāntián) and the four Yīn vessels that control Qì storage and manifestation. Therefore, if you know how to use this piston/pump skillfully, naturally, and smoothly, you will be able to govern the Qì in Muscle/Tendon Changing and Marrow/Brain Washing Qìgōng practices efficiently and effectively.

The way of controlling this gate's opening or closing is through control of the anus. When the anus is pushed out the gate is opened and Qì is released. When the anus is held up, the gate is closed and the Qì is retained. The anus and perineum share the same muscles.

Ground Gate Breathing (Huìyīn Breathing Grand Circulation) (Dìhù Xí, Hùyīn Xí Dàzhōutiān, 地戶息（會陰息大周天）)

Ground Gate Breathing (Dìhù Xí, 地戶息) is also called Huìyīn Breathing (Huìyīn Xí, 會陰息). This breathing training has four purposes:

1. **To Condition and Train Muscles Around the Huìyīn and Anus Area.** If you are able to use your mind to control these muscles efficiently, you will be able to govern the in-out flow of Qì smoothly and naturally.

2. **To Train How to Use Your Mind to Lead Qì in and Out Smoothly and Naturally.** The mind is the key to leading Qì. Without a firm mind, in coordination with correct breathing, the Qì will be weak and the leading will be ineffective.

3. **To Learn How to Absorb Earth Qì from the Huìyīn and Lead It Up to Store It in the Real Lower Dāntián.** From this practice, you will be able to draw the Qì from the ground and store it in the Real Lower Dāntián.

4. **For Rooting.** To a Chinese martial artist, this practice is the key training of leading the Qì to the feet for rooting. Once you are able to lead the Qì to your feet, the sensitivity of your feet will be increased, thus establishing firm stability and rooting.

Practice (Solo):

In this practice, you inhale and hold up your anus and lead the Qì from the Huìyīn to the Real Lower Dāntián and when you exhale you push out your anus and lead your Qì out of the Huìyīn. You should use Reverse Abdominal Breathing since you have an intention to lead the Qì. When you inhale, you should feel that the Qì is led up through the center line of your body to the Real Lower Dāntián, and when you exhale, you should feel the Qì is led out from Real Lower Dāntián to the Huìyīn and out (Figure 6-2).

Exchange Qì with the Ground (Dìrén Qìjiāo, 地人氣交)

After you have reached a stage at which you feel comfortable and natural using Huìyīn Breathing, you will extend the Qì downward and outward beyond the Huìyīn like a cone. Practice Huìyīn Breathing first for a few minutes till you feel comfortable, then gradually extend and grow the Qì cone bigger and lower to the ground.

First inhale and lead the Qì to the center of your Real Lower Dāntián and then exhale to lead the Qì to the Huìyīn and beyond (Figure 6-3). Naturally, you should use Reverse Abdominal Breathing since it is more effective in leading the Qì. Remember, when you lead the Qì to the Huìyīn and beyond, you need to gently push out the Huìyīn. The

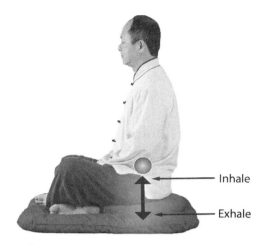

Figure 6-2. Ground Gate Breathing.

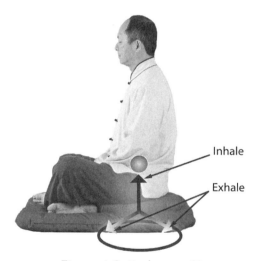

Figure 6-3. Exchange Qì with Ground (Solo).

mind remains the crucial key to a successful practice. After you practice for some time, you will feel the Qì exchange between your Real Lower Dāntián and the ground (i.e., Nature).

You may practice at least fifty times at the beginning. After you practice for a period of time, you will feel the Qì around the entire groin area breathe with you and generate a nice sensational tinkling feeling.

This solo practice can be done while standing, lying down, or sitting.

Practice (Dual):

In this dual practice, you and your partner sit facing the same direction and follow the same steps as in the solo practice. Both hands of the front person should overlap and gently touch their Yīnjiāo (陰交), the cavity that is about one inch under the navel. The Láogōng Cavity (勞宮) at the center of palms should line up. The rear person will place

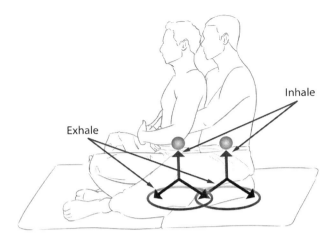

Figure 6-4. Ground Gate Breathing (Dual).

their hands on the top of thefront person's hands with the Láogōng lining up. The important part of this training is to synchronize the breathing smoothly with each other. If it is done correctly, both persons will feel the unification of Qì from both at the groin areas. This dual cultivation can only be practiced in the sitting position (Figure 6-4).

Pick Up Earth Qì (Cǎi Dìqì, 採地氣)

After you are able to exchange Qì with nature through the Huìyīn, you should then learn how to adopt the natural Ground Qì and absorb it into your Real Lower Dāntián (biobattery) for storage or into the Upper Dāntián to nourish your brain.

If you wish to store the Qì at the Real Lower Dāntián, when you inhale, lead the Qì from the ground (i.e., nature) through the Huìyīn to the Real Lower Dāntián. Once the Qì has reached the Real Lower Dāntián, hold your breath for five seconds and then just relax and allow the air out. You should gently lift your Huìyīn (anus) all the time in this practice. This will help you to store the Qì at the Real Lower Dāntián effectively (Figure 6-5). Repeat the practice till you decide to stop.

If you absorb Earth Qì to nourish your brain, you should first inhale and take in Qì from the ground through the Huìyīn and lead it up following the central Qì line (i.e., Thrusting Vessel or spinal cord) to the center of your head (i.e., limbic system). Then, you hold your breath for five to ten seconds, then exhale and just relax and allow the Qì to be absorbed and dissipated into the entire brain for nourishment (Figure 6-6). Naturally, the coordination of your breathing with your mind and Huìyīn remains the crucial key to success.

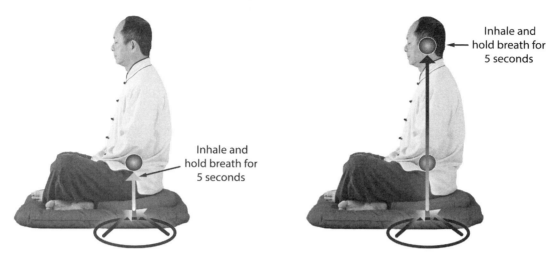

Inhale and
hold breath for
5 seconds

Inhale and
hold breath for
5 seconds

Figure 6-5. Pick Up Earth Qì and Store It at
the Real Lower Dāntián (Inhalation Only).

Figure 6-6. Pick Up Earth Qì to
Nourish the Brain (Inhalation Only).

6.4 HEAVEN GATE GRAND CIRCULATION BREATHING (TIĀNMÉN DÀZHŌUTIĀN XĪ, 天門大周天息)

There are two locations that are considered in Daoist society to be the "Heaven Gate" (Tiānmén, 天門). One is located at the crown (Bǎihuì, Gv-20) (百會) where the spirit enters and exits naturally. When a fetus is formed, the spirit enters the physical body through this gate, and when a person dies, the spirit also exits from this gate and the physical body and spiritual body are separated (Figure 6-7).

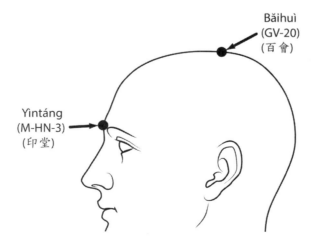

Bǎihuì
(GV-20)
(百會)

Yìntáng
(M-HN-3)
(印堂)

Figure 6-7. Bǎihuì (Gv-20) and
Yìntáng (M-HN-3) (The Third Eye).

The second gate, often called "Heaven Eye" (Tiānyǎn, 天眼) (Tiānmù, 天目), is located at the Third Eye. The Third Eye is also called "Yìntáng" (M-HN-3) (印堂) (Seal Hall) in Chinese medicine and Qìgōng society. Buddhist and Daoist monks believe that those who are able to train themselves to reopen this Third Eye through meditation will reach spiritual enlightenment, the first step toward achieving Buddhahood (Chéngfó, 成佛) or Immortality (Chéngxiān, 成仙). Once they have accomplished this, their spirit will be able to exit and re-enter through this gate while the physical body is still alive. In this section, we will only discuss the Bǎihuì Heaven Gate practice. We will discuss the Third Eye Heaven Gate practice later in this chapter.

This Heaven Gate Breathing (Tiānmén Xí, 天門息) is also called Bǎihuì Breathing (Bǎihuì Xí, 百會息). In Chinese martial society it is also called Fifth Gate Breathing (Dì Wǔxīn Xí, 第五心息). There are a number of purposes for this practice:

1. **To Practice Opening and Closing Heaven Gate.** The Bǎihuì (Gv-20), located on the top of the head, is where the spirit enters and exits naturally. However, we have not been connected to this exchange since our childhood. It is important to recognize and feel this gate again and know how to lead the Qì in and out of this gate. Only then can the spirit enter and exit freely.

2. **To Raise the Spirit of Vitality** (Tíshén, 提神). This practice is called "insubstantial energy leads the Jìng upward" (Xūlǐng Dǐngjìng, 虛領頂勁) in Taijiquan. Jìng (勁) means "to use the mind to lead the Qì for manifestation." When the Qì is led upward, the spirit can be raised, the life force will be strong, and the power can be manifested effectively.

3. **To Exchange Qì with Heaven.** After you know how to lead the Qì in and out through the Bǎihuì, then you learn how to exchange your Qì with nature.

4. **To Absorb Heaven Qì from Nature through the Bǎihuì.** Once you know how to exchange Qì with heaven, next you need to learn how to adopt Heaven Qì (i.e., Natural Qì) and lead it down to your body.

Heaven Gate Breathing (Bǎihuì Breathing Grand Circulation) (Tiānmén Xī, Bǎihuì Xī Dàzhōutiān, 天門息（百會息大周天）)

In this practice, again you should first recognize the body's Two Poles through Embryonic Breathing (Tāixí, 胎息). Once you have felt these two energy centers of the body, pay attention to the upper center (Upper Dāntián) (i.e., limbic system), the spirit residence (Shénshì, 神室). Inhale deeply and lead the Qì from the Bǎihuì to the Upper Dāntián and then exhale to lead the Qì to the Bǎihuì and out (Figure 6-8). You should use Reverse Abdominal Breathing and use your Huìyīn and mind to lead the Qì in and out.

This is the first step of Heaven Gate Breathing Grand Circulation. From this training, you learn how to lead the Qì to and from the Upper Dāntián and Bǎihuì freely and naturally.

Exchange Qì with Heaven (Tiānrén Qìjiāo, 天人氣交)

After you have reached a stage where you feel comfortable and natural with Bǎihuì Breathing, you then extend the Qì upward and outward, like a cone, beyond the Bǎihuì. Practice Bǎihuì Breathing for a few minutes till you feel comfortable, then gradually extend and grow the Qì cone bigger and higher above your head.

First, inhale and lead the Qì from the Bǎihuì while also leading the Qì from the Real Lower Dāntián following the central Qì line upward to the center of your head (Upper Dāntián). Next, exhale and lead the Qì to the Bǎihuì and beyond (Figure 6-9). Again, you should use Reverse Abdominal Breathing and the Huìyīn to lead the Qì. The mind remains the crucial key to a successful practice. After you practice for some time, you will feel the Qì exchange between your Upper Dāntián and Heaven (i.e., nature).

Like Ground Gate Breathing, you may also practice with a partner to enhance the effectiveness of your practice. Since the theory and practice are similar to Ground Gate Breathing, we will not repeat them here.

Pick Up Heaven Qì (Cǎi Tiānqì, 採天氣)

After you are able to exchange your Qì with nature through the Bǎihuì, you should then learn how to adopt the natural Heaven Qì and absorb it into your Real Lower Dāntián (biobattery) for storage or into the Upper Dāntián to nourish your brain.

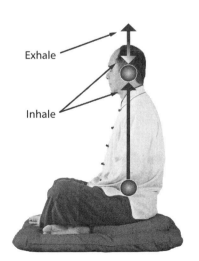

Figure 6-8. Heaven Gate Breathing.

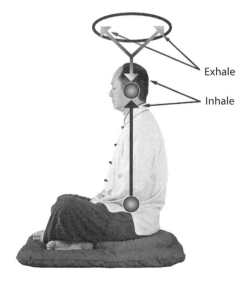

Figure 6-9. Exchange Qì with Heaven.

If you wish to store Qì at the Real Lower Dāntián, when you inhale, lead the Qì from Heaven (i.e., nature) through the Bǎihuì to the Upper Dāntián and follow the Thrusting Vessel (i.e., spinal cord) down to the Real Lower Dāntián. Once the Qì has reached the Real Lower Dāntián, hold your breath for five seconds and then just relax to let the air out by itself and allow the Qì to dissipate into the entire Real Lower Dāntián for storage. *You should gently lift your Huìyīn (anus) all the time in this practice.* This will help you to store the Qì at the Real Lower Dāntián effectively (Figure 6-10). Repeat the practice till you decide to stop.

If you absorb Heaven Qì to nourish your brain, you should then place your mind at the Upper Dāntián. First, inhale and take in all the Qì above your crown and lead it in to the center of your head (i.e., limbic system) while also leading the Qì from the Real Lower Dāntián upward to the same center. Hold your breath for five to ten seconds. Then you exhale, relax, and allow the Qì absorbed and dissipated into the entire brain for nourishment (Figure 6-11). Naturally, the coordination of your breathing with your mind and Huìyīn remains the crucial key to success.

Raise the Spirit (Tíshén, 提神)

In all the above three practices, the breath is gentle, soft, and slender. But in martial arts society, there is another Heaven Gate Breathing practice which is used to raise the Spirit of Vitality (Jīngshén, 精神). From this practice, a person's awareness and alertness can be lifted to a high level. A high level of awareness and alertness is a crucial key for surviving and winning in a battle. As mentioned earlier, this practice is called "insubstantial energy leads the Jìng upward" (Xūlǐng Dǐngjìng, 虛領頂勁).

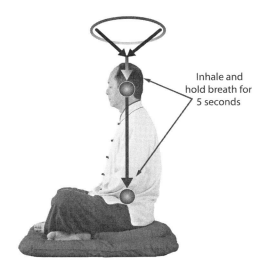

Figure 6-10. Pick Up Heaven Qì and Store It at the Real Lower Dāntián (Inhalation Only).

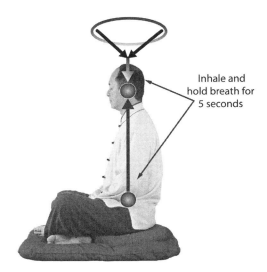

Figure 6-11. Pick Up Heaven Qì to Nourish Upper Dāntián (Inhalation Only).

After you have mastered the four gates breathing (Sìxīn Xí, 四心息) introduced in Section 3.5, you should add the fifth gate and practice Five Gates Breathing (Wǔxīn Xī, 五心息) (Figure 6-12). When the spirit of this gate is lifted, the Qì circulation in the other four gates will be stronger and manifestation will be more effective.

There are two common methods of practice: Scholar Fire (Wénhuǒ, 文火) and Martial Fire (Wǔhuǒ, 武火).

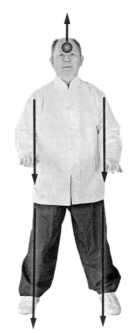

Figure 6-12. Five Gates Breathing (Exhalation Only).

- **Scholar Fire** (Wénhuǒ, 文火): In this practice, the breathing is slow and soft and the mind leading the Qì is firm and strong. When you inhale, lead the Qì to the center of your head, and when you exhale, lead the Qì straight upward as far as possible. It should be as if there is a thread lifting your head to lead your spirit upward. While you are doing so, also lead the Qì to the other four gates: Láogōng (勞宮) in the center of your palms and Yǒngquán (湧泉) at the bottom of your feet. You can practice while sitting or standing. Once you have practiced and reached a high level, add Skin Breathing (or Girdle Vessel Breathing) to expand the Qì sideways. This is a crucial key to balance and maintaining your center. Remember the success of all of these practices depends on your Huìyīn control and the coordination of your breathing and mind.

- **Martial Fire** (Wǔhuǒ, 武火): In combat you want to boost your spirit to a high level in a short time, and this practice helps to cultivate that ability. Inhale and lead the Qì to the center of your head. When you exhale, lead the spirit upward instantly by shouting the "Hā" (哈) sound. Repeat the practice till your body is warm and your spirit is raised to a very high level. The keys to making this happen effectively are to coordinate with the other four gates, Girdle Vessel Breathing, Skin Breathing, the Huìyīn, the mind, and the breathing.

6.5 Heaven/Ground Gates Grand Circulation (Tiānmén/Dìhù Dàzhōutiān, 天門／地戶大周天)

The Upper Dāntián and Real Lower Dāntián are the Two Poles or Qì centers of the body connected by the spinal cord. Since the spinal cord (i.e., Thrusting Vessel) is constructed of highly electric conductive tissue, both poles synchronize with each other simultaneously. If you know how to control the energy between them, you will be able to manipulate the central energy system. This central energy system is very powerful. Once you know how to manage this central energy system, you will be able to significantly regulate your body's energy. In this section, we will introduce a few practices for this purpose. However, before you practice further, you should first practice the Grand Circulations previously introduced until you have reached a stage of "regulating of no regulating" (Diàoér Wúdiào, 調而無調).

Heaven/Ground Gates Two Poles Breathing—Foundation

After you have calmed your mind and stabilized your thoughts, simply inhale deeply, slowly, and slenderly and lead the Qì from Heaven down through your Bǎihuì to your Upper Dāntián (limbic system) while also simultaneously leading the Qì from the ground up through the Huìyīn to the Real Lower Dāntián (physical center). Naturally, you should also gently lift your Huìyīn (i.e., anus or perineum) (i.e., Qì pump) (Figure 6-13).

Next, exhale slowly and slenderly and allow the air out smoothly while using your mind to lead the Qì up to the Heaven and also down to the Earth as far as you can. While you are doing so, also gently push out your perineum (anus). Continue your practice until you decide to stop.

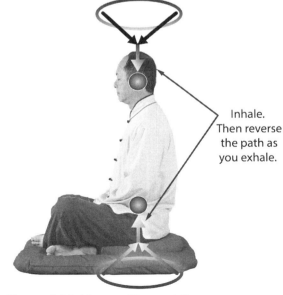

Inhale.
Then reverse the path as you exhale.

Figure 6-13. Heaven/Ground Gates Two Poles Breathing (Inhalation Only).

If you wish to use this practice to adopt the Qì from Heaven to nourish your brain and the Earth to store it at the Real Lower Dāntián, when you reach the end of your inhalation, simply hold your breath for five seconds. However, if you wish to lead out the body's excess Qì and raise your spirit, hold your breath for five seconds when you reach the end of the exhalation.

Heaven/Ground Gates Cleansing Body Breathing—Yáng

Once you synchronized the Heaven and Ground Gates, you can use these Two Poles to cleanse your body, raise your spirit, adopt natural Qì and store it in your Real Lower Dāntián, and also adopt the natural Qì to nourish your brain to a higher energy state. Here we will introduce cleansing body breathing.

First, calm your mind and regulate your breathing to a high harmonious state, then inhale deeply and adopt Heaven Qì in through your Bǎihuì and lead it down to the Real Lower Dāntián. You should also gently lift your Huìyīn (anus) so the Qì can be led effectively. While you are doing so, you may also experience that the Ground Qì has also been absorbed through the Huìyīn. However, you should pay attention to taking in the Heaven Gate Qì and allow the Ground Gate Qì to enter naturally.

Once you have led the Heaven Qì down to the Real Lower Dāntián, exhale and gently push out your Huìyīn (i.e., anus), and lead the Qì out of the Huìyīn and expand it upward around your body (Figure 6-14). You may feel the Qì naturally flow through the two inner leg vessels in each leg and extending farther to the ground. But you should not pay attention to it. When you have led the Qì to chest height, inhale to repeat the same process. Practice till you decide to stop.

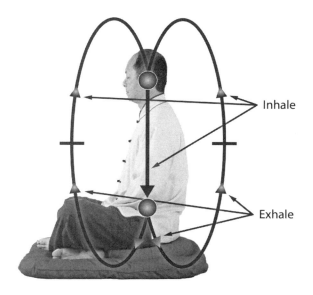

Inhale

Exhale

Figure 6-14. Heaven/Ground Gates
Cleansing Body Breathing–Yáng.

You can practice this Grand Circulation while standing, sitting on a chair or cushion, or even lying down. Since you will intentionally use your mind to lead the Qì down to the Real Lower Dāntián and farther, this practice can be used to lower blood pressure and ease anxiety and insomnia.

Heaven/Ground Gates Raise Up Spirit Breathing—Yīn

In this practice, you reverse the direction in which you lead the Qi along the path and use the Upper Dāntián as the turning point of the breath. This practice will raise your spirit and energize you. It is a crucial practice for proficiency in martial arts. This is because when the spirit is raised, the level of awareness and alertness will be enhanced. Also, when the spirit is raised, the manifestation of power and speed can be more efficient.

After you have regulated your mind and breathing to a calm and focused level, inhale and lead the Qì from the Huìyīn upward following the Thrusting Vessel to the Upper Dāntián. When you do this, you should gently lift your Huìyīn (i.e., anus). Once the Qì has reached the Upper Dāntián, exhale and lead the Qì out through the Bǎihuì and continue to expand it as high and as wide as possible (Figure 6-15). Naturally, when you exhale, you should gently and firmly push out your Huìyīn (i.e., anus).

This practice can raise your spirit and energy and thus it is good for those who have low blood pressure, depression, and fear.

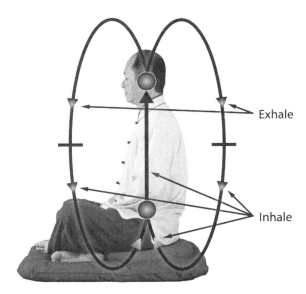

Exhale

Inhale

Figure 6-15. Heaven/Ground Gates
Raise Up Spirit Breathing–Yīn.

Heaven/Ground Gates Storing Qì Breathing—Yáng

In this practice, you want to adopt Heaven and Earth Qì and store it in your Real Lower Dāntián. This practice is a very effective way to store the Qì to an abundant level.

Once you have regulated your mind and breathing to a profound stage, keep your mind in the Real Lower Dāntián (i.e., Embryonic Breathing). Next, inhale deeply, softly, slowly, and slenderly while using your mind to lead the Qì from the Heaven down through the Bǎihuì and then to the Real Lower Dāntián. While you are doing so, also lead the Ground Qì upward through the Huìyīn and then upward to the Real Lower

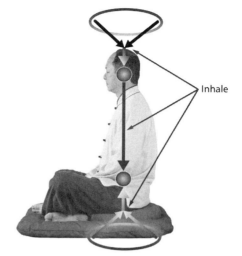

Figure 6-16. Heaven/Ground Gates Storing Qì Breathing–Yáng (Inhalation Only).

Dāntián. Both downward and upward Qì should be gathered at the Real Lower Dāntián and stored there at the same time (Figure 6-16). Next, hold your breath for five seconds and then relax your breathing and allow your respiration to recover automatically.

Heaven/Ground Gates Nourishing Brain Breathing—Yīn

This practice is the opposite of Heaven/Ground Gates Storing Qì Breathing—Yáng. In this practice you lead the Qì from both Heaven and Earth to the Upper Dāntián for

nourishment of the brain. Again you begin by first regulating your mind and breathing to a profound stage and keeping your mind at the Real Lower Dāntián to firm your center. Next you shift your mind to the Upper Dāntián, inhale deeply and lead the Qì from Heaven, through the Bǎihuì, to the center of your head (i.e., limbic system) (Ni Wan Gong, 泥丸宮). At the same time, lead the Qì from the Earth, through the Huìyīn, and then upward through the spinal cord (i.e., Thrusting Vessel) to the center of the head (Figure 6-17). Hold your breath for five seconds. When you are doing so, you should gently lift your Huìyīn (anus) and breath softly slowly and slenderly.

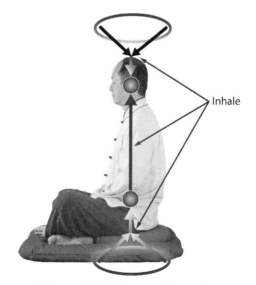

Figure 6-17. Heaven/Ground Gates Nourishing Brain Breathing– Yīn (Inhalation Only).

Next, exhale naturally and allow your respiration to recover. When this happens, the Qì will gently spread and be absorbed by the brain cells. Repeat the same process and continue to gently hold up your Huìyīn.

6.6 Buddhahood Grand Circulation (Spiritual Immortality) (Chéngfó Dàzhōutiān—Chéngxiān, 成佛大周天（成仙）)

The final goal of Buddhist and Daoist spiritual cultivation is called Buddhahood (Chéngfó, 成佛) or Spiritual Immortality (Chéngxiān, 成仙). In Chinese monasteries, monks aim for this final goal of "unification of heaven and human" (Tiānrén Héyī, 天人合一). That means you and the natural spirits are united into one and cannot be separated. Once you have reached this final stage, you will have an eternal spiritual life.

To understand this, you must first understand the concept of two dimensions or spaces that co-exist in this nature, the Yáng World (Yángjiān, 陽間) and Yīn World (Yīnjiān, 陰間). The concept of these two dimensions was the main discussion in *The Book of Changes* (*Yìjīng*, 易經).

According to legend, *The Book of Changes* was first developed by Fú Xī (伏羲) about seven thousand years ago. Later, King Wen of Zhōu (周文王) (1152–1056 BCE) interpreted the writings and compiled the book. According to this work, nature contains two spaces that coexist with each other. Though they are two, actually in function they are one. Later these two spaces were again interpreted in the *Dào Dé Jīng* (道德經) by Lǎozi (around 571—471 BCE) where the Dào (道) is the Yīn space while the Dé (德) is the Yáng space. The Yīn space (i.e., spiritual space) or the Dào is the origin (mother) of everything existing. We still don't understand what the spirit is, though we do have a better understanding of the Yáng space (i.e., material space) or Dé (i.e., the manifestation of the Dào). For physical life forms, the boundary line of these two spaces (or dimensions) is life and death. Many believe, from a scientific standpoint, that the boundary line between these two spaces is gravity (material world) and antigravity (spiritual world or dark energy).

When this concept is applied to humans, the physical life is the Dé that exists in Yáng space while the spiritual life is the Dào that belongs to Yīn space. Physical life is of limited duration and we eventually die. When you are alive, your body contains these two lives, physical life and spiritual life, at the same time. Your mind is between these two spaces and manages your life. The mind is again divided into the conscious mind and subconscious mind. The conscious mind connects to the Yáng world while the subconscious mind connects to the Yīn world (Figure 6-18). The conscious mind thinks and the thoughts are generated from the brain cells while the subconscious mind feels what is generated from the limbic system (i.e., spiritual residence) (Shénshì, 神室) (Figure 6-19). The conscious mind generates ideas that play tricks and are not truthful while the subconscious mind connects to the natural spirit and is more truthful. From the conscious mind, we have generated a matrix or façade of human society and we all live within society wearing masks. In this matrix, we have defined everything and created masks of glory, honor, dignity, money, and power. To maintain this matrix we need to control and dominate our environment, and we have often acted with violence in order to maintain that false control. From the subconscious mind, we connect to the truth and nature.

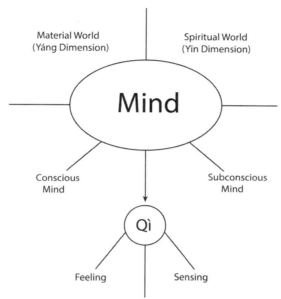

Figure 6-18. Yīn/Yáng Worlds and Mind.

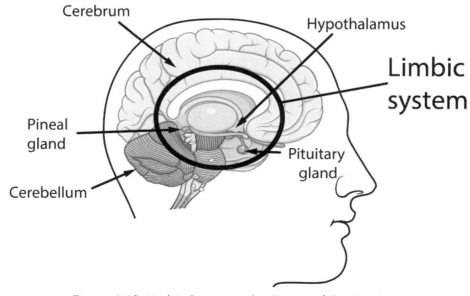

Figure 6-19. Limbic System at the Center of the Head.

In Buddhist and Daoist societies, it is understood that when a person dies, their physical and spiritual bodies will be separated. While the physical body returns to the earth (i.e., dust or dirt), the spirit re-enters the spiritual world (i.e., as a ghost). If the spirit does not find a new residence in nature, the spiritual energy will be slowly dissipated and neutralized into natural spirit. However, if the spirit is able to find a new residence (i.e., through spiritual vibration), a new life will be born. This is the concept of reincarnation. In Chapter 6 of the *Dào Dé Jīng*, it says: "The Valley Spirit (Gǔshén, 谷神) does not die, (then) it is called 'Xuánpìn' (玄牝) (i.e., profound female animal)."[1]

That means the spirit residing in the Spiritual Valley (Shéngǔ, 神谷) (spirit residence) (the space between two lobes of brain) continues to survive even after the physical body is dead, and this spirit can be reborn for another physical life.

In order for our spirit to evolve, it repeatedly returns to a physical life. Through our sensing organs such as the eyes, ears, nose, tongue, and touch, we continue to collect information and learn. Through suffering and joy we continue to experience life. The more we understand life, the more our spirit evolves. However, Buddhist and Daoist monks are searching for the way to spiritual independence so they don't have to return to physical life again. They have experienced the stage where the spirit is able to find the way to absorb the spiritual energy from nature and become independent, and they don't have to re-enter the reincarnation process. They are able to live forever spiritually. This is the stage of Buddhahood, Immortality, or unification of heaven and human.

The first crucial key to a successful practice is knowing how to increase the Qì quantity in the body. The second is knowing how to focus the Qì into a tiny strong beam and emit energy through the Third Eye (i.e., Heaven Eye) (Tiānmù, 天目) to reopen it. Without both quantity and quality of Qì manifestation, the Third Eye (i.e., Heaven Eye) will not open.

From past experience, both Daoists and Buddhists realized that in order to activate more brain cells and improve their function, they would need a lot of Qì. The related scientific explanation is the discovery that we may have developed only a small percentage of the brain's potential function. The scientific understanding is that each brain cell may consume twelve times the amount of oxygen than that of regular cells. To supply the brain this much oxygen, the body has evolved to have four arteries in our neck for blood circulation to the brain. In comparison, a leg, though larger than the brain, has only one major artery. Since the blood cells are carriers of oxygen and Qi, in order to activate more brain cells and increase function, an abundant quantity of Qì supply is needed. The most common way of increasing the quantity of Qì is through abdominal exercises.

However, there is one important question you should ask yourself: how do you expect to charge your biobattery (i.e., Real Lower Dāntián) to a level twelve times higher than normal if you have the same battery as others? Therefore, in addition to building an abundant supply of Qì, you need to condition your biobattery for storage. The method for increasing the storage of Qì in the Real Lower Dāntián is called "Dāntián Zhújī" (丹田築基), which means to build a firm foundation in the Dāntián.

When the quantity of Qì is abundantly stored, it can then be led upward to activate more brain cells (i.e., increase the capacity) and bring the brain to a higher energy level. Through Embryonic Breathing training, you will be able to focus the Qì into a strong beam, like a lens focusing sunbeams, and use that focused Qi to finally reopen the Third Eye. The top brain, the lower brain, and the Girdle Vessel (Dàimài, 帶脈) will thus have become a spiritual cultivation triangle. When the quantity is abundant, the Qì expanding in Girdle Vessel horizontally will be wide and powerful; consequently, the Guardian Qì (Wèiqì, 衛氣) (i.e., aura) will be strong. A strong Guardian Qì is a crucial key to strengthening the immune system. The Qì expansion of the Girdle Vessel provides horizontal foundation and balance. When you are more balanced, the abundant central Qì can be led upward through the spinal cord (i.e., Thrusting Vessel) (Chōngmai, 衝脈) to the brain to raise the spirit. This will offer you the crucial key to reopening the Third Eye (Figure 6-20).

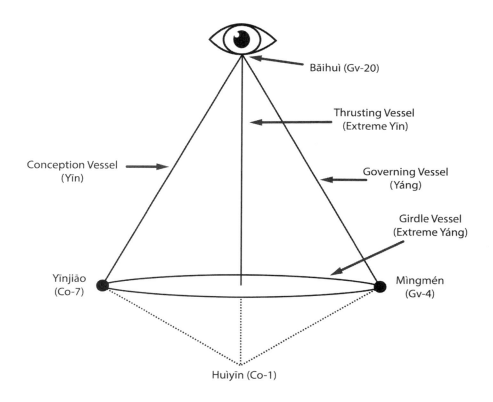

Figure 6-20. Spiritual Triangle.

However, you must also recognize another important and crucial key to reopening the Third Eye, and that is to be truthful. If you continue to be untruthful and wear a mask on your face, then the Third Eye cannot be opened. This is because you will not wish others to know the dark side of you through telepathy. Subconsciously, you will keep it shut. Daoists called themselves "Zhēnrén" (真人) which means "truthful person," since they know this is a crucial key to reaching spiritual immortality.

From past experience, the cultivation of reaching Buddhahood or immorality can be divided into four stages. Here we will explain these four stages of cultivation.

Four Stages/Four Refinements of Cultivation

Many Daoists like to metaphorize the four stages of cultivation as the four phases of a developing baby, from conception to birth. To reopen the Third Eye, you must first have an abundant storage of Qì in your Real Lower Dāntián. This can be done through conditioning your biobattery (i.e., Real Lower Dāntián) to a higher potential of storage of Qì and also from converting original essence (Jīng, 精) into Qì. This stage is called "refine the essence and convert it into Qì" (Liànjīng Huàqì, 練精化氣). It is also called "one hundred days of building the foundation" (Bǎirì Zhújī, 百日築基).

Once you have stored the Qì to an abundant level, then you step into the second stage, "purify Qì and convert it into Shén (i.e., spirit)" (Liànqì Huàshén, 練氣化神). In this stage, you must regulate your thoughts to be truthful and natural till your spirit has returned to the embryonic state. Without this innocent and truthful new spirit, you will not be able to reopen the Third Eye. This refined spirit is called "spiritual embryo" (Shéntāi, 神胎) (Língtāi, 靈胎). This stage is also called "ten months of pregnancy" (Shíyuè Huáitāi, 十月懷胎).

Once the spiritual baby is formed and has matured, then you lead the spirit upward to the Upper Dāntián. Through correct practice with abundant Qì and focus, the spiritual baby will be born. This implies that the Third Eye is reopened. This baby is called "holy spiritual infant" (Shéngyīng, 聖嬰). This is the stage of "refine Shén and return it to nothingness (i.e., naïve and empty of thoughts)" (Liànshén Fǎnxū, 練神返虛). It is also called "three years of nursing" (Sānnián Bǔrǔ, 三年哺乳). In this stage, the new spiritual baby must stay around the mother body for nourishment for at least three years.

The final stage is called "crush the nothingness" (Fěnsuì Xūkōng, 粉碎虛空). That means the spiritual baby must learn how to be independent and survive without the mother body. In this stage, the baby has grown up and knows how to absorb the Qì from the great nature directly so he does not need to re-enter into reincarnation. Naturally, he will not need his physical body anymore. This stage is also called "nine years of facing the wall" (Jiǔnián Miànbì, 九年面壁). It implies you need to face simplicity and nothingness. In this stage, the mental and physical attachments with human affairs will be completely eliminated. It is believed that as long as this spirit still has an attachment to human thoughts, the spirit will reincarnate to the physical world for re-cycling. The final stage of "unification of heaven and human" (Tiānrén Héyī, 天人合一), Buddhahood (Chéngfó, 成佛) or Spiritual Immortality (Chéngxiān, 成仙), is the stage at which you no longer need to reincarnate into the physical world.

You can see that the Dào of reaching enlightenment or becoming a Buddha requires years of training. After the Marrow/Brain Washing (Xǐsuǐjīng, 洗髓經) training secret was revealed to lay society, a new change in training from that of monasteries took place. The final goal of enlightenment or Buddhahood was no longer the main goal of practice for laymen. Also, because the final step of training was hard to understand and to reach, many practitioners who were looking only for longevity considered that there were only the first three steps of training and ignored the final step.

1. Refine the Essence and Convert It into Qì (Liànjīng Huàqì, 練精化氣) One Hundred Days of Building the Foundation (Bǎirì Zhújī, 百日築基)

The first stage of spiritual cultivation is to build up an abundant storage of Qì at the Real Lower Dāntián. The way of reaching this goal is to refine (i.e., to convert) original essence (Jīng, 精) into Qì.

In order to produce energy in your body, you must first have matter or fuel that can be converted into energy. In the past, it was believed that all lives have original essence (Yuánjīng, 元精) that is inherited from the parents. Then, what is the original essence? It was said, "The original essence is stored in the kidneys." To understand this clearly, you must first understand how the Chinese define the kidneys. The kidneys on both sides of your lower back are called internal kidneys (Nèishén, 內腎) while the testicles or ovaries are called external kidneys (Wàishén, 外腎). From modern science we understand that these kidneys are the glands that produce hormones. As is well known, the function of hormones is to regulate the body's metabolism. In other words, hormones can be considered as a catalyst that expedite the body's biochemical reactions. When the hormone level is high, the body's metabolism is high and smooth, so abundant energy is produced. As we age, hormone production declines and the energy produced is lower. Therefore, we can extrapolate that what was called original essence in the past actually meant the hormones in our body. However, we should recognize the fact that the catalyst in a chemical reaction, though it involves and expedites the chemical reaction, does not change its original chemical structure. It is the same in our bodies. Then, what is the essence or fuel that can be converted into Qì?

If we look at the ancient documents again, it is said: "The way of converting the original essence into Qì is through abdominal breathing." Abdominal breathing is also called "back to childhood breathing" (Fǎntóng Hūxī, 返童呼吸). Practically, what it implies is that when you move your abdominal area up and down in coordination with your breathing, you are converting the original essence into Qì. However, if we ponder it carefully, we can see that actually we are converting the fat stored in the abdominal area into Qì. In Chinese Qìgōng, this place is called the Elixir Field (Dāntián, 丹田) or Elixir Furnace

(Dānlú, 丹爐). Elixir means the Qì that is able to extend your life. This place is also called Qì Sea (Qìhǎi, 氣海) (Co-6) in Chinese medicine. Qìgōng society and medical societies both recognize that the Qì can be produced abundantly or unlimitedly in this area.

Then, what is the structure here and how can its fat be converted into Qì? If you were to dissect the abdominal area, you would see that there are six layers of muscle, fat, and fasciae (Figure 6-21). We know muscles are good conductors of electricity while fat and fasciae are poorer conductors. When these different conductive materials are sandwiched together, they take on the structure of a battery. That is why this place is called Dāntián since it can produce and store Qì.

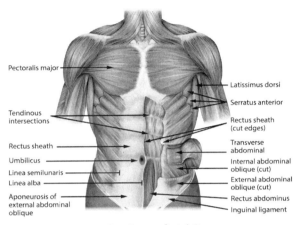

Figure 6-21. Superficial Structure of the Abdominal Area.

Next, why do all animals, including us, have the same structure at the abdominal area? If we trace humans back one million years, we were the same as animals. We hunted and ate whenever food was available. However, it was not often that you received food regularly, especially in wintertime. All animals including humans have evolved a structure that allows them to store extra food as fat in the body. Whenever we lacked food, this fat could be converted into energy to keep us alive. Remember, fat is the extra food essence stored in our body and fat can be converted into energy efficiently and effectively.

Naturally, there are also many other places that can store fat. Unfortunately, most of the Qì converted from non-abdominal fat through exercises will be dissipated outside of the body. Only a small portion of it can be led inward to the body for nourishment. In Qìgōng practice this is called External Elixir (Wàidān, 外丹). However, the situation in the abdominal area is very different. The abdominal area is on the pathway of the Conception Vessel (Rènmài, 任脈) (i.e., Qì Reservoir). Through Small Circulation, the Qì converted in this area can then be distributed into the twelve meridians and reach the entire body. That is why the abdominal area is so important in fat storage.

Practically, through abdominal up-and-down exercises, you can enhance the conversion of fat into Qì. That is why this place is also called "Elixir Furnace" (Dānlú, 丹爐). However, Daoists consider this Dāntián to be a "False Dāntián" (Jiǎ Dāntián, 假丹田). This is because when the Qì produced and stored in this area has reached a certain level, the Qì will be circulated and consumed in the Conception and Governing Vessels. This

False Dāntián serves the purpose of health and longevity. But it will not serve the goal of spiritual enlightenment.

In order to reach enlightenment, you must store the Qì in the Real Lower Dāntián (i.e., guts or second brain), the main biobattery of the body. Only when the Qì stored in the Real Dāntián reaches an extraordinary level can this Qì be led upward to nourish the brain and reopen the Third Eye.

In this stage, you should know how to condition your Real Lower Dāntián so it is capable of storing the Qì to at least twelve times more than normal. Next, you must know how to convert the fat into Qì and store it in the Real Lower Dāntián. If you wish to know more about how to condition your biobattery, please refer to the book, *Qìgōng—Secret of Youth*, by published by YMAA. Remember, you should be very careful. There are some dangerous consequences if you are not cautious and don't know the theory behind the training.

Here, I would like to summarize the known methods for increasing the quantity of Qì.

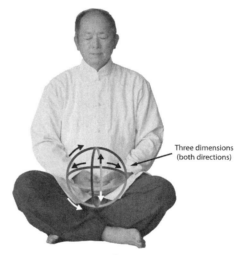

Figure 6-22. Three Directions of Abdominal Exercises.

A. **Convert Fat at the False Lower Dāntián into Qì.** As mentioned, the False Lower Dāntián is called the Elixir Furnace (Dānlú, 丹爐). Through abdominal exercises, you can convert the fat stored there into Qì. There are a few ways to exercise your abdominal area (Figure 6-22).

1. **Forward and Backward Circling.** In this exercise, you circle your abdominal muscles forward twenty times and then backward for another twenty circles.

2. **Sideways Clockwise and Counterclockwise Circling.** Next, circle your abdominal muscles in the second dimension, sideways, clockwise, and counterclockwise. Again, circle in one direction twenty times and then twenty in the other direction.

3. **Horizontal Clockwise and Counterclockwise Circling.** Next, circle your abdominal muscles in the third dimension, horizontally, clockwise, and counterclockwise. Again, circle in one direction twenty times and then in the other direction twenty times. Through these three-dimensional exercises, you will cover most of the muscle exercises around the abdominal area and gradually

convert the fat into Qì. Once you have conditioned your muscles to a certain level, you may then increase the number of repetitions.

   4. **Up-Down Bouncing of Abdominal Muscles.** This is another way of exercising your abdominal muscles so the fat can be converted into Qì. You simply bounce your abdominal muscles up and down fifty times. After you have trained for a period of time and feel comfortable with this exercise, you may increase the number of repetitions.

B.   **Increase Essence (i.e., Hormone) of Testicles and Ovaries.** As we have seen, the quantity of hormones is another crucial key to converting the fat into Qì efficiently (i.e., biochemical reaction). It has been experienced in Chinese monasteries that through massage stimulation of the testicles and ovaries, the hormone production can be increased. This will increase the sexual Qì and store it in the legs' two Yīn Qì vessels, the Yīn Heel and Yīn Linking Vessels (Yīnqìao/Yīnwéi Mai, 陰蹻 / 陰維脈). The Qì stored in these two vessels can then be led up to nourish the brain. If you are interested in stimulating massage techniques (male only), please refer to the book: *Qìgōng—Secret of Youth,* by YMAA.

C. **Deep Abdominal Breathing with Coordination of Perineum.** As explained in Chapter 4, the abdomen and perineum (Huìyīn, 會陰) are the two major pumps of the central Qì system. This central Qì system is constructed by two poles (Upper Dāntián or limbic system, and Real Lower Dāntián or center of gravity)

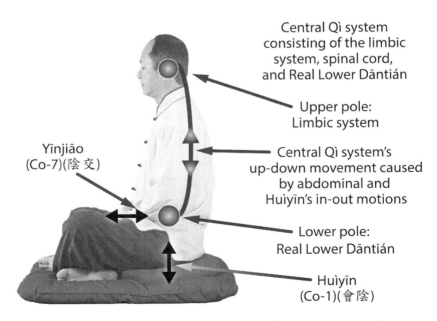

Figure 6-23. Two Important Pumps: Yīnjiāo (Abdomen) and Huìyīn (Perineum).

and connected by the spinal cord (Thrusting Vessel) (Figure 6-23). When these two pumps are manipulated correctly and skillfully, the central Qì system will be strong. In addition, it is understood that through deep abdominal breathing with the coordination of the perineum, the glands such as the pineal, pituitary, adrenal, and testicles (or ovaries) can be stimulated. Thus, the production of hormones can be maintained or enhanced. When hormones are abundant, the Qì production can be increased.

D. Adopt Qì from Nature. It has also been discovered that through correct practices, we are able to adopt Qì from nature, such as the sun, moon, earth, trees, animals, or cosmic Qì falling on us. We have discussed this subject earlier in this chapter so we will not repeat it here.

E. Taking Herbs. Many herbs, such as ginseng (Rénshén, 人参), codonopsis (Dǎng-shén, 黨参), astragali radix (Huángqí, 黃耆), and a few others, are known to nourish the body's Qì. I am not an herbalist and not qualified to discuss this topic. Please refer to Chinese herbal books for more information.

2. Purify Qì and Convert It into Spirit (Liànqì Huàshén, 練氣化神)—Ten Months of Pregnancy (Shíyuè Huáitāi, 十月懷胎)

After a hundred days of the first stage of building the foundation, the Spiritual Embryo will be conceived in the Huángtíng (黃庭) (Yellow Yard, i.e., guts or the second brain). This is the seed from which the spiritual baby grows. Now, in this second stage, you will need ten months of pregnancy (twenty-eight days for each Chinese month). During these ten months you must continue to provide purified Qì for the baby, just as a mother supplies nutrition and oxygen to the embryo. You must also train to convert the semen into Qì more efficiently while the Spiritual Embryo is growing continuously. If the conversion process is insufficient, the embryo will wither and die before its birth or else will be born unhealthy and may not continue to grow well. During this stage, you are growing the embryo into a complete baby that has its own life.

In this period, you must make your mind as truthful and innocent state as a baby's. This will help you trace back to the beginning of life. In order to do so, you need to clean (i.e., wash off) your emotional thoughts in both the conscious and subconscious minds. Conscious thoughts include those emotions and dogmas that we have created in our human matrix society. The subconscious mental content is in the dark side of the genetic memories from human history.

In this stage, through Embryonic Breathing Meditation, you first find, recognize, and feel the Two Poles, the spiritual center and Qì center. Next, you need to regulate your conscious mind and minimize its activities, especially emotional dogmas. This will allow your subconscious mind to merge and see what is hidden in the dark side of your genetic memory. You have to face your dark side and clean your thoughts. In this step, you drop your mask, face yourself, and be truthful. Only then will your spirit return to its infant stage, innocent and naïve. This will help you to increase your feeling and sensing of nature.

In addition, you must also firm and find the way to store abundant Qì at your Real Lower Dāntián (i.e., Qì residence) (Zhēn Xià Dāntián, 真下丹田) (Qìshè, 氣舍). Once you have done this, you will bring the spirit (i.e., son) down to unite with Qì (i.e., mother) and become a singularity. In Qìgōng meditation this is called "unification of mother and son" (Mǔzǐ Xiànghé, 母子相合) and is the final stage of Embryonic Breathing. This is what the *Dàodejing* calls "Embracing Singularity" (Bàoyī, 抱一).

After you have practiced long enough to feel the Qì and the spirit gathered in the Real Lower Dāntián and you have reached a certain level, you may feel like you are pregnant and have a baby developing in your Real Lower Dāntián (i.e., womb). Traditionally, many Daoists believed that in order to have developed a Spiritual Embryo (Shèntāi, 聖胎) you must bring the Fire Qì (Huǒqì, 火氣) stored in the Middle Dāntián down and Water Qì (Shuǐqì, 水氣) from Real Lower Dāntián up to meet each other at the stomach area (Huángtíng, 黃庭) (Yellow Yard). This process is called Kǎn-Lí (坎離) (water-fire). Only through Yīn and Yáng's intercourse can the new Spiritual Embryo be conceived.

However, from my personal belief and understanding based on scientific analysis, as long as you have plenty of Qi stored that unites with the new spirit, the Spiritual Embryo can be conceived. The most difficult part of this training, as mentioned earlier, is conditioning your Real Lower Dāntián (i.e., biobattery) so it has the capability of storing the Qì to at least twelve times more than normal. If this is the case, without conditioning our biobattery, how can we expect to store the Qì to a level twelve times higher? Only when you have a high level of storage can the Spiritual Embryo survive and grow.

While you are carrying the Spiritual Embryo, you must also do one important thing. As the Embryo is growing, the spirit in this embryo is also being formed. Therefore, in this second stage of training, in addition to the Qì nourishment, you also need to lead your spirit to this embryo. It is like a mother whose spirit and concentration must be in the embryo while it is growing in order to obtain a spiritually healthy baby. In this stage, the mother's habits and what she thinks will be passed on to the baby.

This means that in this stage, with the mother's help, the Spiritual Embryo will also grow its own spirit. That is why this stage is called "Purifying the Qì and converting it into Shén" (Liànqì Huàshén, 練氣化神). Remember, only when the embryo has its own Shén (spirit) can it be born as a healthy, whole being. The Daoist Lǐ, Qīng-Ān (李清菴) said: "Shén and Qì combine to originate the super spiritual quality. Xīn (心) and breath are mutually dependent to generate the Holy Embryo."[2] That means that in order to grow a Holy Embryo you must first learn to combine your Shén and Qì in the Huángtíng. Only then will the Holy Embryo have a supernatural, spiritual quality. Xīn is your emotional mind, and breathing is the strategy of the training. Only when you are able to regulate your emotions and coordinate them with your breathing in this Holy Embryo will it be able to grow and mature.

Many Qìgōng practitioners believe that once the embryo is formed, it should be moved upward to the Upper Dāntián to grow. As a matter of fact, it does not matter where your embryo grows. First you must have plenty of Qì, then you must learn how to use this Qì to nourish the embryo, and finally you must help the embryo to build up its own Shén. As long as you are able to store an abundance of Qì to activate and energize your brain cells and raise up your Shén, where the embryo grows is not important. It is said in a Daoist document, *Real Commentaries of the Golden Elixir* (*Jīndān Zhēnzhuán*, 金丹真傳), that "when the elixir is accomplished in ten months, the Holy Embryo is completed. (At this time,) the truthful person will appear."[3] After you have meditated for ten months and the Qì is abundantly stored in the Huángtíng, you then lead the Qì upward to nourish your brain. When this happens, the mask on your face drops off. You will then be facing your true self—the real you in truth. This is the stage of self-recognition.

This step is also called "Returning the Essence to Nourish the Brain" (Huánjīng Bǔnǎo, 還精補腦) or "Refine Qì to Sublimate" (Liànqì Shénghuá, 煉氣昇華). Return means to convert the essence into Qì and use it to activate more brain cells so the Qì-storage capacity of the brain can be increased. This is the step of "Nourishing Shén" (Yǎngshén, 養神).

When more brain cells are activated, the brain's ability to function will also be increased. Current scientific studies acknowledge we only know about 12 percent of how the brain functions. That implies that we still don't know much about what power and capability the brain is able to manifest. It is called "sublimate" (Shénghuá, 昇華) because when you lead your Qì to nourish the brain, it feels like ice sublimating into vapor.

The goal of activating more brain cells and increasing the capacity for Qì storage is to build up a high quantity of Qì. However, when Qì quantity is stored at an abundant level and more brain cells are activated, your thoughts will be in a more chaotic situation. This is because, though you have brought your brain to a higher energized state, you are not able control the elevated power and that causes Qì to manifest into a chaotic situation. Therefore, you also need to know how to control the increased level of Qì and manifest it efficiently.

In addition to opening the Third Eye, you will need to gather the Qì into a tiny beam just like a lens focuses sunbeams. This is the quality of manifestation. In order to reach this goal, you must first learn "Embryonic Breathing Meditation" (Tāixí Jìnguò, 胎息静坐). In this meditation, you learn how to minimize the action of brain cells (i.e., conscious mind) and allow the subconscious mind to be awakened. Naturally, to reach this goal, you must regulate your conscious thoughts and also those evil thoughts merged from the dark side of genetic memory (brain washing). When you do this, the Qì trapped in the brain cells can be led to your limbic system (i.e., center of your head, or Qì cavity) (Qìxuè, 氣穴). This is the step of "Stabilize Spirit" (Dìngshén, 定神).

Once the spirit is stabilized, then you will be able to keep it in its residence (Shénshì, 神室) (i.e., limbic system). This is the step of "Firm or Solidify the Spirit" (Gùshén, 固神). In this stage, you are not just firming your spirit but also nourishing it to a higher energized state.

When your spirit has been raised and the Qì can be focused to a high level (threshold voltage), the step of "Condense Shén" (Níngshén, 凝神), through the Spiritual Valley (Shéngǔ, 神谷) (the gap between two lobes of brain), the Third Eye can be reopened.

Practice:

This is the final stage of practice I can offer. After this stage, I have not had any experience and, furthermore, there are not many available written documents, so I will not be able to offer you any guidelines. However, I know that if you are able to pass this stage and have reopened the Third Eye, you will be enlightened and have the capability of "Spiritual Communication" (Shéntōng, 神通) with nature. That means you will not need any teacher or any document to lead you since you will be able to acquire all knowledge recorded in the Spiritual World.

In this practice, remember that you must first have:

A. High Qì storage capacity of your biobattery or guts (i.e., Second Brain).
B. Produced an abundant level of Qì for storage.
C. A regulated subconscious mind able to focus the Qì stored in the brain into a tiny beam. As mentioned, this can be achieved through Embryonic Breathing Meditation.
D. You must be truthful to yourself and others.

If you have achieved all the above requirements, you can then lead the Qì up to the limbic system (i.e., center of your head) and then forward to the Third Eye. Over time, you will feel the potential difference begin to build up. You will also feel pressure that gets stronger each time. Since bone is a semi-conductor, one day, when the potential difference has reached to the threshold voltage (V_{th}), the bone blocking the Third Eye will suddenly switch from being an insulator to a conductor of energy. Your Third Eye will have reopened and the Holy Spirit (Shéngyīng, 聖嬰) will be born (Figure 6-24).

3. Refine Shén and Return It to Nothingness (Liànshén Fǎnxū, 練神返虛)—Three Years of Nursing (Sānnián Bǔrǔ, 三年哺乳)

This is the stage of reopening your Third Eye. To achieve this training, you must get rid of temptation or emotional attachments to human society. If these attachments are still hanging with you, your spirit will remain in the emotional bondage of human society.

Remember, emotions are the origin of the dark side of your spiritual development. You must train yourself to be compassionate but not emotional. Understand this condition, and your spirit can grow stronger and stronger in a peaceful environment.

According to scientific studies, the electric property of the bone is like a semi-conductor.[4] When the electric potential difference built up between two sides of the bone in the Third Eye is still under threshold voltage, the bone is an insulator. However, once the potential difference has reached to threshold voltage (V_{Th}), it will suddenly change into a conductor. When this happens, the energy in your brain can communicate with the outer world without blockage. The Third Eye is considered as "Xuánguān" (玄關), which means "tricky gate." When the Qì is condensed in this gate to open it up through concentration, the process is called "Kāiqìào" (開竅), or "opening the tricky gate." According to the Chinese Qìgōng society, once this gate has opened, it remains open.

Once the spiritual baby is born, your Third Eye has reopened and you are enlightened. This is called "Spirit Orifice" (Chūqìao, 出竅) in Qìgōng society. That means your spirit and the natural spirit are able to communicate with each other directly without obstacles and you are able to sense the natural Qì and its variations clearly. In addition, you will have resumed the capability of telepathy. This is the stage of "spiritual communication" (Shéntōng, 神通), the first step of "unification of heaven and human" (Tiānrén Héyī, 天人合一).

However, even when the spiritual baby is born and is able to separate from the mother body, he must stay with the mother body for a period of time so he can learn the

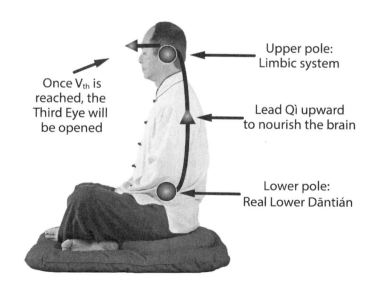

Once V_{th} is reached, the Third Eye will be opened

Upper pole:
Limbic system

Lead Qì upward
to nourish the brain

Lower pole:
Real Lower Dāntián

Figure 6-24. Opening the Third Eye.

environment under mother's protection. This is because the new spirit can be induced onto the wrong path by the natural evil spirits around. Therefore, this is the stage of "Three Years of Nursing" (Sānnián Bǔrǔ, 三年哺乳) or "Refine Spirit to End the Human Temperament" (Liànshén Liǎoxìng, 煉神了性).

Nursing means to watch, to take care of, and to nourish continuously. This process in enlightenment or brain washing Qìgōng practice is called "Yǎngshén" (養神), or "to nurse the Shén." In this stage you are continuously nursing the baby as it grows stronger and stronger. In other words, you are increasing the Qì there so that you can sense nature more easily. When you have reached this stage, since you are training your spirit (Shén, 神) to sense nature, it will gradually become used to staying with the natural energy and it will slowly forget the physical body. Since the natural spirit cannot be seen, it is nothingness. Nothingness also refers to the absence of emotional feelings and desires. This is why this stage of training is called "Refining Shén and Returning It to Nothingness" (Liànshén Fǎnxū, 練神返虛). Since your spiritual body originated from physical and emotional nothingness, in this training, you are returning to nothingness. The Buddhists call this "Sìdà Jiēkōng" (四大皆空) or "Four Large are Empty." This means that the four elements (earth, fire, water, and air) are absent from the mind so that you are completely indifferent to worldly temptations.

4. Crushing the Nothingness (Fěnsuì Xūkōng, 粉碎虛空)—Nine Years of Facing the Wall (Jiǔnián Miànbì, 九年面壁)

This is the final stage of spiritual cultivation in both Buddhist and Daoist societies. It is called "Buddhahood" (Chéngfó, 成佛) or "Immortality" (Chéngxiān, 成仙). To achieve this goal, you need to grow your spirit stronger and stronger and also know how to absorb the Qì from nature so you don't have to rely on your mother body to survive. This is the stage of "Nine Years of Facing the Wall" (Jiǔnián Miànbì, 九年面壁) or "Crushing the Nothingness," and it means destroying the illusion that connects the physical world with the spiritual plane.

After you are able to survive in spiritual form independently without the mother body, then you can discard your physical body (i.e., human form). This is the stage called "Buddhahood of Eternity" (Chéngfó Yǒngshēng, 成佛永生) by Buddhists or "Shelling and Become Immortality" (Tuōké Chéngxiān, 脫殼成仙) by Daoists, the stage of final cultivation of "unification of heaven and human" (Tiānrén Héyī, 天人合一). Once you have reached this stage, you will not have to re-enter the cycle of reincarnation.

To conclude this section, I would like to point out again that this book can only teach you about the first three stages of enlightenment or brain washing Qìgōng training, which can give you a long and healthy life. There are many documents about the first three stages of training, but very little is known about the last stage of attaining Buddhahood or spiritual Immortality. However, I believe that once you have accomplished the first three stages and achieve enlightenment, you will be able to find the path to reach the final stage.

6.7 Recovery from the Meditative State (Jìngzuòhòu Zhī Huīfù, 靜坐後之恢復)

Each time after you finish your meditation you should conduct some recovering exercises. The purposes of these exercises are:

1. **Lead the Qì to Its Origin** (i.e., Real Lower Dāntián) so there is no Qì residue remaining in the wrong path or places that can cause problems. When you finish your meditation and before you resume your normal activities, you must first bring the Qì back to the Real Lower Dāntián. This is to prevent any Qì residue remaining stagnant on the Qì paths and causing problems. For example, if there is some excess Qì still hanging around your head after meditation, it can cause you to get a headache or trigger episodes of high blood pressure. If you lead the Qì back to its origin, you will remove the excess Qì from the head.

2. **Bring the Mind to the Balanced and Awakened State from the Semi-Sleeping State.** When you finish, you should bring your Qì to its origin and you should also bring your mind to an awakened state so your conscious mind is able to take over smoothly.

3. **Recover Blood and Qì Circulation from Sitting in the Same Posture Too Long.** After you have been seated for a period of time, the blood and Qì circulation on your legs will be stagnant and may trigger a numb feeling. In addition, your torso will also be tensed, especially your lower back. Through stretching, you can loosen the tightened muscles and resume the normal circulation of your blood and Qì.

4. **Vibrate the Central Qì Line.** The last step of the recovering exercises is to bring your Qì to the central line and then downward to the Real Lower Dāntián.

The methods of recovering from meditation are both mental and physical. The trick is to reverse the normal regulating process of meditation. First regulate your mind, then your breathing, and finally your body. Here I introduce the general methods of recovery that have been passed down traditionally or gained through my personal experience. Naturally, after you practice for a while, you may also create and recompile the recovery routines that suit you the best.

Regulate the Mind, Qì, and Breathing

The first step in recovery from meditation is keeping your mind calm and slowly awakening from your semi-hypnotic state. You may feel as if you have just awoken from a deep sleep. Gradually allow your conscious mind to take control again.

Bring your mind to the Real Lower Dāntián. This is very important. The Real Lower Dāntián is the residence of the Qì, so the first step is to return it there to prevent disturbance. If you are suddenly awakened from deep meditation, the treatment is the same as in cases of shock.

Keep your mind in the Real Dāntián and resume Embryonic Breathing for a couple minutes until you feel that Qì has returned. After Embryonic Breathing, you may practice a few minutes of Skin Breathing if you know it well. Try to exhale longer than you inhale. This leads the Qì to the skin surface and rouses the body from the sleeping state.

Then move your mind to the Upper Dāntián and relocate your spiritual center. Sit there for a couple of minutes. When you do this mentally, you wake yourself up completely and comfortably.

Remember, when you recover mentally from your meditative state, you should not resist or speed up the process. You should take your time and be natural and comfortable. This way you maintain the satisfaction, peace, and harmony.

Regulate the Body

After bringing your mind back to the concrete world, you should then regulate your body and arouse it from sleep. Effective movements and stretches are recommended. Through correct movement, you disperse any stagnant Qì that may be caused by a long period of sitting or improper posture.

1. STRETCH AND LOOSEN UP YOUR LEGS

First, extend your legs forward and sway them from side to side. Next, bend your upper body forward at the hip joint to stretch your lower back and legs (Figure 6-25). You may repeat this a few times till you feel comfortable.

2. UPWARD TORSO STRETCHING

Next, stretch your torso. Interlock your hands and push the palms upward (Figure 6-26). This stretch loosens any tightness in the torso or spine caused by sitting for a long time. After your hands have reached their highest position, stay there, inhale deeply, and then exhale. Inhale again and lower your arms. Repeat twice.

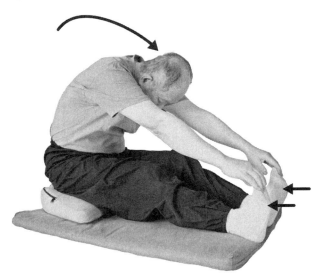

Figure 6-25. Stretch and Loosen Up Legs.

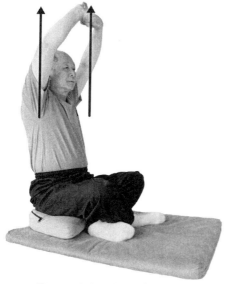

Figure 6-26. Stretch Torso.

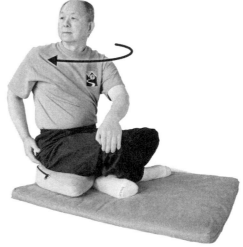

Figure 6-27. Twist Torso.

3. SIDEWAYS TORSO TWIST

After the upward stretch, twist your torso sideways. First, turn your body to the left and use your right hand to pull your left knee while pushing your left shoulder backward (Figure 6-27). Stay in this position, inhale, and then exhale. Next, repeat on the other side. Repeat two more times on each side.

4. SPINE WAVING

Next, loosen your vertebrae with a spine waving motion. Move section by section from the sacrum up to the neck. Place your hands on your knees and pull them as you generate a waving spine motion (Figure 6-28). When you begin to pull, the lower torso is

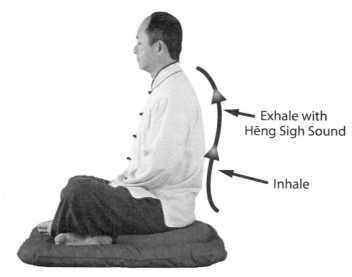

Exhale with
Hēng Sigh Sound

Inhale

Figure 6-28. Spine Waving.

thrust forward and you inhale deeply. When the waving motion reaches the upper spine, you exhale. Move comfortably and naturally, with the spine movement of a sigh. When you are depressed or feel a strong emotion stuck in your body, you innately inhale deeply with the "Hēng" (哼) sound and generate a waving motion from the lower back. When the motion reaches the upper torso, you exhale with a sigh. This is a natural torso movement that allows you to relax the torso and release any trapped emotional energy.

5. Loosening the Shoulders

Next, loosen the upper spine and shoulders, and remove any stagnant Qì there. Slowly move your shoulders clockwise in a big circle at least six times (Figure 6-29). When they circle forward, inhale deeply, and when they circle backward, exhale deeply. After you complete the clockwise circling, reverse direction and repeat for the same number of times. However, this time you should inhale deeply when you circle backward and exhale when you circle forward. To lead stagnant Qì down and loosen up the torso, you may alternately circle one shoulder forward and the other one backward (Figure 6-30). Repeat six times, then reverse direction. You may coordinate your breathing any way you choose.

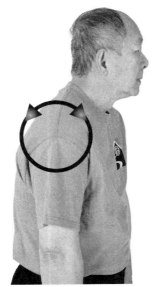

Figure 6-29. Circle Shoulders.

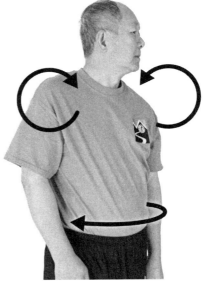

Figure 6-30. Circle Shoulders with Torso Twisting.

6. TURNING THE HEAD

To loosen the neck, gently push your head downward and backward ten times (Figure 6-31). Next, tilt your head from side to side ten times (Figure 6-32). Finally, twist your neck by turning your head from side to side ten times (Figure 6-33). You may coordinate with deep breathing to provide a relaxed condition for stretching.

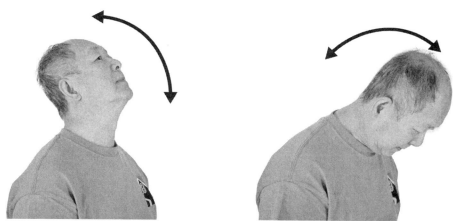

Figure 6-31. Head Downward and Backward.

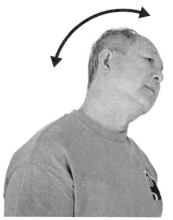

Figure 6-32. Tilt Head Sideways.

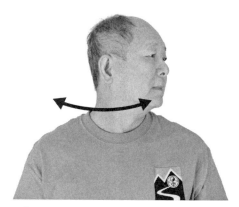

Figure 6-33. Turn Head Sideways.

7. MASSAGING THE HEAD

After loosening the neck, circle your tongue in the mouth to generate saliva and rub your palms together until they are warm (Figure 6-34). Next, inhale and hold your breath to keep the Qì trapped in your palms. Then touch both palms to your face and exhale to allow the release of the Qì from the palms. Finally, inhale deeply to absorb the Qì released from your palms into the face and then exhale and brush both palms down to the abdominal area while swallowing your saliva (Figure 6-35). You may repeat as many times as you wish. This exercise is called Washing the Face (Xǐliǎn, 洗臉). It rejuvenates the skin with enhanced Qì and improves the blood circulation on your face.

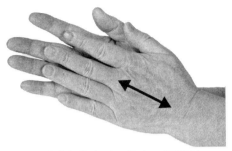

Figure 6-34. Rub the Palms Till Warm.

Immediately after Washing the Face, use the palms to brush the hair from the forehead backward to the neck twenty-four times (Figure 6-36). This is called Combing the Hair (Shūtóu, 梳頭). It keeps your hair healthy and looking young.

Next, rub your hands until they are warm. Hold your breath and cover your eyes with the palms (Figure 6-37). Exhale to allow the release of the Qì trapped in your palms. Inhale deeply to absorb the Qì into your

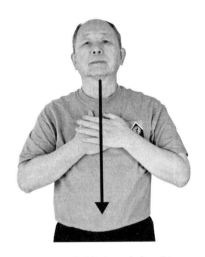

Figure 6-35. Lead the Qì Down to the Abdomen.

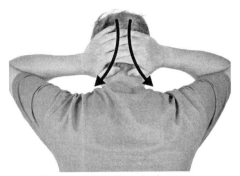

Figure 6-36. Comb the Hair.

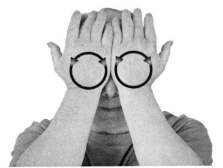

Figure 6-37. Iron the Eyes.

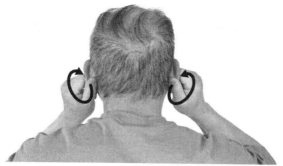

Figure 6-38. Massage the Ears.

eyes. Hold the breath for five seconds and then exhale to allow distribution of the Qì to the entire eye area. This is called Ironing the Eyes (Tàngyăn, 3), which nourishes degenerating eyes. After that, you may massage your eyes gently with a circular motion to improve the Qì circulation.

Next, use your thumb and index fingers to massage your ears for a few minutes (Figure 6-38). Different parts of the ears are related to different organs (Figure 6-39). Massaging them keeps the internal organs healthy. Then cover your ears with your palms and circle forward ten times and backward ten times (Figure 6-40). This improves the circulation of Qì and blood in the deeper parts of the ears. Finally, press the ears and pop them several times (Figure 6-41). This

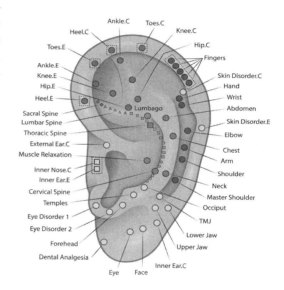

Figure 6-39. Ear Connecting to Body Parts.
(Illustration by Shutterstock)

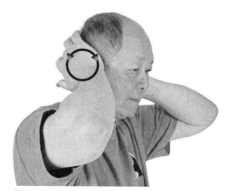

Figure 6-40. Circle Ears with Palms.

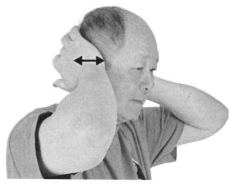

Figure 6-41. Pop Ears.

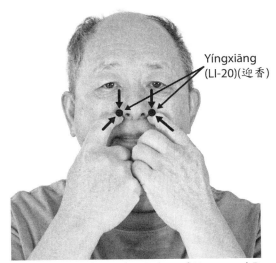

Figure 6-42. Pressing Down Along the Sides of Nose and Pressing Yíngxiāng.

stimulates the eardrums and improves the circulation in them. All these are simple ways of maintaining the ears in a healthy condition.

Next, use your index finger or thumb to rub and press down along the sides of your nose and then use your middle finger to press the Yíngxiāng Cavity (LI-20) (迎香) (Figure 6-42). This releases pressure built up in the frontal sinus.

Finally, use the fingertips to tap your head from front to back and from the center to the sides for a few minutes (Figure 6-43) This tapping action leads the Qi accumulated inside the head to the skin surface. After tapping, use both hands to brush your head lightly from the front backward (Figure 6-44).

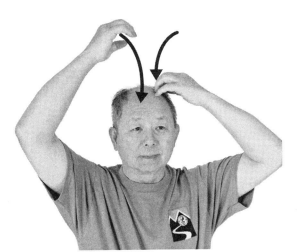

Figure 6-43. Tap Head
with Finger Tips.

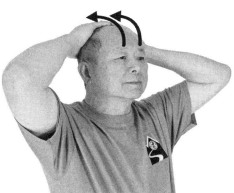

Figure 6-44. Brush Qì to Rear Head.

8. Massaging the Three Yīn Channels on the Legs—Spleen, Liver, and Kidneys

Massage your legs from the thighs to the bottom of the feet, especially the insides of the legs where the three Yīn channels are located. After massaging for a couple of minutes, use your thumb to press the Sānyīnjiāo (Sp-6) (三陰交) cavity (Figure 6-45). Sānyīnjiāo means Three Yīn Junctions and is the junction of the three Yīn channels: spleen, liver, and kidneys. Press for five seconds and then release. Repeat three times. This leads Qi down from the hips.

Next, massage the inside of your feet where the two Yīn vessels (Yīn Heel and Yīn Linking Vessels, 陰蹻脈・陰維脈) end. Finally, massage the Yǒngquán (K-1) (湧泉) cavity for a few minutes (Figure 6-46).

9. Chanting

Right after meditation, a meditator often makes specific chanting sounds. This leads the Qi down to the Lower Dāntián. These chanting sounds are commonly used for healing purposes as well. Three of the most common ones used are Ǎn (唵), Ā (阿), and Hōng (吽). The use of these three sounds has been recorded in a Buddhist classic, which I would like to translate for your reference.

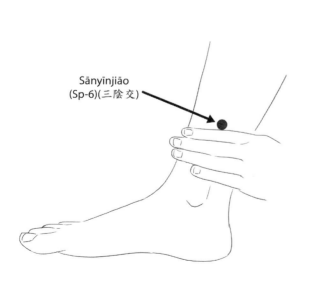

Figure 6-45. Sānyīnjiāo (Sp-6) (三陰交).

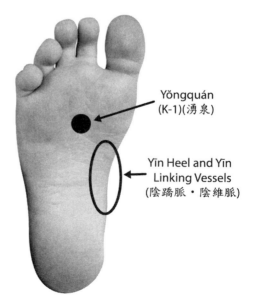

Figure 6-46. The End of Yīn Heel and Linking Vessel Plus Yǒngquán (K-1) (湧泉).

Classic of Positioning the Image into the Extreme Calmness
《安象三昧儀經》

After chanting these real words (Buddhist classic), imagine the perfection of the Buddha's image. Then use Ǎn, Ā, and Hōng, three words, and place them on the image. Place the word Ǎn on the crown, place the word Ā on the mouth, and place the word Hōng in the heart.

誦此真言已，復想如來如真實身諸相圓滿，然以唵阿吽三字，安在像身三處，用唵字安頂上，用阿字安口上，用吽字安心上。

It is common for a Buddhist to imagine a likeness of Buddha in his mind and then chant or meditate. This brings him to a profound level of peace and calmness. The three words Ǎn, Ā, and Hōng are also commonly used right after chanting of the Buddhist scriptures or deep meditation.

Many meditators use the fourth word to lead Qi down to the Lower Dāntián. The fourth word does not have sound and the word itself does not exist. It only exists in the mind right after chanting the third word, as you lead the Qi downward to return to its residence at the Lower Dāntián. That means returning your being to the Wuji state.

First, inhale deeply while raising your arms from the sides of your body with the palms facing upward. When both hands reach their highest point, start to exhale, lowering the hands with your palms facing downward while making the sound of Ǎn (唵) (Figure 6-47). You will feel a strong vibration at the back of your brain when the sound of Ǎn is made. Continue to exhale, lowering your hands until they reach the level of the mouth, then change the sound into Ā (阿) and continue to lower them. When the Ā sound is made, the throat vibrates strongly. Continue exhaling as you lower your hands until they reach the sternum, then change the sound to Hōng (吽). When this happens, you will feel a strong vibration in your upper chest. Finally, keep quiet while still exhaling and use the mind to lead the Qi down to the Lower Dāntián to complete the chanting process. You may repeat the whole process three times.

The positions where you change the words of your chanting are at the Yīntáng (M-HN-3) (印堂) (Upper Dāntián), Tiāntū (Co-22) (天突), Jiūwěi (Co-15) (鳩尾), and Qìhǎi (Co-6) (氣海). These four cavities are four of the seven major corresponding gates of the body.

10. If Necessary, Walk for a Few Minutes

If you wish, after you have finished the recovery massage and exercises, you may walk or simply lie down to rest for a few minutes.

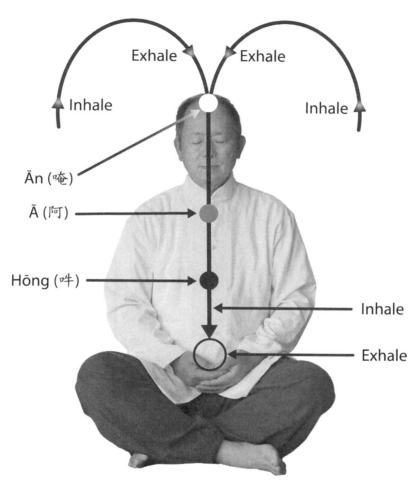

Figure 6-47. Chanting Sounds.

References

1. "谷神不死，是謂玄牝。"
2. 李清菴詩云：〝神氣和合生靈質，心息相依結聖胎。〞
3. 《金丹真傳・溫養》：〝丹成十月聖胎完，自有真人出現。〞
4. Robert O. Becker, MD, and Gary Selden, *The Body Electric* (New York: Quill, 1985).

PART IV

Combination of Muscle/ Tendon Changing and Marrow/Brain Washing Grand Circulations

Combined Practice of Muscle/Tendon Changing and Marrow/Brain Washing Grand Circulations

7.1 INTRODUCTION (JIÈSHÀO, 介紹)

Once you comprehend the theory and have practiced both Muscle/Tendon Changing and Marrow/Brain Washing Grand Circulations for a period of time, you may find various possible Grand Circulations that combine both and serve your purposes.

In this chapter, we will offer you three different examples for your reference. From these examples, you will be able to grasp the concepts and the significant benefits. In the next section, we will introduce how to combine these two Grand Circulations to solve the problems of high blood pressure and insomnia. Then, in Section 7.3, we will discuss how Taijiquan practitioners can use both Grand Circulations for rooting (Zhāgēn, 紮根) and Five Gates Breathing (Wǔxīn Xí, 五心息) training. Finally, we will introduce in Section 7.4 some combined Grand Circulation practices for self-sexual energy cultivation (Dānxiū, 單修) and dual sexual energy exchange (Shuāngxiū, 雙修).

7.2 LEADING QÌ DOWNWARD—PREVENT HIGH BLOOD PRESSURE, HEADACHE, AND INSOMNIA (YǏNQÌ XIÀXÍNG—FÁNGZHÌ GĀOXUĔYĀ, TÓUTÒNG, SHĪMIÁN, 引氣下行 – 防治高血壓、頭痛、失眠)

Leading Qì Downward—Prevent High Blood Pressure, Headache, and Insomnia

This is an example of a typical combination of Marrow/Brain Washing Small Circulation and Muscle/Tendon Changing Grand Circulation. This Qìgōng Grand Circulation will help you lower high blood pressure, ease headaches, and solve the problem of insomnia.

As we explained in Chapter 1, from the Chinese medical and Qìgōng point of view, the diaphragm is considered the dividing area between the upper and lower parts of the body. This is because the Qì circulation of the three Yīn organs, lungs, heart, and pericardium (above diaphragm) are connected to the arms and reach to the fingers while the Qì circulation of other three Yīn organs, liver, kidneys, and spleen reach down to the bottom of the feet.

You should also recognize that the biobattery (guts) is located under the diaphragm. Whenever the Qì is led down to the battery, the body will remain calm and cool since there is no Qì (energy) being led outward for manifestation. However, if there is extra Qì led upward and above the diaphragm, the heartbeat will be faster and the breathing will be heavier. This will trigger high blood pressure and cause insomnia. When the Qì is led down to the biobattery (i.e., Real Lower Dāntián, or second brain or guts), the body will be calm and cool. Consequently, you will be able to lower your blood pressure and sleep more deeply.

Often, in order to lead the Qì down further so the upper body can be cooled down more effectively, the Qì is led all the way down to the bottom of the feet. When you are doing so, you are mixing the Marrow/Brain Washing Small Circulation and Muscle/Tendon Changing Grand Circulation.

If you practice this Qìgōng for headaches and high blood pressure, you may stand, sit, or lie down. However, if you practice for insomnia, you should be lying down in a relaxed and comfortable position.

First, inhale deeply and lead the Qì down from the head to the Real Lower Dāntián, then exhale gradually and slowly to lead the Qì downward to the bottom of the foot and toes (Figure 7-1). Repeat the same process till the headache is gone and the heartbeat returns to normal. To use this for insomnia, simply repeat this practice while lying on a bed and pay attention to the breathing and leading Qi. In no time you will feel relaxed and fall asleep without even noticing it.

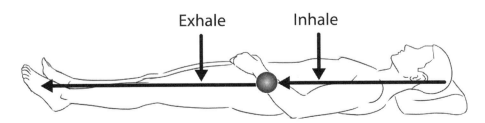

Figure 7-1. Lead the Qì Down from the Head.

However, if you have a low blood pressure, you simply reverse the path and the way of breathing. When you inhale, lead the Qì upward from your feet to the Real Lower Dāntián and when you exhale, lead it up to your head.

Three Power Qì Exchange (Sānchái Qìjiao, 三才氣交)

Once you have mastered the skill of rooting practice in Muscle/Tendon Changing Grand Circulation by leading the Qi from the Huìyīn (anus) to the bottom of the feet through the Yīn Heel Vessel ((Yīnqìaomài, 陰蹻脈) and Yin Linking Vessel (Yīnwéimài, 陰維脈), then you may want to combine this rooting training with Sky Gate Breathing of Brain/Marrow Washing Grand Circulation. You may call it the Three Power Qì Exchange. Three Power (Sānchái, 三才) means the power of the heaven (Tiān, 天), the earth (Dì, 地), and the human (Rén, 人) (Figure 7-2). This practice has commonly been used in Tàijíquán (太極拳) practice for center, balance, and rooting training. This exercise can also be used to lead the Qì down from the head to the ground for easing headaches, lowering high blood pressure, or dealing with insomnia.

The best way to practice is standing since when you stand upright, you have a better feeling of being centered, balanced, and rooted. When you practice, first inhale and use your mind to lead the heaven Qí in through your Bǎihuì (Gv-20) (百會) and down to the Real Lower Dāntián, then exhale to lead the Qì to the Huìyīn, following the Yīn Heel Vessel and Yin Linking Vessel down to the bottom of the feet and into the ground.

Three Power to Cleanse the Body (Sānchái Jìngshēn, 三才淨身)

If you wish to use the above technique to remove unhealthy Qì (Evil Qì) (Xiéqì, 邪氣) or stagnant Qì, all you need to do is focus on your exhalation and make it longer than your inhalation. Once you have reached to the end of an exhalation, hold your breath for five seconds to allow the releasing of the Qì to reach its maximum and go farther into the ground. When you inhale, just relax and

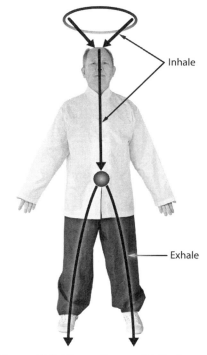

Inhale

Exhale

Figure 7-2. Three Power Qi Exchange.

allow it to happen naturally. Remember to gently push out your Huìyīn (會陰) (anus) during the whole exercise (Figure 7-3).

This practice has also commonly been used for rooting training in Chinese martial arts society. A practitioner usually practices on bricks to increase the difficulty of Qì exchange with the ground.

Pick Up Earth Qì (Cǎi Dìqì, 採地氣)

If you wish to adopt Earth Qì to increase your Qì storage in the Real Lower Dāntián, first inhale and absorb the Earth Qì through the Yǒngquán (K-1) (湧泉) cavities on the soles of your feet and then lead it upward to the Real Lower Dāntián. Once the Qì is led to the Real Lower Dāntián, hold your breath for five seconds. When you exhale, simply relax and allow the absorbed Qì to

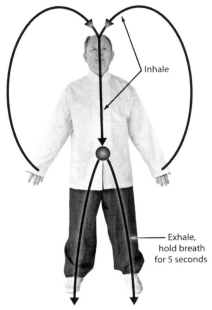

Figure 7-3. Three Power to Cleanse the Body.

be naturally dissipated to the guts. *Remember to keep your Huìyīn (會陰) (anus) gently held upward throughout this practice.* In order to stabilize the Qì storage, your mind should be at the center of your Real Dāntián (Figure 7-4).

7.3 ROOTING TRAINING/FIVE GATES BREATHING (ZHĀGĒN/WǓXĪN XĪ, 紮根/五心息)

Rooting training and Five Gates Breathing are very important in all Chinese martial arts. Rooting practice is used to build up a firm root. With a firm root, the power emitted can be strong. This training is also important for seniors to improve the sensitivity of the feet in relationship to the ground. When the sensitivity of the feet is increased, the firm rooting feeling can prevent seniors from falling.

Five Gates Breathing is used to train the raising of the Spirit of Vitality (Jīngshén, 精神). When the spirit is raised, the fighting spirit and morale will be high. With the

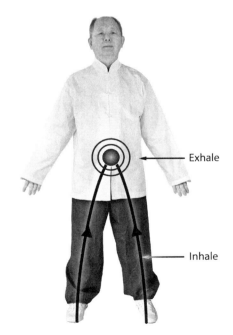

Figure 7-4. Pick Up Earth Qì.

balance of the other four gates, two Láogōng (P-8) (勞宮) cavities at the center of palms, and two Yǒngquán (K-1) (湧泉) cavities at the bottom of the feet, the power emitted will be balanced, strong, and rooted. This training can also be used for improving health, especially depression, low energy, and lack of motivation.

ROOTING (ZHĀGĒN, 紮根)

In this practice, first stand on the ground with your legs about shoulder width apart. Practice your Reverse Abdominal Breathing until the breath is regulated and comfortable. Next, inhale deeply and use your mind to lead the Qì upward following the spinal cord (i.e., Thrusting Vessel) to the Limbic System at the center of your head. Next, exhale and lead the Qì upward through the Bǎihuì (Gv-20) (百會) cavity and up. While you are doing so, also lead the Qì from the Real Lower Dāntián downward through the legs and down to the ground (Figure 7-5). From this training, you are creating a Qì balance from the two poles, upward and downward. To enhance the leading of Qì, you may squat down slightly while you are exhaling. You should lead the Qì from the head from as high as you can reach, and from your feet from as low as possible. The root can thereby grow deeper and the spirit can be raised higher. Often, to enhance the Qì manifestation, once you reach the end of the exhalation, simply hold your breath for five seconds. After that, inhale deeply and bring your Qì to the two poles again. In order to lead the Qì further, it is also common for a practitioner to stand on bricks and practice. This is because once you are standing on bricks, to keep from falling your mind must be on the bottom of the bricks and feel beneath the brick. After you have mastered standing on one brick under each foot, increase to two, three, and so on. The more bricks, the more profound your mind and feeling must be. Once you remove the bricks and stand on the ground again, you will be able to use your mind to lead the Qì and feel deeply under the ground.

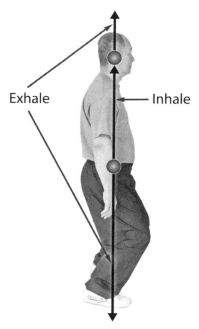

Exhale — Inhale

FIVE GATES BREATHING (WǓXĪN XĪ, 五心息)

This practice is very similar to rooting training. However, there are important additions to the rooting training. First, you add two more gates to the breathing: the gates in the center of your palms. Since you are leading the Qì to your palms, you should use martial Grand Circulation (Section 3.6). Therefore, when you inhale, you are leading the Qì upward, following the spinal cord to the upper pole, and you are also opening

Figure 7-5. Rooting Practice.

the Mìngmén (Gv-4) (命門) cavity and leading the Qì up your back outside of the spine, following the Governing Vessel (Dūmài, 督脈) to the Dàzhuī (Gv-14) (大椎) cavity. Anatomically, the Dàzhuī is located on the body's posterior in the depression below the spinous process of the seventh cervical vertebrae, approximately at the level of the shoulder.

When you exhale, squat down and lead the Qì from the Real Lower Dāntián downward to the feet and beyond while also leading the Qì from Dàzhuī to the center of the arms and further. You should also lead the Qì up from the Upper Dāntián (Limbic System), through the Bǎihuì (Gv-20) (百會) and upward (Figure 7-6). Your palms should face downward to balance the upward spiritual gate.

Again, you may practice on bricks to enhance your training. After you finish your training, you should bring your Qì and mind back to the Real Lower Dāntián and take several deep breaths for recovery.

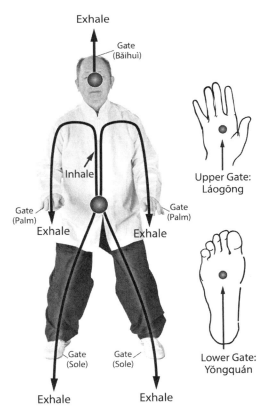

Figure 7-6. Five Gates Breathing.

7.4 Sexual Energy Cultivation (Xìngnéng Zhī Péiyǎng, 性能之培養)

Sexual activity is the most common and natural animal behavior in nature. Through sex, the minds of animals are stimulated and lifted to a high sensory level. This mental and physical satisfaction and excitement results in reproduction of the species. It is no different for humans.

In order to understand this common behavior, you should first recognize a few important facts:

1. During intercourse, a male will usually lose his sperm and his Qì when he ejaculates. The female will receive both the sperm and the Qì for the nourishment of her egg. According to Chinese Qìgōng, a male is more Yáng on the surface and Yīn at the center line while the female is more Yīn on the surface and Yáng at the centerline. That means the Qì in a male is more manifested to the surface while in a female the Qì is stronger at the central line. That is why a male is more muscular and has more hair while the female is able to carry a baby in her womb. During intercourse, the penis will be at the most Yáng and excited. When this Yáng penis enters the Yīn vagina, the Qì will flow from Yáng to Yīn naturally.

   As matter of fact, many male animals or insects such as Furcifer Labordi chameleons, Antechinus, Phascogale, Brazilian slender opossums, dark fishing spiders, honeybees, and many others die after impregnating the female. Human males do not die, but they do lose a lot of Qì during intercourse. Therefore, if a male wants to have a healthy sex life, he should establish a regulated sexuality and know how to conserve the energy instead of abusing it.

2. There are a few places in the body that can be touched and stimulated to excite the brain to a higher sensational level. These places are commonly the tongue, nipples, penis (male), labia (female), and anus. Among these, the Qì exchanges through the penis, labia, and anus are the strongest because through penetration, the Qì can reach the central energy line (i.e., spinal cord or Thrusting Vessel) and go directly to the brain. However, from Qìgōng concepts and practices, there is another place that is sensitive and able to stimulate the Qì in the central line. That is the perineum (Huìyīn, 會陰), the junction of the four Yīn vessels. Since this cavity is connected to the brain directly without any obstacle, it can also cause some excitement and stimulation of the brain.

3. Depending on the individual and also the training, a male is able to train himself to sustain an erection (Yáng condition) during intercourse. In addition, through training, a male will be able to prevent himself from ejaculating. Even though a male may be able to control his ejaculation, he will still lose Qì once his penis enters the vaginal canal. However, if he ejaculates, the Qì release will be just like a dam breaking.

4. There is one way that a male will not lose his Qì, and that is if he is able to get his partner more excited than him. This will reverse the Yīn and Yáng status. In the past, a male sex expert was not only able to stop his Qì from being lost to a female during intercourse; he was also able to absorb the Qì from a female. This practice is called "pick up (the Qì) from Yīn to nourish the Yáng" (Cǎiyīn Bǔyáng, 採陰補陽).

Since I am not an expert in sexual energy exchange, I will not be able to offer my opinion or experience. However, I will briefly summarize some solo male practices, based on the Muscle/Tendon Changing and Marrow/Brain Washing Qìgōng documents, for stimulating your sexual organs to increase your sexual hormone and semen production. Unfortunately, there is no female training explained in the text, and I don't have any idea about a woman's practice. However, I believe that once a female is able to comprehend the theory, she will be able to figure out the practice. As with men, sexual stimulation also increases women's hormone production. Also, storing Qi is a biologically natural condition for women. Perhaps the only additional area of focus not considered in masculine practice is being aware of how compressing the Dāntián also includes the vaginal canal and the urethra. If you are interested to learn more about such training, please refer to the book, *Qìgōng, The Secret of Youth*, by YMAA.

Solo Practice for Male

You should be aware that all the trainings are combinations of both Muscle/Tendon Changing and Marrow/Brain Washing. Other than brain washing for spiritual enlightenment, these practices were also used for sexual training.

1. **To Fill Up the Qì in Two Vessels, Yīn Heel and Yīn Linking Vessels (Yīnqìao/ Yīnwéi Mài, 陰蹻/陰維脈) in Each Leg**

If the Qì stored in these two reservoirs is abundant, you can either lead it up to nourish your brain for enlightenment or increase your sexual capability. In Chinese medicine, these two vessels connect to the perineum (Huìyīn), and the perineum is connected to the sexual organs at the groin area. Through stimulating the sexual organs, sexual hormones will be produced. This will expedite the biochemical reaction (metabolism) and thus Qì will be produced.

> In the Yīnqīao vessel, Qì is misty. How many real originals are (hidden) inside; (if you can) pick (them up) and (lead them to) enter into the emptiness and refine into Qì, (even) Pénglái is myriad miles away, the road is open (to you).

陰蹻脈上氣濛濛，多少真元在此中；採入虛無煉成氣，蓬萊萬里
路相通。

When you stimulate the groin and generate semen, the Qì first fills up the Yīnqiāo vessel. It is called misty because it is as heavy as a thick fog. This Qì is considered semen Qì (Jīngqì, 精氣) since it is converted from semen. Semen is considered part of the Original Essence. The original here refers to Original Jīng (Yuánjīng, 元精), Original Qì (Yuánqì, 元氣), and Original Shén (Yuánshén, 元神). If you know how to pick up (i.e., use) and lead this Qì and to refine it into your Shén (spirit), you will be able to live forever like the immortals. Pénglái (蓬萊) is an island in ancient Chinese folk legends where the immortals were said to live.

Through stimulating practice, you will increase semen production. Then, you must convert it into Qì. If you do not convert it efficiently, the extra semen will stimulate your sexual desire to a high level. Therefore, after you have completed the groin stimulation process, you must continue with the conversion process. The trick of increasing the efficiency of the conversion is to lead the Qì from the four vessels in the legs upward to the Huángtíng (黃庭) (or Real Lower Dāntián) and the head. When the Qì in the four leg vessels is led upward, the semen-Qì conversion will increase to refill the four vessels.

Naturally, when the Qì is full in the two vessels of each leg, you will have plenty of Qì to support your sexual activities. Without abundant Qì support, you will not be able to do anything.

2. Thirteen Secret Key Training Words—Stimulate Sexual Organs (Male)

As mentioned earlier, since there is no ancient document for female training, I will not be able to introduce the training for female readers. However, if you understand the theory behind the practice, you should be able to find or create some stimulation to serve this purpose. Here we will review these thirteen key words for males from two ancient documents, *Yìjīnjīng* (易筋經)(i.e., *Muscle/Tendon Changing Classic*) and *Xǐsuǐjīng* (洗髓經)(i.e., *Marrow/Brain Washing Classic*).

Thirteen Key Words (十三字訣)

(Of) the methods of training this Gōng (Fū), one is with the testicles (Zhūlún) and one is with the penis (Héngmó).

行此功法，一在珠輪，一在橫磨。

The poetry uses euphemisms here, referring to the testicles as "Zhūlún" (珠輪), or "rotating pearls," and the penis as "Héngmó" (橫磨), a "cylindrical grindstone." This sentence states that when you train Marrow/Brain Washing (Xǐsuǐjīng) Gongfu you must start with your testicles and penis.

Thread together into one, say Yì, say Xǐ.

一以貫之，曰易曰洗。

The Chinese in this sentence is very idiomatic and colloquial. The first part expresses the idea of putting Chinese coins on a string. Since ancient times Chinese coins have been made with a hole in them so that they could be strung together. The coins are together yet still separate, individual coins. When Chinese refer to a list of several items, they will sometimes use the word "say" before each item. Yì means the exercises of the Muscle/Tendon Changing (Yìjīnjīng, 易筋經), and Xǐ means the exercises of the Marrow/Brain Washing (Xǐsuǐjīng, 洗髓經). This sentence means that when you train, you should train both methods together instead of only training one and ignoring the other. As explained earlier, Yìjīnjīng is a Lí (離) (Fire) training while Xǐsuǐjīng is a Kǎn (坎) (Water) training. Together they bring Yīn and Yáng into balance. This is the way of the Dào.

For the testicles, the secret training words are: say Slip Out (Zhēng), say Massage (Róu), say File (Cuō), say Hang (Zhuì), say Slap (Pāi).

在珠輪行功字訣：曰掙、曰揉、曰搓、曰墜、曰拍。

The word "Zhēng" (掙) means to struggle to get free. For example, if someone has grabbed your wrist, if you break free with force it is called "Zhēngkāi" (掙開), which means "struggle to open." This means that when you train, you hold your testicles with your hand and let them slip out of your grasp. Naturally, you only hold them lightly at the beginning so as not to injure them. "Róu" (揉) means to massage. When you Róu, your finger(s) stay in one place on the skin and circle around. Because the skin is loose, you can massage the area under the skin without rubbing your finger against the skin. "Cuō" (搓) means to rub or to file. When you Cuō, you use your hands or fingers to rub the skin and generate heat. "Zhuì" (墜) means to hang something and let the object drop naturally. The last word, "Pāi" (拍), means slap. That means you use your hand to slap the testicles gently. Except for Zhuì (hang), which is used to convert the semen into Qì, the other four words refer to common ways of stimulating the testicles.

For the penis, the secret training words are: say Hold (Wò), say Bind (Shù), say Nourish (Yǎng), say Swallow (Yàn), say Draw In/Absorb (Shè), say Hold Up (Tí), say Close (Bì), say Swing (Shuāi).

在橫磨行功字訣：曰握、曰束、曰養、曰咽、曰攝、曰提、曰閉、曰摔。

"Wò" (握) means to use your hand to hold something. "Shù" (束) means to bind or tie up something. "Yǎng" (養) means to nourish, to enhance, to make grow. "Yàn" (咽) means to swallow. "Shè" (攝) has the meaning of draw in, absorb, or take. "Tí" (提) means to hold up or raise. "Bì" (閉) means to close, and "Shuāi" (捽) means to swing from one side to the other. All of the above are ways of stimulating or training with the penis, although, in fact, not all of them apply directly to the penis.

As matter of fact, all above methods are used to stimulate your sexual organs so the hormone production can be enhanced. You may also develop your own ways for this kind of stimulation. However, your mind must be firm and strong. If your mind is allured from these stimulations, you may end up with ejaculation and lose your sperm.

Sexual Qì Exchange Dual Cultivation Grand Circulation (Xìngjiāo Shuāngxiū Dàzhōutiān, 性交雙修大周天)

Sexual Qì Exchange Dual Cultivation is one of the most powerful mutual Qì nourishment practices. Sexual energy exchange is a normal and natural behavior for humans and other animals. However, one of the potential problems that can hinder the purpose of this practice is that practitioners may become emotionally entangled. If you practice Dual Cultivation for sexual enjoyment, you will not have a problem with your lover. However, if you train sexual Dual Cultivation for enlightenment, then any emotional entangling will trap you in emotional bondage and hinder the opening of the Third Eye.

Sexual Qì exchange can be beneficial using heterosexual or homosexual practice. As long as both persons know how to practice, the Qì exchange can be achieved.

It is said in ancient documents:

Yīn and Yáng are not necessarily male and female; the strength and the weakness of Qì in the body are Yīn and Yáng.

陰陽不必分男女，體氣強弱即陰陽。

Two men can plant and graft and a pair of women can absorb and nourish.

兩個男人可栽接，一對女人能採補。

In this practice you exchange and nourish Qì with your partner through your sensual organs such as the tongue, nipples, penis, vagina, or anus. As mentioned earlier, these organs connect to the central Qì system (i.e., central nervous system). Exchanging Qì through this method can stimulate the mind to a highly excited level and increase the production of hormones beneficial to health and wellbeing.

There are many commonly known ways to contact and stimulate these organs: mouth to mouth (or tongue to tongue, the most common one being the kiss), mouth to nipple, mouth to penis/vagina, and finally penis to vagina/anus. The main purpose of this practice is to harmonize the Qì with your partner. In this practice, both you and your partner will exchange the Qì through the sexual organs. Each one has two options for application: lead the Qì up to the Upper Dāntián to raise the Spirit of Vitality or lead the Qì to the Real Lower Dāntián for storage. It is rare to have two persons who have the same quantity of Qì. Through this practice, whoever has too much will share and give so the body's excess Yáng can be regulated while the one who is weaker will receive Qì for nourishment.

There are a few simple guidelines for this practice:

1. Both should coordinate their breathing so it is smooth, comfortable, and natural. When one inhales, the other exhales. The key to releasing or absorbing the Qì is the Huìyīn (anus). Remember, when the anus is pushing out, the Qì is released, and when the anus is lifted, the Qì is taken in or kept. Since both persons have an intention to lead the Qì, Reverse Abdominal Breathing should be used.

2. If person A is offering the Qì and B is taking the Qì, then person A should exhale longer than they inhale while B should inhale longer than they exhale. Naturally, person A should gently push out the anus (Huìyīn) while person B gently holds it up. When both reach the end of a breath, simply hold the breath and the Huìyīn position for five seconds.

3. The person who gets more excited emotionally will usually lose Qì while the calm person will receive Qì.

4. If during Qì exchange, the one who pushes out their anus (Huìyīn) all the time will continue to lose Qì. However, the one who holds up the anus all the time will continue to absorb Qì.

Historically, this exchange was done by a couple; one younger and one older partner, since a younger person—until we reach our thirties or forties—has more abundant hormones and Qì to contribute while the older person has experience, theoretical understanding, and skill. In modern times, this is a very personal matter involving the mutual consent of legal-aged practitioners. Outside of monasteries, people tend to become interested in meditation and this type of practice later in life.

Since these are common human activities, we will not discuss them further. You may follow the guidelines and practice by yourself. Soon, you will gain experience. Please remember that this kind of practice can trigger significant emotional disturbance if the work is not done to first regulate the mind and emotions. That is the reason that many Daoists are against this practice. You must practice with total respect for each other.

Part V

Conclusions

CHAPTER 8

Conclusions

8.1 INTRODUCTION (JIÈSHÀO, 介紹)

This book only offers you some concepts to inspire your thinking and hopefully encourage you to pursue and create your future. The meaning of our lives is to understand nature and untie all its mysteries. It is a long and timeless journey to reach the final goal of enlightenment. However, it is why we are here.

Humans have spent countless years to reach the current stage of both material and spiritual development. However, though our material science has reached an advanced level, our understanding of the spiritual world is still very shallow. The last century was one of material science, and hopefully this century will be the spiritual century, for if we cannot advance and evolve our spirituality to the next level, by the end of this century, we may have to face catastrophic self-destruction and possibly be the cause our own extinction.

We need to face many questions for us to advance our spirituality to the next level. Can we rid ourselves of human emotional bondage, especially that which stems from the dogma we create about glory, dignity, pride, greediness, and power? Can we as a society move to a higher spiritual level and share our fortunes with others who are not as fortunate?

Chinese Buddhist and Daoist understanding and experience conclude that there are four stages of spiritual evolution. The first step is "self-recognition" (Zìshì, 自識). In this step, the mask on your face starts to drop off, which allows you to see your spiritual being more clearly. Mistakes you have committed and untruths you have hidden in your subconscious mind will gradually appear in your conscious mind. In Chinese Qìgōng society, it is believed that the subconscious mind is associated with your spiritual connection with nature and is more truthful than the conscious mind. Once your mask drops off, you must face your real self. You must face your past and analyze it. In addition, in order to gain permanent emotional balance, you must search for ways to free yourself from the feeling of guilt hidden deep inside you. This process will make you humble, enable you to understand yourself better, and finally help you find the center of your being.

The next step is "self-awareness" (Zìjué, 自覺). In this step, if you pay attention, you will be aware of your deep inner spirit and your problems. You will also start to recognize the existence of other spiritual beings. You will slowly and gradually start paying attention to your thinking and behavior as well as that of others. From this awareness, you will be able to realize your existence and understand the role you should play in this society. Through this "self-awareness" meditation process, you will establish a calm and peaceful mind that allows you to harmonize with others and nature.

From awareness, you gradually enter the third stage of cultivation. This stage is "self-awakening" (Zìxǐng/Zìwù, 自醒/自悟). In the self-awareness stage, you pay attention, collect information, and learn to understand yourself and your environment. In this third stage of self-awakening, you gradually begin to awaken and see things more clearly. After awakening, many people come to see how ugly human spiritual beings are and decide to keep away from lay society and become hermits or monks. Others change their thinking about the meaning of life after awakening. Many others are able to build up their confidence and make their lives more meaningful.

Once awakened, we will recognize how we have been abused and manipulated into wars and spiritual control by political and spiritual leaders. You start to search for ways to set yourself free from bondage. This stage of "freedom from bondage" (Jiětuō, 解 脫) means searching for freedom both physically and spiritually so you are able to reach "spiritual independence." When you have reached this stage, your spiritual being can be independent and does not have to rely on someone else. Having reached this condition, you will not be easily abused.

Buddhist and Daoist monks looked for a way to escape from re-entering the cycle of reincarnation. They were searching for a way to build an independent spirit that could survive without the physical body. This was the final goal of their spiritual eternality and freedom from spiritual bondage.

If we look at human history, we can see that the entire human race is in the third stage of self-awakening. We have awakened and realized how ugly and materially ambitious humans have historically been. However, it will still take a long period of time to reach the final stage of freedom from bondage. Spiritual development is the key to evolve to the next stage.

8.2 PAST, PRESENT, AND FUTURE (GUÒQÙ, XIÀNZÀI, YǓ WÈILÁI, 過去，現在，與未來)

To advance ourselves to the next stage of spiritual development, we must face the dark side of ourselves that is hidden deeply in our genetic memory, in our subconscious mind. Next, we must comprehend and pursue awakening to the present. Only then will we be able to create a future "free from bondage" and reach a stage of harmony and peace in the human world.

Past

Historically, in order to survive, we separated ourselves into various groups or races. Leaders were chosen and a pecking order was established. This grouping helped us survive natural challenges, but we also used our group isolation to justify conquering, killing, and enslaving the other. The values of domination, power, glory, dignity, and pride were developed and indoctrinated into each generation. A dominating and manipulated society or matrix was established. After thousands of years of this bloody dark history, we have established a deep genetic memory in our conscious mind. These dogmas still circulate in our blood.

If we continue to allow ourselves to become trapped by these dark impulses, the human spirit will not evolve to the next level. If we wish to evolve, we cannot ignore or downplay the positive aspects of genetic memory such as compassion, love, fairness, forgiveness, mercy, sharing, and mutual assistance. This positive side of us will bring the world into a harmonious and peaceful state that will allow our spirit to grow.

Present

Once we understand the past, then we must analyze it and bring ourselves to a stage of awareness. Unfortunately, as we have seen, we are heavily influenced today by marketing and the allure of making money. Many movies and computer games focus on the dark side of our nature and ignore the development of the bright side.

We must also recognize that today's spiritual science is still in its infancy even though in the last century we have developed material science to an unprecedented level. Unfortunately, due to the dark side of our nature, we have also developed weapons so powerful they could wipe out the entire human race more than a hundred times over. There are well over thirteen thousand nuclear bombs in the world today, prepared and ready to launch in an instant. The next war will be completely destructive.

If you look at the development of the spiritual sciences, we see that it remains at the same level it was two centuries ago. Human spiritual evolution (Yīn side) and material development (Yáng side) have become imbalanced. If scientists continue to focus on just material science, they will not be able to break through to the spiritual side. Spiritual science cannot be seen but must be felt.

We are still mired in the spiritual bondage and dogmas that were created long ago. Will we be able to open our minds and are we ready to accept the new developments in spiritual science? In order to develop the spiritual sciences, we must develop our subconscious feeling. To reach a profound feeling, we have to encourage the next generation to meditate and develop deep inner cultivation.

If we really wish to understand or untie the mystery of our lives, we must know the material world (Yáng) and also the spiritual world (Yīn). Only then can we really comprehend the meaning of our lives.

We have to cease the development of more advanced and destructive weapons. We are entering a most crucial and important era. The future we create depends on how we cultivate our mind today.

Future

After we face the past and present, hopefully through awakening, we will be able to finally set ourselves free from material and spiritual bondage. The question is, are we ready to accept the challenge? Can we conquer ourselves and cleanse our past of the darkness that is still stuck in our genetic memory?

We should not be afraid. Dare to face the truth! Dare to accept the challenge! Dare to dream and create a new hope! We must find an effective way to cleanse the negativity that still dominates our thinking. Human mentality and education must be aimed toward future universal knowledge, understanding, and communication. I believe that once our spirit has evolved to a higher intelligent, peaceful, and harmonious level, we will be able to establish a wide scale of communication with advanced spiritual beings in the universe.

Here are some questions for you to ponder:

1. In order to bring our spirit to a higher level, must the entire human race reopen their Third Eye so evil thoughts and deeds cannot be hidden and initiated?
2. If the entire human race evolves spiritually and reopens the Third Eye, will we have telepathy? If we do, then no evil thought can be hidden.
3. Can we reopen the Third Eye through modern technology or must it be reopened through spiritual self-cultivation?
4. Once our brain has been developed to a more functional and powerful level, can we use our mind to move physical objects?
5. When the mind is strong, can we levitate our body (through anti-gravitational force)?
6. Will we be able to live seven hundred to eight hundred years, as it is said, like aliens?

This information is based on my study of ancient documents and modern scientific research and many years of experience in Qìgōng, but even I am blind and do not wish to limit your practice or bind you to my way of thinking. As I always say, this is for you to ponder. The practice is yours.

There are still many interesting questions that need to be asked and answered. We are in a challenging world and challenging times. The future is in our hands.

Acknowledgements

Axie Breen for her cover design.

Tim Comrie for typesetting.

Axie Breen and Quentin Lopes for the illustrations.

David Silver for content editing.

Leslie Takao and Doran Hunter for copy editing.

Colin Borsos and Javier Rodrigues for general help.

Appendix: Translation and Glossary of Chinese Terms

Bā 八 Eight.

Bāduànjǐn 八段錦 The Eight Pieces of Brocade. A popular medical Qìgōng set for health maintenance.

Bāguà 八卦 The Eight Trigrams.

Bái 白 White.

Bǎihuì (Gv-20) 百會 An acupuncture cavity belongs to Governing Vessel, located on crown.

Bǎihuì Xī Dàzhōutiān 百會息大周天 "Bǎihuì Breathing Grand Circulation." Also called "Heaven Gate Breathing" (Tiānmén Xī, 天門息).

Bǎirì Zhújī 百日築基 "One Hundred Days of Building the Foundation." It also means "Refine the Essence and Convert It into Qì" (Liànjīng Huàqì, 練精化氣).

Bāmài 八脈 Eight vessels (Qì reservoirs).

Bàn 伴 Partner.

Bào Pǔ Zi 抱朴子 *Embracing Simplicity*, by Gé Hóng (葛洪) (283–343 A.D.).

Bàoyī 抱一 Embracing the singularity.

Bìhù 閉戶 "The closed door." It means that the Mingmén (Gv-4) (命門) cavity between L2 and L3 has been closed.

Bǔ 補 Nourishing.

Cái 財 Money.

Cǎidìqì 採地氣 Pick up earth Qì.

Cǎitiānqì 採天氣 Pick up heaven Qì.

Cǎiyīn Bǔyáng 採陰補陽 Pick up (the Qì) from Yīn to nourish the Yáng.

Chán 禪 A form of Buddhist meditation created by Dámó (達摩) (i.e., Dharma). Later it was exported to Japan, where it became known as Rěn (忍).

Chángqiáng (Gv-1) 長強 An acupuncture cavity belongs to Governing Vessel. Also known as tailbone (Wěilǔ, 尾閭).

Chángshòu 長壽 Long life span.

Chéngfó 成佛 Becoming Buddha; means that Buddhahood is achieved.

Chéngxiān 成仙 Becoming Immortal. Daoist term for Buddhahood.

Chōngmài 衝脈 Thrusting Vessel, one of the body's eight vessels (Bāmài, 八脈).

Chòupínáng 臭皮囊 "Notorious skin bag."

Chuántǒng Guǎngyì 傳統廣義 A general traditional definition.

Chuántǒng Xiáyì 傳統狹義 A narrow traditional definition.

Chūqiào 出竅 "Open spirit orifice." It means that the spiritual baby is born and your Third Eye has reopened. You are enlightened.

Dàimài 帶脈 Girdle (or Belt) Vessel, one of the body's eight vessels (Bāmài, 八脈).

Dàimài Xī 帶脈息 Girdle (Belt) Vessel Breathing.

Dàmíng Xīnzhòu 大明心咒 Great Bright Heart Mantra.

Dámó 達摩 Dharma. The Indian Buddhist monk who is credited with creating the *Yìjīnjīn* (易筋經) and *Xǐsuǐjīng* (洗髓經) while at the Shaolin monastery. His last name was Sardili, and he was also known as Bodhidarma. He was once the prince of a small tribe in southern India.

Dámó Yìjīnjīng/Xǐsuǐjīng 達磨易筋經/洗髓經 Dharma's Muscle/Tendon Changing and Marrow/Brain Washing.

Dāndǐng Dàogōng 丹鼎道功 "The Dào Training in the Elixir Crucible."

Dǎngshén 黨參 Codonopsis.

Dānlú 丹爐 Elixir furnace."

Dāntián 丹田 "Elixir Field" (i.e., biobattery) that produces and stores Qì.

Dāntián Zhújī 丹田築基 Building the foundation of Dāntián.

Dānxiū 單修 Cultivate alone.

Dào 道 "The Natural Way."

Dàojiā 道家 Dào's family or style.

Dàowài Cǎiyào 道外採藥 Picking herbs from outside of the Dào.

Dàoxué 道學 Traditional scholar Daoism.

Dǎoyǐn 導引 Direct and lead.

Dàzhōutiān 大周天 Grand Circulation

Dàzhuī (Gv-14) 大椎 Acupuncture name for a cavity on the Governing Vessel. It means "Big Vertebra."

Dàzìrán 大自然 Great nature.

Dǎzuò 打坐 Sitting meditation.

Dì 地 Earth.

Dì 地 Place (Dìfāng, 地方).

Dì Wǔxīn Xí 第五心息 Fifth gate breathing.

Diànqì 電氣 Electric Qì.

Diǎnxué 點穴 Point cavity; means cavity press or acupressure.

Diǎnxué Ànmó 點穴按摩 Cavity press massage (i.e., acupressure).

Diàodāng 吊襠 Hanging groin.

Dìhù 地戶 Ground Gate.

Dìhùxí 地戶息 Ground Gate Breathing Grand Circulation. Also called "Huìyīn Breathing Grand Circulation" (Huìyīn Xí Dàzhōutiān, 會陰息大周天).

Dìlǐshī 地理師 Dìlǐ (地理) means geomancy, and Shī (師) means teacher. Therefore, Dìlǐshī is a master who analyzes geographic locations according to the formula in the Yìjīng (易經, The Book of Changes) and the energy distribution in the Earth. Also called Fēngshuǐshī (風水師).

Dìng 定 To stabilize and to calm.

Dìngshén 定神 To stabilize or firm. The goal is to reach steadiness and firmness of the body, mind, and spirit.

Dìngyì 定義 Definition.

Dìqì 地氣 Earth Qì.

Dìrén Qìjiāo 地人氣交 Exchange Qì of human with earth.

Dūmài 督脈 Governing Vessel. One of the Eight Extraordinary Vessels.

Éméi Dàpéng Gōng 峨眉大鵬功 Éméi big roc gōng.

Éméishān 峨嵋山 Name of a mountain in Sìchuān province (四川).

Fǎ 法 Techniques.

Fǎnjīng Bǔnǎo 返精補腦 "To return the Jīng to nourish the brain," a special Daoist Qìgōng term.

Fǎntóng Hūxī 返童呼吸 Back to Childhood Breathing, also called Abdominal Breathing. A Nèiān practice through which one regains control of the muscles in the lower abdomen.

Fēngfǔ (Gv-16) 風府 Wind's Dwelling. An acupuncture cavity on the Governing Vessel (Dūmài, 督脈)

Fēnglù 風路 Wind path.

Fēngshuǐ 風水 Wind Water. Geomancy. Divination of natural energy relationships in a location, especially the interrelationships of wind and water; hence the name.

Fēngshuǐshī 風水師 Wind Water Teacher. Master of divination. Also called Dìlǐshī (地理師).

Fěnsuì Xūkōng 粉碎虛空 Crushing the Nothingness. The training of "Nine Years of Facing the Wall" (Jiǔnián Miànbì, 九年面壁).

Fójiā 佛家 Buddhist family or religion.

Fú Xī 伏羲 According to legend, *The Book of Changes* was first developed by Fú Xī (伏羲) about seven thousand years ago.

Fúqì 伏氣 Tame the Qì.

Fūsuǐ Xī (Tǐxī) 膚髓息（體息） Skin/Marrow breathing (body breathing).

Fūxī 膚息 Skin breathing. Also called "body breathing" (Tǐxī, 體息) in Qìgōng practice.

Fùxí 複習 Review.

Gāngmén 肛門 Anus.

Gōng 功 Energy or hard work.

Gōngfū (or Kūng Fū) 功夫 Energy Time. Any study, learning, or practice that requires patience, energy, and time to accomplish. Chinese martial arts require a great deal of time and energy, so they are commonly called Gōngfū.

Gòngzhèn Zhōngxīn 共振中心 Resonance centers.

Gù 固 To solidify and to firm.

Guānjié Xí 關節息 Joint breathing.

Guānyīn Púsà 觀音菩薩 Guānyīn Bodhisattva.

Guǐ 鬼 Ghost. When you die, if your spirit is strong, your soul's energy does not decompose and return to nature. This soul energy is a ghost.

Guīké Xī 龜殼息 Turtle Shell Breathing.

Guǐqì 鬼氣 Ghost Qì.

Gùjīng 固精 To make solid, to firm the essence"; it means to firm Original Jīng.

Gùshén 固神 To firm the spirit.

Gǔshén 谷神 The Valley Spirit.

Gǔsuǐ 骨髓 Bone marrow.

Gǔsuǐ Díxǐ 骨髓滌洗 Bone Marrow Washing.

Hā 哈 Laughing sound.

Hǎidǐ 海底 Sea Bottom. Martial arts name for the Huìyīn (Co-1, 會陰), or perineum.

Háijīng Bǔnǎo 還精補腦 To Return the Essence to Nourish the Brain. A Daoist Qìgōng process wherein Qì produced from essence is led to nourish the brain.

Hàn Shū Yì Wén Zhì 漢書藝文志 *Han's Book of Art and Literature*, by Bāngù (班固) during the Chinese East-Hàn Dynasty (25–220 CE).

Hēi 黑 Black.

Hēng 哼 Sad sound.

Hóng 紅 Red.

Hòutiān Qì 後天氣 Post-Birth Qì or Post-Heaven Qì. This is converted from the essence of food and air and classified as Fire Qì since it makes your body Yáng.

Huáng 黃 Yellow.

Huángdì Nèijīng Sùwèn 黃帝內經素問 *Plain Questions: Yellow Emperor's Internal Canon of Medicine*, by Líng Shū (靈樞) (Miraculous Pivot); composed during Chinese Hàn Dynasty (circa 100–300 BCE).

Huángqì 黃者 Astragali Radix.

Huángtíng 黃庭 "Yellow Yard." A special Daoist term that means guts (i.e., the second brain).

Huànqìfǎ 換氣法 Exchange Qì technique.

Huìyīn (Co-1) 會陰 "Meet Yīn." The perineum, an acupuncture cavity on the Conception Vessel. It is also called "Sea Bottom" (Hǎidǐ, 海底).

Huìyīn Xī Dàzhōutiān 會陰息大周天 Huìyīn Breathing Grand Circulation. Also called Ground Gate Breathing Grand Circulation (Dìhù Xí, 地戶息).

Hún 魂 The Soul. Commonly used with the word Líng (靈), which means spirit. Daoists believe one's Hún (魂) and Pò (魄) originate with his Original Qì (Yuánqì, 元氣) and separate from the physical body at death.

Huǒlù 火路 Fire Path. The regular path of Small Circulation that follows the natural Qì circulation of the body.

Huóqì 活氣 Living Qì or Vital Qì. When something is alive, it has Vital Qì.

Huǒqì 火氣 Literally, "Fire Qì. Also called "Post-Birth Qì."

Jiǎ Dāntián 假丹田 False Lower Dāntián. Called Qìhǎi (Co-6, 氣海) (Qì sea) in Chinese medicine. Daoists believe that the Lower Dāntián in front of the abdomen is not the Real Dāntián.

Jiànkāng 健康 To maintain a healthy physical body.

Jiāodiǎn 焦點 Focal points.

Jīchǔ 基礎 Foundation.

Jiē 接 To join, to connect, or to graft.

Jiěshì 解釋 Explanation.

Jiětuō 解脫 Liberate yourself from spiritual bondage.

Jīn 筋 Muscles and tendons.

Jīndān Dàdào 金丹大道 Golden elixir large way.

Jīng 經 Classic or bible.

Jīng 經 Channels or meridians. Twelve organ-related rivers that circulate Qì throughout the body.

Jīng 精 Essence. The most refined part of anything. What is left after something has been refined and purified. In Chinese medicine, Jīng can mean semen, but it generally refers to the basic substance of the body enlivened by the Qì and Shén (spirit).

Jǐngjuéxìng 警覺性 Awareness.

Jìnglì 勁力 Martial power.

Jīngliàn 精煉 To refine or purify a liquid to a high quality.

Jīngliáng 精良 "Pure and good"; means "excellent quality."

Jīngmíng 精明 "Keen and clever"; when someone is smart or wise, he or she is called "Jīngmíng."

Jīngqì 精氣 Essence Qì or semen Qì, converted from Original Essence (Yuánjīng, 元精).

Jīngshāo Qìgōng 經梢氣功 Meridian Qìgōng.

Jīngshén 精神 Essence Spirit. Means Spirit of Vitality; raised Qì but restrained by Yì (意).

Jǐngtìxìng 警惕性 Alertness.

Jīngxì 精細 Delicate and painstaking (literally, "pure and fine"). When a piece of art work is well done, it is called "Jīngxì."

Jīngzǐ 精子 Son of essence; means sperm.

Jìngzuó 靜坐 To sit quietly in meditation; means sitting meditation.

Jiūwěi (Co-15) 鳩尾 Wide Pigeon's Tail. An acupuncture cavity at the lower sternum on the Conception Vessel. Called Xīnkǎn (心坎) (i.e., Heart Pit) by martial society.

Juéyīn 厥陰 Absolute Yīn.

Jùjīng Huìshén 聚精會神 "Gathering your Jīng to meet your Shén"; implies that your mind is concentrating on doing something.

Kāiqìao 開竅 Open the crux or tricky gate.

Kǎn 坎 In the Eight Trigrams, Kǎn represents "water" while Lí represents "fire."

Kēxué Gēnjī 科學根基 Scientific foundation.

Kōngqì 空氣 Air.

Láogōng (P-8) 勞宮 Labor's Palace. A cavity on the Pericardium Primary Channel in the center of the palm.

Lí 離 In the Eight Trigrams, Kǎn represents "water" while Lí represents "fire."

Liàn 練 To refine, to train, or to discipline.

Liànjīng Huàqì 練精化氣 "Refine the Essence and Convert It into Qì." It is the practice of "One Hundred Days of Building the Foundation" (Bǎirì Zhújī, 百日築基).

Liànqì 練氣 Training the Qì.

Liànqì Huàshén 練氣化神 "Purify Qì and convert it into Shén." It is the practice of "Ten Months of Pregnancy" (Shíyuè Huáitāi, 十月懷胎).

Liànqì Shénghuá 煉氣昇華 To train Qì and sublimate it. Xǐsuǐjīng (洗髓經) training to lead Qì to the Huángtíng (黃庭) or the brain.

Liànshén 練神 To train the Shén (i.e., spirit). To refine, strengthen, and focus the Shén.

Liànshèn 練身 To train the body.

Liànshén Fǎnxū 練神返虛 To train the spirit to return to nothingness, to attain freedom from emotional bondage. An advanced stage of enlightenment and Buddhahood training to lead the spirit to separate from the body. It is called "Three Years of Nursing" (Sānnián Bǔrǔ, 三年哺乳).

liànshén liǎoxìng 練神了性 To refine the spirit and end human emotional nature. The final stage of enlightenment training where you keep your emotions neutral, undisturbed by human nature.

Lǐjiě 理解 To comprehend.

Líng 靈 1. The spirit of being, which acts upon others. Líng only exists in highly spiritual animals such as humans and apes. It represents an emotional comprehension and understanding. When you are alive, it is your intelligence and wisdom. When you die, it is the spirit of the ghost. Líng also means divine or supernatural. Together with Shén (Língshén, 靈神) it means supernatural spirit. Qì is the source that nourishes it and is called Língqì (靈氣), meaning supernatural energy, power, or force. Líng is often used to describe someone who is sharp, clever, nimble, and able to quickly empathize with people and things. 2. Supernatural Shén is called Líng. Líng describes someone who is sharp, clever, nimble, and able to quickly empathize with others. Líng can also be a supernatural psychic capability that allows you to communicate with nature or other spiritual beings. Often it means divine inspiration that allows you to comprehend and understand changes or variations in nature.

Língguǐ 靈鬼 Spiritual ghost.

Línghún 靈魂 Spiritual soul.

Língshén 靈神 Supernatural Shén or divine.

Língtāi 靈胎 Spiritual baby or embryo.

Língtái (Gv-10) 靈臺 Spiritual Platform. An acupuncture cavity on the Governing Vessel. Called Jiájí (夾脊) (Squeeze the Spine) by Daoists and Mìngmén (命門) (Life Door) by martial arts society.

Lìqì 力氣 Strength.

Lóngmén (M-CA-24) 龍門 Groin. A miscellaneous acupuncture cavity.

Lǜ 綠 Green.

Lúnyǔ 論語 Confucius' *Analects*.

Luò 絡 Countless secondary channels (i.e., streams) branched out from meridians (i.e., rivers) that allow the Qì to reach the skin and the bone marrow.

Mài 脈 Vessel or Qì channel. The eight vessels (Bāmài, 八脈) involved with transporting, storing, and regulating Qì.

Miǎnyìlì 免疫力 Immunity.

Mìngmén (Gv-4) 命門 Life Door. An acupuncture cavity that belongs to the Governing Vessel (Dūmài, 督脈) located between L2 and L3 vertebrae. It is also called "Bìhù" (閉戶) and means "the closed door."

Mǔzǐ Xiànghé 母子相合 Unification or mutual harmonization of mother and son. The final stage of Embryonic Breathing in that the spirit (i.e., son) and the Qì (i.e., mother) are united at the Real Lower Dāntián.

Nàilì 耐力 Endurance.

Nànjīng 難經 *Classic on Disorders* by Biǎn Què (扁鵲) during Qín and Hàn Dynasties (221 BCE–220 CE) (秦、漢).

Nǎohù (Gv-17) 腦戶 Brain's Household. An acupuncture cavity on the Governing Vessel. Also called Jade Pillow (Yùzhěn, 玉枕) by Daoist society.

Nǎosuǐ 腦髓 Refers to the brain, including limbic system, cerebrum, cerebellum, and medulla oblongata.

Nǎoxiàchuítǐ 腦下垂體 The pituitary gland.

Nèidān 內丹 Internal Elixir. A form of Qìgōng in which Qì (elixir) is built up in the body and spread out to the limbs.

Nèidān Gōng 內丹功 Internal elixir Qìgōng or Gōngfū.

Nèigōng 內功 Internal Gōngfū. All training in which the mind leads the circulation of Qì, either for manifestation or enlightenment.

Nèijīng 內經 A chapter of the book *Huángdì Nèijīng Sùwèn* (*Plain Questions: Yellow Emperor's Internal Canon of Medicine*, 黃帝內經素問) (Hàn Dynasty, circa 100–300 BCE) by Líng Shū (靈樞) (*Miraculous Pivot*).

Nèiqì 內氣 Internal Qì. The bioelecticity circulation in the body is considered internal Qì.

Nèishèn 內腎 Internal kidneys. The same kidneys defined by Western medicine.

Nì Fùhūxī 逆腹呼吸 Reverse Abdominal Breathing. Also called Fǎn Fùhūxī (反腹呼吸) or Daoist Breathing (Dàojiā Hūxī, 道家呼吸).

Níng 凝 To concentrate, to condense, to refine, to focus, and to strengthen.

Níngshén 凝神 Condense or focus the spirit. Once you can keep your spirit in one place, you can condense it into a tiny spot to make it stronger.

Níwángōng 泥丸宮 Mud Pill Palace. Located at the center of your head. The limbic system.

Pài 派 Style or division.

Péng, Zǔ 彭祖 Péng, Zǔ was a legendary Qìgōng practitioner during the period of Emperor Yáo (堯) (2356–2255 BCE), who was said to have lived for eight hundred years.

Pénglái 蓬萊 Pénglái Immortal Island (Pénglái Xiāndǎo, 蓬萊仙島). An island in the East Sea where the immortals resided, according to Chinese legend.

Pínghéng 平衡 Balance.

Qí 奇 Odd, strange, or mysterious.

Qì 氣 The general definition of Qì is universal energy, including heat, light, and electromagnetic energy. A narrower definition refers to the energy circulating in human or animal bodies. A current popular model is that Qì in the body is bioelectricity.

Qì Ànmó 氣按摩 Qì massage. One of the high levels of massage techniques in which a massage doctor uses his own Qì to remove Qì stagnation in the patient's body. Also called Wàiqì Liáofǎ (外氣療法), which means healing with external Qì.

Qiángjiān (Gv-18) 強間 Between Strength. An acupuncture cavity on the Governing Vessel. This and the Third Eye are located at the exit point of the Spiritual Valley (Shéngǔ, 神谷).

Qiángshēn 強身 To condition the physical body (include internal organs).

Qiǎnyìshì 潛意識 The subconscious mind.

Qiàomén 竅門 Means "knack gate." Huìyīn (會陰) is called "Qiàomén" since it is the crucial gate to manipulate Qì function in the body.

Qìbà 氣壩 The Qì reservoirs; means Eight vessels (Bāmài, 八脈).

Qìchǎngxuè 氣場穴 Qì field cavity.

Qìchén Dāntián 氣沉丹田 Sink the Qì to Dāntián.

Qìgōng 氣功 Gōng (功) means Gōngfū (功夫). Qìgōng is the study and training of Qì.

Qìguān Xī 器官息 Organ's breathing.

Qìhǎi (Co-6) 氣海 Sea of Qì. Qì Ocean. An acupuncture cavity on the Conception Vessel, about two inches below the navel.

Qìhuàlùn 氣化論 *Theory of Qì's Variation* by Zhuāngzi (莊子) (370–369 BCE).

Qǐhuǒ 起火 To start the fire. To build up Qì at the Lower Dāntián (Xià Dāntián, 下丹田).

Qìjié 氣結 Qì knot; means the stagnation or blockage of Qì's circulation.

Qíjīng Bāmài 奇經八脈 Odd Meridians and Eight vessels; the extraordinary meridian (EM).

Qíjīng Bāmài Kǎo 奇經八脈考 *Deep Study of the Extraordinary Eight Vessels* by Lǐ, Shí-Zhēn (1518–1593 CE, 李時珍).

Qīng 清 Clear, clean, and peaceful.

Qīng 青 Blue.

Qīng Xiū Pài 清修派 Peaceful Cultivation Division. A branch of Daoist Qìgōng.

Qīngchénshān 青城山 Qīngchén Mountain, located in Sìchuān province (四川省).

Qìshè 氣舍 "Qì dwelling," located at the center of the gut.

Qìshì 氣勢 Energy or momentum.

Qìxuè 氣血 Qì Blood. According to Chinese medicine, Qì and blood cannot be separated, and the two words are commonly used together.

Qìxuè 氣穴 Qì cavities.

Qìzhōngshū 氣中樞 Central Qì system (i.e., central nervous system; spinal cord).

Rén 人 Man.

Rěn 忍 Japanese name of Chán meditation.

Rènmài 任脈 Conception Vessel. One of the eight vessels (Bāmài, 八脈).

Rénqì 人氣 Human Qì.

Rénshén 人參 Ginseng.

Rénshì 人事 Human relations. Human events, activities, and relationships.

Rénzhōng (Gv-26) 人中 Philtrum. An acupuncture cavity on the Governing Vessel (Dūmài, 督脈). Also called Shuǐgōu (水溝), meaning water ditch.

Rèqì 熱氣 Heat Qì.

Ruǎn Qìgōng 軟氣功 Soft Qìgōng.

Sānbǎo 三寶 Three Treasures, meaning Jīng (essence, 精), Qì (energy, 氣), and Shén (spirit, 神). Also called Sānyuán (三元, three origins) or (Sānběn, 三本).

Sānběn 三本 Three Foundations. Also called Sānyuán (三元) (three origins) or (Sānbǎo, 三寶) (three treasures).

Sāncái 三才 The Three Powers. Heaven (Tiān, 天), Earth (Dì, 地), and Man (Rén, 人).

Sàngōng 散功 Energy dispersion. Premature degeneration of the body where Qì cannot effectively energize it. Generally caused by excessive training. A known problem for those who overtrain hard Gōngfū.

Sānguān 三關 Three gates or three obstacles of Small Circulation meditation. They are Wěilú (尾閭), Jiājí (夾脊), and Yùzhěn (玉枕).

Sānjiāo 三焦 Triple Burners. One of the twelve primary Qì channels (i.e., meridians).

Sānnián Bǔrǔ 三年哺乳 Three Years of Nursing. The training of "Refining Shén and return it to Nothingness" (Liànshén Fǎnxū, 練神返虛).

Sānshēng 三聲 The three sounds.

Sānyīnjiāo (Sp-6) 三陰交 Three Yīn Junctions. An acupuncture cavity on the spleen channel. The junction of the three Yīn channels, namely spleen, liver, and kidneys.

Sānyuán 三元 Three origins. Also called Sānbǎo (三寶) (Three Treasures).

Sēngbīng 僧兵 Monk soldiers. Shaolin martial monks.

Shàng dāntián 上丹田 Upper Dāntián, the center of the brain, which connects to the lower center of the forehead (or the Third Eye). In fact, often the entire brain is considered to be the Upper Dāntián.

Shānzhōng (Co-17) 膻中 The central area between the nipples. Some Qìgōng practitioners consider Shanzhong to be the Middle Dan Tian. Its acupuncture name is Penetrating Odor.

Shàolínsì 少林寺 Shàolín Temple. A Buddhist temple in Hénán province (少林寺), famous for its martial arts.

Shàoyáng 少陽 Lesser Yáng.

Shàoyīn, 少陰 Lesser Yīn.

Shèjīng 攝精 Absorb the essence.

Shén 神 "Divine spirit."

Shén Bù Shǒushè 神不守舍 "The spirit is not kept at its residence." It is called "Shén Bù Shǒushè" when someone's mind is scattered and confused; his Shén wanders.

Shēngmén 生門 Means "the door of life" and implies Yīnjiāo (Co-7, 陰交) or navel.

Shēngmìng 生命 Life.

Shēngmìng Zhújī 生命築基 To build a foundation of life.

Shéngǔ 神谷 The Spiritual Valley. Formed by the two hemispheres of the brain, with the Upper Dāntián (i.e., The Third Eye) at the exit point.

Shénhún 神魂 Refers to the spirit of a dying person since his spirit is between "Shén" and "Hún."

Shénjiāo 神交 Spiritual communication.

Shénmíng 神明 Spiritually divine or enlightened beings.

Shénqì Xiānghé 神氣相合 Mutual harmony or unification of spirit and Qì. The final regulating of spirit.

Shénshì 神室 Shén Dwelling. The Limbic System at the center of your head is where the spirit resides. It is also called "Mud Pill Palace" (Níwángōng, 泥丸宮).

Shènshuǐ 腎水 Kidneys' water.

Shéntāi 神胎 Spiritual embryo.

Shénting (Gv-24) 神庭 Spirit's Hall. An acupuncture cavity that belongs to the Governing Vessel (Dūmài, 督脈).

Shéntōng 神通 Spiritual enlightenment or spiritual communication. It means that one has reopened "The Third Eye" and has the capability for spiritual communication with natural spirit.

Shéntōng Dàzhōutiān Jìngzuò 神通大周天靜坐 Spiritual enlightenment grand circulation.

Shénxí 神息 Spirit breathing. The stage of Qìgōng training where the spirit is coordinated with the breathing.

Shénxí Xiāngyī 神息相依 Mutual dependence of spirit and breathing.

Shénxiān 神仙 Immortal Spirit.

Shēnxīn Pínghéng 身心平衡 The balance of the body and the Xīn (i.e., emotional mind).

Shénzhì 神志 The mind generates the will, which keeps the Shén firm. The Chinese commonly use Shén (spirit) and Zhì (will) together because they are so related.

Shénzhì Bùqīng 神志不清 Means "the spirit and the will (generated from Yì) are not clear."

Shíèrjīng 十二經 The twelve primary Qì channels or meridians (i.e., Qì rivers).

Shíyuè Huáitāi 十月懷胎 Ten Months of Pregnancy. The training of "Purify Qì and convert it into Shén" (Liànqì Huàshén, 練氣化神).

Shǒu 守 To keep and to protect.

Shǒushén 守神 To protect and to keep spirit in its residence.

Shuāngxiū 雙修 Dual cultivation. A Qìgōng training method in which Qì is exchanged with a partner to balance the Qì of both. It also means dual cultivation of the body and the spirit.

Shuǐlù 水路 Water Path. One Qì path in which Qì is led up through the Thrusting Vessel (Chōngmài, 衝脈) to the brain for nourishment. It can calm down the excitement of your body. It is also the path of the cultivation of spiritual enlightenment.

Shuǐqì 水氣 Water Qì. It is also called "Pre-Birth Qì" that is able to cool down the Post-Birth Qì (Hòutiānqì, 後天氣), which is called "Fire Qì" (Huǒqì, 火氣).

Shūtóu 梳頭 Combing the hair.

Sìdà Jiēkōng 四大皆空 Four large are empty. This means that the four elements (earth, fire, water, and air) are absent from the mind so that you are completely indifferent to worldly temptations.

Sǐqì 死氣 Dead Qì. The Qì remaining in a dead body. Also called ghost Qì (Guǐqì, 鬼氣).

Sìxīn Xí 四心息 Four Gates Breathing.

Sōngguǒtǐ 松果體 The pineal gland.

Sōngshān 嵩山 Sōng Mountain.

Sōngshēn 鬆身 Loosen and relax the body.

Suànmìngshī 算命師 Calculate Life Teacher. A fortune teller who calculates your future and destiny.

Suǐ 髓 Includes "Gǔsuǐ" (骨髓), which means "bone marrow," and "Nǎosuǐ" (腦髓), which refers to the brain, including the limbic system, cerebrum, cerebellum, and medulla oblongata.

Suǐqì 髓氣 Marrow Qì.

Tàijí Qìgōng 太極氣功 Qìgōng practice for Tàijíquán practitioners.

Tàijíqiú Qìgōng 太極球氣功 Tàijí Ball Qìgōng.

Tāixī 胎息 Embryonic Breathing.

Tàiyáng 太陽 Greater Yáng.

Tàiyīn 太陰 Greater Yīn.

Tàngyǎn 燙眼 Iron the Eyes. A Qìgōng practice that keeps the eyes in a healthy condition.

Tiān 天 Heaven or sky. One of the "Three Powers" (Sāncái, 三才). In ancient China, people believed heaven to be the most powerful force in the universe.

Tiānmén 天門 Heaven Gate.

Tiānmén Xī 天門息 Heaven Gate Breathing. Also called Bǎihuì Breathing Grand Circulation (Bǎihuì Xī Dàzhōutiān, 百會息大周天).

Tiānmén Xí Dàzhōutiān 天門息大周天 Heaven Gate Breathing Grand Circulation.

Tiānmén/Dìhù Bǔnǎo Xí 天門／地戶補腦息 Heaven/Ground Gates Nourishing Brain Breathing.

Tiānmén/Dìhù Chōngqì Xí 天門／地戶充氣息 Heaven/Ground Gates Nourishing Qì Breathing.

Tiānmén/Dìhù Jìngshēn Xí 天門／地戶淨身息 Heaven/Ground Gates Cleansing Body Breathing.

Tiānmén/Dìhù Liǎngyí Xí Dàzhōutiān 天門／地戶兩儀息大周天 Heaven/Ground Gates Two Poles Breathing.

Tiānmén/Dìhù Tíshén Xí 天門／地戶提神息 Heaven/Ground Gates Raise Up Spirit Breathing.

Tiānmén/Dìhù Xí Dàzhōutiān 天門／地戶息大周天 Heaven/Ground Gates Grand Circulation.

Tiānmù 天目 Heaven Eye; means the "Third Eye." The Chinese believe that prior to our evolution into humans, our race possessed an additional sense organ in our forehead. This third eye provided a means of spiritual communication between one another and with the natural world. As we evolved and developed means to protect ourselves from the environment, and as societies became more complex and human vices developed, this Third Eye gradually closed and disappeared.

Tiānqì 天氣 Heaven Qì. Commonly refers to the weather, which is governed by Heaven Qì.

Tiānrén Héyī 天人合一 The Unification of the Heaven and Human. A high level of Qìgōng meditation in which one can communicate with the Qì of Heaven.

Tiānrén Qìjiāo 天人氣交 Human and heaven (i.e., nature) exchange Qì with each other.

Tiānshí 天時 Heavenly timing. The repeated natural cycles generated by the heavens, such as seasons, months, days, and hours.

Tiāntū (Co-22) 天突 Heaven's Prominence. An acupuncture cavity on the Conception Vessel (Dūmài, 督脈). This cavity connects with the Dàzhuī cavity (Gv-14, 大椎) on the back, and they are regarded as a pair of corresponding cavities.

Tiānyǎn 天眼 Literally, "Heaven Eye"; means the "Third Eye." Called Yìntáng (M-HN-3, 印堂) in acupuncture.

Tiáo 調 Translates as "regulating." Tiáo (調) is constructed of two words: Yán (言), which means "speaking" or "negotiating," and Zhōu (周), which means "to be complete," "to be perfect," or "to be round." A gradual regulating process, resulting in that which is regulated achieving harmony with others.

Tiáoér Wútiáo 調而無調 Regulating without regulating.

Tiáoqì 調氣 Regulating the Qì.

Tiáoshén 調神 Regulating the spirit (i.e., Shén).

Tiáoshēn 調身 Regulating the body.

Tiáoxí 調息 Regulating the breathing.

Tiáoxīn 調心 Regulating the emotional mind.

Tiěbùshān 鐵布衫 Iron Shirt. A special hard Qìgōng training in Chinese martial arts.

Tiěshāzhǎng 鐵砂掌 Iron Sand Palm. A special hard Qìgōng palm conditioning in Chinese martial arts.

Tíshén 提神 Raise up spirit.

Tǐxī, 體息 Body breathing. Also called "skin breathing" (Fūxī, 膚息) in Qìgōng practice. This Qìgōng breathing technique enables you to lead Qì to the skin surface, to strengthen Guardian Qì (Wèiqì, 衛氣).

Tōngsānguān 通三關 Widen to pass the passages of three gates. The three gates are Wěilú (尾閭), Jiājí (夾脊), and Yùzhěn (玉枕).

Tuīná 推拿 To push and grab. Chinese massage for healing and treating injuries.

Tǔnà 吐納 Qìgōng is commonly called Tǔnà, which means "to utter and admit." This implies uttering and admitting the air through the nose in respiration.

Wàidān 外丹 External Elixir. External Qìgōng exercises to build up Qì in the limbs or skin surface and lead it into the center of the body for nourishment.

Wàidān Gōng 外丹功 External Elixir Qìgōng or Gōngfū.

Wàiqì 外氣 External Qì. Air Qì is considered to be external Qì.

Wàiqì Liáofǎ 外氣療法 External Qì healing. A high level of Qì massage in which you use your own Qì to remove Qì stagnation in the patient.

Wàishèn 外腎 Chinese define the kidneys as internal kidneys and external kidneys. Internal kidneys (Nèishèn, 內腎) are the kidneys defined by Western medicine. External kidneys are the testicles or ovaries.

Wěilú 尾閭 Tailbone (i.e., coccyx). Called Chángqiáng (Gv-1, 長強) (Long Strength) in acupuncture.

Wèiqì 衛氣 Protective Qì or Guardian Qì. The Qì at the surface of the body forms a shield to protect the body from negative external influences such as cold.

Wénhuǒ 文火 Scholar fire. Means to build up the Qì at the Lower Dāntián gradually through soft and slender breathing.

Wǔdāngshān 武當山 Wǔdāng Mountain. Located in Húběi province (湖北省).

Wǔhuǒ 武火 Martial fire. Means to build up the Qì at the Lower Dāntián quickly through fast abdominal breathing.

Wújí Qìgōng 無極氣功 Wújí standing meditation.

Wǔqì Cháoyuán 五氣朝元 Literally means "five Qìs toward their origins." Means to use the energized Shén to direct the Qì into your five Yīn organs (heart, lung, liver, kidney, and spleen) so that they can function more efficiently.

Wǔqínxì 五禽戲 The Five Animal Sports. A popular medical Qìgōng that imitates the movements of the tiger, deer, bear, ape, and bird for health maintenance. It was created by Jūn Qiàn (君倩) during the Jìn Dynasty (265–420 CE, 晉朝), though others say it was created by Dr. Huá Tuó (華佗).

Wǔtiáo 五調 Five regulatings, including regulating the body, breathing, emotional mind, Qì, and spirit.

Wútiáo Értiáo 無調而調 Regulating without regulating. All actions are so natural that no more regulating is necessary.

Wúwéi 無為 Means "the regulating without regulating."

Wǔxīn Xī 五心息 Five Gates Breathing. A Nèidān Qìgōng (內丹氣功) practice in which one uses the mind in coordination with breathing to lead Qì to the center of the palms, feet, and Bǎihuì (Gv-20, 百會).

Wǔxíng 五行 Five Elements or Five Phases; includes Metal (Jīn, 金), Wood (Mù, 木), Water (Shuǐ, 水), Fire (Huǒ, 火), and Earth (Tǔ, 土).

Wǔxué Dàzhōutiān 武學大周天 Martial Grand Circulation—Power and Endurance.

Wǔxué Qìgōng 武學氣功 Martial Qìgōng.

Xǐ 洗 "To wash" or "to clean."

Xià dāntián 下丹田 Lower Dāntián. Located at the abdominal area, one or two inches below the navel.

Xiān 仙 Immortal.

Xiāntāi 仙胎 Holy Embryo.

Xiāntiān Qì 先天氣 Literally, "Pre-Heaven Qì." It is also called Yuánqì (元氣) or Dāntián Qì (丹田氣). It is the Qì that is converted from Original Essence (Yuánjīng, 元精) and stored in the Lower Dāntián. Considered to be Water Qì, it calms the body.

Xiǎozhōutiān 兩儀小周天 Two Poles Small Circulation. It can also be called Marrow/Brain Washing Small Circulation (Xǐsuǐjīng Xiǎozhōutiān, 洗髓經小周天).

Xiǎozhōutiān 小周天 Small Cyclic Heaven or Small Circulation Meditation. Called Microcosmic Orbit in Yoga, or Turning the Wheel of the Natural Law (Zhuǎn Fǎlún, 轉法輪) by Buddhist society. It is a Nèidān Qìgōng (內丹氣功) training in which Qì is generated at the Lower Dāntián (下丹田) and then moved through the Conception and Governing Vessels.

Xiàyīn 下陰 Low Yīn. The groin. Also called Lóngmén (M-CA-24, 龍門) (Dragon's Gate) in Chinese medicine.

Xiè 洩 Releasing.

Xièqì 洩氣 Releasing Qì.

Xiéqì 邪氣 Evil Qì.

Xǐliǎn 洗臉 Washing the face.

Xīn 心 Heart. The mind generated from emotional disturbance; considered to be the fire mind.

Xìng Shuāngxiū 性雙修 Sexual Dual Cultivation (i.e., sexual Qì exchange).

Xìngmìng Shuāngxiū 性命雙修 Dual cultivation of temperament and physical life.

Xìngnéng 性能 Sexual energy.

Xīnshén Bùníng 心神不寧 Literally, "the (emotional) mind and spirit are not at peace and steady."

Xīnxí Xiāngyī 心息相依 The Xīn and the breathing mutually rely on each other.

Xīnyuán Yìmǎ 心猿意馬 Xīn (is) an ape, and Yì (is) a horse. Xīn (heart) represents the emotional mind, which acts like a monkey, unsteady and disturbing. Yì is the wisdom mind generated from calm, clear thinking and judgment. The Yì is like a horse, calm and powerful.

Xǐsuǐjīng 洗髓經 Marrow and Brain Washing Classic. It is Qìgōng training meant to lead Qì to the marrow to cleanse it or to the brain to nourish the spirit for enlightenment and is regarded as the key to longevity and spiritual enlightenment.

Xǐsuǐjīng Xiǎozhōutiān 洗髓經小周天 Marrow/Brain Washing Small Circulation. It can also be called Two Poles Small Circulation (Liǎngyí Xiǎozhōutiān, 兩儀小周天).

Xiū 修 Cultivation, study, and training.

Xiūqì 修氣 Cultivating the Qì.

Xiūshēn 修身 Cultivating the body.

Xuánguān 玄關 Tricky gate. Key places in Qìgōng training. The Third Eye is considered one of the "Xuánguān."

Xuánpìn 玄牝 Profound female animal. The marvelous and mysterious Dào, mother of creation of millions of objects.

Xuè 穴 Cavity.

Xuèwèi Xí 穴位息 Cavity breathing.

Xūlǐng Dǐngjìng 虛領頂勁 Insubstantial energy leads the Jìng upward.

Yán 言 Speaking or negotiating.

Yáng 陽 One of the two poles (Liǎngyí, 兩儀). The other is Yīn. In Chinese philosophy, the active, positive, masculine polarity is classified as Yáng. In Chinese medicine, Yáng means excessive, overactive, or overheated. The Yáng (or outer) organs are the Gall Bladder, Small Intestine, Large Intestine, Stomach, Bladder, and Triple Burner.

Yǎng 養 To nourish, increase, raise up, or to cultivate.

Yángjiān 陽間 Yǎng World. The material world in which we live.

Yángmíng 陽明 Yáng Brightness.

Yángqiāomài 陽蹻脈 Yáng Heel Vessel. One of the eight vessels.

Yángquán 陽泉 Yáng fountain.

Yángshén 陽神 Yang spirit; a confused and excited spirit.

Yǎngshén 養神 To nourish and raise the spirit.

Yángwéimài 陽維脈 Yáng Linking Vessel. One of the eight vessels.

Yì 意 Mind. (Pronounced "ee"). Specifically, the mind generated by clear thinking and judgment, which can make you calm, peaceful, and wise. It is considered the water mind or wisdom mind

Yì 易 To change, to replace, or to alter.

Yìjīng 易經 *The Book of Changes*. Considered the preeminent ancient Chinese classic (Qúnjīng Zhīshǒu, 群經之首) in Chinese history and has influenced Chinese culture heavily.

Yìjīnjīng 易筋經 *The Muscle/Tendon Changing Classic*, credited to Dá Mó (達磨) around 550 CE. It describes Qìgōng training for strengthening the physical body.

Yìjīnjīng Xiǎozhōutiān 易筋經小周天 Yìjīnjīng Small Circulation.

Yīn 陰 In Chinese philosophy, this is the passive, negative, feminine polarity. In Chinese medicine, Yīn means deficient. The Yīn organs are the Heart, Lungs, Liver, Kidneys, Spleen, and Pericardium.

Yìng Qìgōng 硬氣功 Hard Qìgōng.

Yíngqì 營氣 Managing Qì. Manages or controls the functioning of the body.

Yíngxiāng (LI-20) 迎香 Welcome Fragrance. An acupuncture cavity that belongs to the Large Intestine channel.

Yīnjiān 陰間 Yīn world. The spirit world after death is considered Yīn.

Yīnjiāo (Co-7) 陰交 Yīn junction. The junction of two vessels, the Conception Vessel (Rènmài, 任脈) and the Thrusting Vessel (Chōngmài, 衝脈). Yīnjiāo is on the Conception Vessel. It is also considered a paired cavity with Mìngmén (Gv-4) (命門) (Life's Door), located between the L2 and L3 vertebrae.

Yǐnqì Guīyuán 引氣歸元 Lead the Qì to its origin.

Yīnqiāomài 陰蹺脈 Yīn Heel Vessel. One of the eight vessels.

Yīnshén 陰神 Concealed Yīn spirit. The spirit is nourished and raised by Water Qì; it is firm and steady.

Yīnshuǐ 陰水 Yīn water.

Yīntáng (M-HN-3) 印堂 Seal Hall. A miscellaneous acupuncture cavity, located at the Third Eye area.

Yīnwéimài 陰維脈 Yīn Linking Vessel. One of the eight vessels.

Yìqì Xiānghé 意氣相合 Harmonization of mind and Qì.

Yìshì 意識 The conscious mind.

Yìshǒu Dāntián 意守丹田 Keep the Yì at the Dāntián. In Qìgōng training, you keep your mind at the Lower Dāntián to accumulate Qì. When you circulate it, you always lead it back to your Lower Dāntián at the end of practice.

Yǐyì Yǐnqì 以意引氣 Use the Yì (i.e., wisdom mind) to lead the Qì.

Yǒngquán (K-1) 湧泉 Gushing Spring. An acupuncture cavity on the Kidney Primary Qì Channel.

Yǒngquán Xí 湧泉息 Yǒngquán breathing.

Yuánjīng 元精 Original Essence. The fundamental, original essential substance inherited from your parents. It is converted into Original Qì (Yuánqì, 元氣). Actually, the hormones produced by our endocrine glands are referred to as "Pre-Birth Essence" or "Original Essence."

Yuánqì, 元氣 Pre-Birth Qì or Original Qì. It is also called "Xiāntiān Qì" (先天氣). which literally means "Pre-Heaven Qì."

Yuánshén 元神 Original Shén. The Shén that is kept in its residence by the Yì and that is nourished by the Original Qì.

Zāi 栽 To plant or to grow.

Zāijiēpài 栽接派 Plant and Graft Division. A style of Daoist Qìgōng training.

Zēngqiáng Miǎnyìlì 增強免疫力 To boost the strength of immune system.

Zhāgēn 紮根 Rooting.

Zhànzhuāng 站樁 Standing meditation.

Zhēn Xià Dāntián 真下丹田 Real Lower Dāntián (i.e., Real Lower Elixir Field). Human biobattery.

Zhèng Fùhūxī 正腹呼吸 Normal Abdominal Breathing. Commonly called Buddhist Breathing (Fójiā Hūxī, 佛家呼吸).

Zhèngqì 正氣 Normal Qì or righteous Qì. When one is righteous, he is said to have righteous Qì, which evil Qì cannot overcome.

Zhēnjiǔxuè 針灸穴 Acupuncture cavity.

Zhēnrén 真人 Real Person or Truthful Person. Daoists call themselves "truthful persons" since they must be truthful to reopen their Third Eye.

Zhōng Dāntián 中丹田 Middle Dāntián, the area of the lower sternum connected to the diaphragm.

Zhōu 周 To be complete, perfect, or round.

Zhuang Zhou 莊周 Also known as Zhuāngzi (莊子). A Daoist scholar who lived during the Warring States Period (403–222 BCE). He wrote a book also called *Zhuāngzi* (莊子).

Zhuāngzi 莊子 The book written by the Daoist scholar Zhuāng Zhōu during the Chinese Warring States Period (403–222 BCE) (Zhànguó, 戰國).

Zhújī 築基 Build a foundation.

Zìjué 自覺 Self-awareness.

Zìshì, 自識 Self-recognition.

Zǐwǔ Liúzhù 子午流注 Zǐ (子) refers to the period around midnight (11 p.m. to 1 am), and Wǔ (午) refers to midday (11 am to 1 pm). Liúzhù (流注) means the tendency to flow. The term refers to a schedule of Qì circulation showing which channel has the predominant Qì flow at any particular time, and where the predominant Qì flow is in the Conception and Governing Vessels.

Zìxǐng/Zìwù 自醒/自悟 Self-awakening.

Zǒuhuǒ Rùmó 走火入魔 Walk into the fire and enter the devil. If you lead your Qì into the wrong path, it is called walking into the fire. If your mind has been led into confusion, it is called entering the devil.

Index

About the Author

Yáng, Jwìng-Mǐng, PhD (楊俊敏博士)

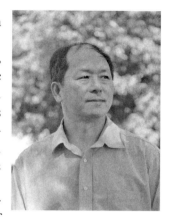

Dr. Yáng, Jwìng-Mǐng was born on August 11, 1946, in Xīnzhúxiàn (新竹縣), Táiwān (台灣), Republic of China (中華民國). He started his Wǔshù (武術) (Gōngfū or Kūng Fū, 功夫) training at the age of fifteen under Shàolín White Crane (Shàolín Báihè, 少林白鶴) Master Chēng, Gīn-Gsào (曾金灶). Master Chēng originally learned Tàizǔquán (太祖拳) from his grandfather when he was a child. When Master Chēng was fifteen years old, he started learning White Crane from Master Jīn, Shào-Fēng (金紹峰) and followed him for twenty-three years until Master Jīn's death.

In thirteen years of study (1961–1974) under Master Chēng, Dr. Yáng became an expert in the White Crane style of Chinese martial arts, which includes both the use of bare hands and various weapons, such as saber, staff, spear, trident, two short rods, and many others. With the same master he also studied White Crane Qìgōng (氣功), Qín Ná or Chín Ná (擒拿), Tuīná (推拿), and Diǎnxué massage (點穴按摩) and herbal treatment.

At sixteen, Dr. Yáng began the study of Yáng Style Tàijíquán (楊氏太極拳) under Master Kāo, Táo (高濤). He later continued his study of Tàijíquán under Master Lǐ, Mào-Chīng (李茂清). Master Lǐ learned his Tàijíquán from the well-known Master Hán, Chìng-Táng (韓慶堂). From this further practice, Dr. Yáng was able to master the Tàijí bare-hand sequence, pushing hands, the two-man fighting sequence, Tàijí sword, Tàijí saber, and Tàijí Qìgōng.

When Dr. Yáng was eighteen years old, he entered Tamkang College (淡江學院) in Taipei Xiàn to study physics. In college, he began the study of traditional Shàolín Long Fist (Chángquán or Cháng Chuán, 少林長拳) with Master Lǐ, Mào-Chīng at the Tamkang College Guóshù Club (淡江國術社), 1964–1968, and eventually became an assistant instructor under Master Lǐ. In 1971, he completed his MS degree in physics at the National Táiwān University (台灣大學) and then served in the Chinese Air Force from 1971 to 1972. In the service, Dr. Yáng taught physics at the Junior Academy of the Chinese Air Force (空軍幼校) while also teaching Wǔshù (武術). After being honorably discharged in 1972, he returned to Tamkang College to teach physics and resumed study under Master Lǐ, Mào-Chīng. From Master Lǐ, Dr. Yáng learned Northern Style Wǔshù, which includes both bare hand and kicking techniques, and numerous weapons.

In 1974, Dr. Yáng came to the United States to study mechanical engineering at Purdue University. At the request of a few students, Dr. Yáng began to teach Gōngfū, which resulted in the establishment of the Purdue University Chinese Kūng Fū Research Club in the spring of 1975. While at Purdue, Dr. Yáng also taught college-credit courses in Tàijíquán. In May of 1978, he was awarded a PhD in mechanical engineering by Purdue.

In 1980, Dr. Yáng moved to Houston to work for Texas Instruments. While in Houston, he founded Yáng's Shàolín Kūng Fū Academy, which was eventually taken over by his disciple, Mr. Jeffery Bolt, after Dr. Yáng moved to Boston in 1982. Dr. Yáng founded Yáng's Martial Arts Academy in Boston on October 1, 1982.

In January of 1984, he gave up his engineering career to devote more time to research, writing, and teaching. In March of 1986, he purchased property in the Jamaica Plain area of Boston to be used as the headquarters of the new organization, Yáng's Martial Arts Association (YMAA). The organization expanded to become a division of Yáng's Oriental Arts Association, Inc. (YOAA).

In 2008, Dr. Yáng began the nonprofit YMAA California Retreat Center. This training facility in rural California is where selected students enroll in a five to ten-year residency to learn Chinese martial arts.

Dr. Yáng has been involved in traditional Chinese Wǔshù since 1961, studying Shàolín White Crane (Báihè), Shàolín Long Fist (Chángquán), and Tàijíquán under several different masters. He has taught for more than forty-six years: seven years in Táiwān, five years at Purdue University, two years in Houston, twenty-six years in Boston, and more than eight years at the YMAA California Retreat Center. He has taught seminars all around the world, sharing his knowledge of Chinese martial arts and Qìgōng in Argentina, Austria, Barbados, Botswana, Belgium, Bermuda, Brazil, Canada, China, Chile, England, Egypt, France, Germany, Holland, Hungary, Iceland, Iran, Ireland, Italy, Latvia, Mexico, New Zealand, Poland, Portugal, Saudi Arabia, Spain, South Africa, Switzerland, and Venezuela.

Since 1986, YMAA has become an international organization, which currently includes more than fifty schools located in Argentina, Belgium, Canada, Chile, France, Hungary, Ireland, Italy, New Zealand, Poland, Portugal, South Africa, Sweden, the United Kingdom, Venezuela, and the United States.

Many of Dr. Yáng's books and videos have been translated into many languages, including French, Italian, Spanish, Polish, Czech, Bulgarian, Russian, German, and Hungarian.

Books by Dr. Yáng, Jwìng-Mǐng
Analysis of Shàolín Chín Ná, 2nd ed. YMAA Publication Center, 1987, 2004

Ancient Chinese Weapons: A Martial Artist's Guide, 2nd ed. YMAA Publication Center, 1985, 1999

Arthritis Relief: Chinese Qìgōng for Healing & Prevention, 2nd ed. YMAA Publication Center, 1991, 2005

Back Pain Relief: Chinese Qìgōng for Healing and Prevention, 2nd ed. YMAA Publication Center, 1997, 2004

Bāguàzhăng: Theory and Applications, 2nd ed. YMAA Publication Center, 1994, 2008

Comprehensive Applications of Shàolín Chín Ná: The Practical Defense of Chinese Seizing Arts. YMAA Publication Center, 1995

Essence of Shàolín White Crane: Martial Power and Qìgōng. YMAA Publication Center, 1996

How to Defend Yourself. YMAA Publication Center, 1992

Introduction to Ancient Chinese Weapons. Unique Publications, Inc., 1985

Meridian Qìgōng, YMAA Publication Center, 2016

Northern Shàolín Sword, 2nd ed. YMAA Publication Center, 1985, 2000

Qìgōng for Health and Martial Arts, 2nd ed. YMAA Publication Center, 1995,1998

Qìgōng Massage: Fundamental Techniques for Health and Relaxation, 2nd ed. YMAA Publication Center, 1992, 2005

Qìgōng Meditation: Embryonic Breathing. YMAA Publication Center, 2003

Qìgōng Meditation: Small Circulation, YMAA Publication Center, 2006

Qìgōng, the Secret of Youth: Dá Mó's Muscle/Tendon Changing and Marrow/ Brain Washing Qìgōng, 2nd ed. YMAA Publication Center, 1989, 2000

Root of Chinese Qìgōng: Secrets of Qìgōng Training, 2nd ed. YMAA Publication Center, 1989, 1997

Shàolín Chín Ná. Unique Publications, Inc., 1980

Shàolín Long Fist Kūng Fū. Unique Publications, Inc., 1981

Simple Qìgōng Exercises for Health: The Eight Pieces of Brocade, 3rd ed. YMAA Publication Center, 1988, 1997, 2013

Tài Chí Ball Qìgōng: For Health and Martial Arts. YMAA Publication Center, 2010

Tài Chí Chuán Classical Yáng Style: The Complete Long Form and Qìgōng, 2nd ed. YMAA Publication Center, 1999, 2010

Tài Chí Chuán Martial Applications, 2nd ed. YMAA Publication Center, 1986, 1996

Tài Chí Chuán Martial Power, 3rd ed. YMAA Publication Center, 1986, 1996, 2015

Tài Chí Chuán: Classical Yáng Style, 2nd ed. YMAA Publication Center, 1999, 2010

Tài Chí Qìgōng: The Internal Foundation of Tài Chí Chuán, 2nd ed. rev. YMAA Publication Center, 1997, 1990, 2013

Tài Chí Secrets of the Ancient Masters: Selected Readings with Commentary. YMAA Publication Center, 1999

Tài Chí Secrets of the Wǔ and Lǐ Styles: Chinese Classics, Translation, Commentary. YMAA Publication Center, 2001

Tài Chí Secrets of the Wú Style: Chinese Classics, Translation, Commentary. YMAA Publication Center, 2002

Tài Chí Secrets of the Yáng Style: Chinese Classics, Translation, Commentary. YMAA Publication Center, 2001

Tài Chí Sword Classical Yáng Style: The Complete Long Form, Qìgōng, and Applications, 2nd ed. YMAA Publication Center, 1999, 2014

Tàijí Chín Ná: The Seizing Art of Tàijíquan, 2nd ed. YMAA Publication Center, 1995, 2014

Tàijíquan Theory of Dr. Yáng, Jwìng-Mǐng: The Root of Tàijíquan. YMAA Publication Center, 2003

Xíngyìquán: Theory and Applications, 2nd ed. YMAA Publication Center, 1990, 2003 Yáng Style Tài Chí Chuán. Unique Publications, Inc., 1981

Videos by Dr. Yáng, Jwìng-Mǐng
Advanced Practical Chín Ná in Depth, YMAA Publication Center, 2010

Analysis of Shàolín Chín Ná. YMAA Publication Center, 2004

Bāguàzhǎng (Eight Trigrams Palm Kūng Fū). YMAA Publication Center, 2005

Chín Ná in Depth: Courses 1–4. YMAA Publication Center, 2003

Chín Ná in Depth: Courses 5–8. YMAA Publication Center, 2003

Chín Ná in Depth: Courses 9–12. YMAA Publication Center, 2003

Five Animal Sports Qìgōng. YMAA Publication Center, 2008

Knife Defense: Traditional Techniques. YMAA Publication Center, 2011

Meridian Qìgōng. YMAA Publication Center, 2015

Neigong. YMAA Publication Center, 2015

Northern Shàolín Sword. YMAA Publication Center, 2009

Qìgōng Massage. YMAA Publication Center, 2005

Saber Fundamental Training. YMAA Publication Center, 2008

Shàolín Kūng Fū Fundamental Training. YMAA Publication Center, 2004

Shàolín Long Fist Kūng Fū: Basic Sequences. YMAA Publication Center, 2005

Shàolín Saber Basic Sequences. YMAA Publication Center, 2007

Shàolín Staff Basic Sequences. YMAA Publication Center, 2007

Shàolín White Crane Gōng Fū Basic Training: Courses 1 & 2. YMAA Publication Center, 2003

Shàolín White Crane Gōng Fū Basic Training: Courses 3 & 4. YMAA Publication Center, 2008

Shàolín White Crane Hard and Soft Qìgōng. YMAA Publication Center, 2003

Shuāi Jiāo: Kūng Fū Wrestling. YMAA Publication Center, 2010

Simple Qìgōng Exercises for Arthritis Relief. YMAA Publication Center, 2007

Simple Qìgōng Exercises for Back Pain Relief. YMAA Publication Center, 2007

Simple Qìgōng Exercises for Health: The Eight Pieces of Brocade. YMAA Publication Center, 2003

Staff Fundamental Training: Solo Drills and Matching Practice. YMAA Publication Center, 2007

Sword Fundamental Training. YMAA Publication Center, 2009

Tài Chí Ball Qìgōng: Courses 1 & 2. YMAA Publication Center, 2006

Tài Chí Ball Qìgōng: Courses 3 & 4. YMAA Publication Center, 2007

Tài Chí Chuán: Classical Yáng Style. YMAA Publication Center, 2003

Tài Chí Fighting Set: 2-Person Matching Set. YMAA Publication Center, 2006

Tài Chí Pushing Hands: Courses 1 & 2. YMAA Publication Center, 2005

Tài Chí Pushing Hands: Courses 3 & 4. YMAA Publication Center, 2006

Tài Chí Qìgōng. YMAA Publication Center, 2005

Tài Chí Sword, Classical Yáng Style. YMAA Publication Center, 2005

Tài Chí Symbol: Yīn/Yáng Sticking Hands. YMAA Publication Center, 2008

Tàiji 37 Postures Martial Applications. YMAA Publication Center, 2008

Tàiji Chín Ná in Depth. YMAA Publication Center, 2009

Tàiji Saber: Classical Yáng Style. YMAA Publication Center, 2008

Tàiji Wrestling: Advanced Takedown Techniques. YMAA Publication Center, 2008

Understanding Qìgōng, DVD 1: What is Qìgōng? The Human Qì Circulatory System. YMAA Publication Center, 2006

Understanding Qìgōng, DVD 2: Key Points of Qìgōng & Qìgōng Breathing. YMAA Publication Center, 2006

Understanding Qìgōng, DVD 3: Embryonic Breathing. YMAA Publication Center, 2007

Understanding Qìgōng, DVD 4: Four Seasons Qìgōng. YMAA Publication Center, 2007

Understanding Qìgōng, DVD 5: Small Circulation. YMAA Publication Center, 2007

Understanding Qìgōng, DVD 6: Martial Arts Qìgōng Breathing. YMAA Publication Center, 2007

Xíngyìquán: Twelve Animals Kūng Fū and Applications. YMAA Publication Center, 2008

Yáng Tài Chí for Beginners. YMAA Publication Center, 2012

YMAA 25-Year Anniversary. YMAA Publication Center, 2009

BOOKS FROM YMAA

101 REFLECTIONS ON TAI CHI CHUAN
108 INSIGHTS INTO TAI CHI CHUAN
A WOMAN'S QIGONG GUIDE
ADVANCING IN TAE KWON DO
ANALYSIS OF SHAOLIN CHIN NA 2ND ED
ANCIENT CHINESE WEAPONS
ART AND SCIENCE OF STAFF FIGHTING
THE ART AND SCIENCE OF SELF-DEFENSE
ART AND SCIENCE OF STICK FIGHTING
ART OF HOJO UNDO
ARTHRITIS RELIEF, 3D ED.
BACK PAIN RELIEF, 2ND ED.
BAGUAZHANG, 2ND ED.
BRAIN FITNESS
CHIN NA IN GROUND FIGHTING
CHINESE FAST WRESTLING
CHINESE FITNESS
CHINESE TUI NA MASSAGE
COMPLETE MARTIAL ARTIST
COMPREHENSIVE APPLICATIONS OF SHAOLIN CHIN NA
CONFLICT COMMUNICATION
DAO DE JING: A QIGONG INTERPRETATION
DAO IN ACTION
DEFENSIVE TACTICS
DIRTY GROUND
DR. WU'S HEAD MASSAGE
ESSENCE OF SHAOLIN WHITE CRANE
EXPLORING TAI CHI
FACING VIOLENCE
FIGHT LIKE A PHYSICIST
THE FIGHTER'S BODY
FIGHTER'S FACT BOOK 1&2
FIGHTING ARTS
FIGHTING THE PAIN RESISTANT ATTACKER
FIRST DEFENSE
FORCE DECISIONS: A CITIZENS GUIDE
INSIDE TAI CHI
JUDO ADVANTAGE
JUJI GATAME ENCYCLOPEDIA
KARATE SCIENCE
KATA AND THE TRANSMISSION OF KNOWLEDGE
KRAV MAGA COMBATIVES
KRAV MAGA FUNDAMENTAL STRATEGIES
KRAV MAGA PROFESSIONAL TACTICS
KRAV MAGA WEAPON DEFENSES
LITTLE BLACK BOOK OF VIOLENCE
LIUHEBAFA FIVE CHARACTER SECRETS
MARTIAL ARTS OF VIETNAM
MARTIAL ARTS INSTRUCTION
MARTIAL WAY AND ITS VIRTUES
MEDITATIONS ON VIOLENCE
MERIDIAN QIGONG EXERCISES
MINDFUL EXERCISE
MIND INSIDE TAI CHI
MIND INSIDE YANG STYLE TAI CHI CHUAN
NATURAL HEALING WITH QIGONG
NORTHERN SHAOLIN SWORD, 2ND ED.
OKINAWA'S COMPLETE KARATE SYSTEM: ISSHIN RYU
PRINCIPLES OF TRADITIONAL CHINESE MEDICINE
PROTECTOR ETHIC
QIGONG FOR HEALTH & MARTIAL ARTS 2ND ED.
QIGONG FOR TREATING COMMON AILMENTS

QIGONG MASSAGE
QIGONG MEDITATION: EMBRYONIC BREATHING
QIGONG GRAND CIRCULATION
QIGONG MEDITATION: SMALL CIRCULATION
QIGONG, THE SECRET OF YOUTH: DA MO'S CLASSICS
REDEMPTION
ROOT OF CHINESE QIGONG, 2ND ED.
SAMBO ENCYCLOPEDIA
SCALING FORCE
SELF-DEFENSE FOR WOMEN
SHIN GI TAI: KARATE TRAINING
SIMPLE CHINESE MEDICINE
SIMPLE QIGONG EXERCISES FOR HEALTH, 3RD ED.
SIMPLIFIED TAI CHI CHUAN, 2ND ED.
SOLO TRAINING 1&2
SPOTTING DANGER BEFORE IT SPOTS YOU
SPOTTING DANGER BEFORE IT SPOTS YOUR KIDS
SPOTTING DANGER BEFORE IT SPOTS YOUR TEENS
SUMO FOR MIXED MARTIAL ARTS
SUNRISE TAI CHI
SURVIVING ARMED ASSAULTS
TAE KWON DO: THE KOREAN MARTIAL ART
TAEKWONDO BLACK BELT POOMSAE
TAEKWONDO: A PATH TO EXCELLENCE
TAEKWONDO: ANCIENT WISDOM
TAEKWONDO: DEFENSE AGAINST WEAPONS
TAEKWONDO: SPIRIT AND PRACTICE
TAI CHI BALL QIGONG: FOR HEALTH AND MARTIAL ARTS
TAI CHI BALL WORKOUT FOR BEGINNERS
THE TAI CHI BOOK
TAI CHI CHIN NA, 2ND ED.
TAI CHI CHUAN CLASSICAL YANG STYLE, 2ND ED.
TAI CHI CHUAN MARTIAL POWER, 3RD ED.
TAI CHI CONCEPTS AND EXPERIMENTS
TAI CHI CONNECTIONS
TAI CHI DYNAMICS
TAI CHI FOR DEPRESSION
TAI CHI IN 10 WEEKS
TAI CHI PUSH HANDS
TAI CHI QIGONG, 3RD ED.
TAI CHI SECRETS OF THE ANCIENT MASTERS
TAI CHI SECRETS OF THE WU & LI STYLES
TAI CHI SECRETS OF THE WU STYLE
TAI CHI SECRETS OF THE YANG STYLE
TAI CHI SWORD: CLASSICAL YANG STYLE, 2ND ED.
TAI CHI SWORD FOR BEGINNERS
TAI CHI WALKING
TAIJIQUAN THEORY OF DR. YANG, JWING-MING
FIGHTING ARTS
TRADITIONAL CHINESE HEALTH SECRETS
TRADITIONAL TAEKWONDO
TRAINING FOR SUDDEN VIOLENCE
TRIANGLE HOLD ENCYCLOPEDIA
TRUE WELLNESS SERIES (MIND, HEART, GUT)
WARRIOR'S MANIFESTO
WAY OF KATA
WAY OF SANCHIN KATA
WAY TO BLACK BELT
WESTERN HERBS FOR MARTIAL ARTISTS
WILD GOOSE QIGONG
WINNING FIGHTS
XINGYIQUAN

AND MANY MORE . . .

VIDEOS FROM YMAA

ANALYSIS OF SHAOLIN CHIN NA
BAGUA FOR BEGINNERS 1 & 2
BAGUAZHANG: EMEI BAGUAZHANG
BEGINNER QIGONG FOR WOMEN 1 & 2
BEGINNER TAI CHI FOR HEALTH
CHEN TAI CHI CANNON FIST
CHEN TAI CHI FIRST FORM
CHEN TAI CHI FOR BEGINNERS
CHIN NA IN-DEPTH SERIES
FACING VIOLENCE: 7 THINGS A MARTIAL ARTIST MUST KNOW
FIVE ANIMAL SPORTS
FIVE ELEMENTS ENERGY BALANCE
INFIGHTING
INTRODUCTION TO QI GONG FOR BEGINNERS
JOINT LOCKS
KNIFE DEFENSE
KUNG FU BODY CONDITIONING 1 & 2
KUNG FU FOR KIDS AND TEENS SERIES
LOGIC OF VIOLENCE
MERIDIAN QIGONG
NEIGONG FOR MARTIAL ARTS
NORTHERN SHAOLIN SWORD
QI GONG 30-DAY CHALLENGE
QI GONG FOR ANXIETY
QI GONG FOR ARMS, WRISTS, AND HANDS
QIGONG FOR BEGINNERS: FRAGRANCE
QI GONG FOR BETTER BALANCE
QI GONG FOR BETTER BREATHING
QI GONG FOR CANCER
QI GONG FOR DEPRESSION
QI GONG FOR ENERGY AND VITALITY
QI GONG FOR HEADACHES
QI GONG FOR THE HEALTHY HEART
QI GONG FOR HEALTHY JOINTS
QI GONG FOR HIGH BLOOD PRESSURE
QIGONG FOR LONGEVITY
QI GONG FOR STRONG BONES
QI GONG FOR THE UPPER BACK AND NECK
QIGONG FOR WOMEN WITH DAISY LEE
QIGONG FLOW FOR STRESS & ANXIETY RELIEF
QIGONG MASSAGE
QIGONG MINDFULNESS IN MOTION
QI GONG—THE SEATED WORKOUT
QIGONG: 15 MINUTES TO HEALTH
SABER FUNDAMENTAL TRAINING
SAI TRAINING AND SEQUENCES
SANCHIN KATA: TRADITIONAL TRAINING FOR KARATE POWER
SCALING FORCE
SEARCHING FOR SUPERHUMANS
SHAOLIN KUNG FU FUNDAMENTAL TRAINING: COURSES 1 & 2
SHAOLIN LONG FIST KUNG FU BEGINNER—INTERMEDIATE—
    ADVANCED SERIES
SHAOLIN SABER: BASIC SEQUENCES
SHAOLIN STAFF: BASIC SEQUENCES
SHAOLIN WHITE CRANE GONG FU BASIC TRAINING SERIES
SHUAI JIAO: KUNG FU WRESTLING
SIMPLE QIGONG EXERCISES FOR HEALTH
SIMPLE QIGONG EXERCISES FOR ARTHRITIS RELIEF
SIMPLE QIGONG EXERCISES FOR BACK PAIN RELIEF
SIMPLIFIED TAI CHI CHUAN: 24 & 48 POSTURES
SIMPLIFIED TAI CHI FOR BEGINNERS 48
SIX HEALING SOUNDS
SUN TAI CHI

SWORD: FUNDAMENTAL TRAINING
TAEKWONDO KORYO POOMSAE
TAI CHI BALL QIGONG SERIES
TAI CHI BALL WORKOUT FOR BEGINNERS
TAI CHI CHUAN CLASSICAL YANG STYLE
TAI CHI FIGHTING SET
TAI CHI FIT: 24 FORM
TAI CHI FIT: ALZHEIMER'S PREVENTION
TAI CHI FIT: CANCER PREVENTION
TAI CHI FIT FOR VETERANS
TAI CHI FIT: FOR WOMEN
TAI CHI FIT: FLOW
TAI CHI FIT: FUSION BAMBOO
TAI CHI FIT: FUSION FIRE
TAI CHI FIT: FUSION IRON
TAI CHI FIT: HEALTHY BACK SEATED WORKOUT
TAI CHI FIT: HEALTHY HEART WORKOUT
TAI CHI FIT IN PARADISE
TAI CHI FIT: OVER 50
TAI CHI FIT OVER 50: BALANCE EXERCISES
TAI CHI FIT OVER 50: SEATED WORKOUT
TAI CHI FIT OVER 60: GENTLE EXERCISES
TAI CHI FIT OVER 60: HEALTHY JOINTS
TAI CHI FIT OVER 60: LIVE LONGER
TAI CHI FIT: STRENGTH
TAI CHI FIT: TO GO
TAI CHI FOR WOMEN
TAI CHI FUSION: FIRE
TAI CHI QIGONG
TAI CHI PUSHING HANDS SERIES
TAI CHI SWORD: CLASSICAL YANG STYLE
TAI CHI SWORD FOR BEGINNERS
TAI CHI SYMBOL: YIN YANG STICKING HANDS
TAIJI & SHAOLIN STAFF: FUNDAMENTAL TRAINING
TAIJI CHIN NA IN-DEPTH
TAIJI 37 POSTURES MARTIAL APPLICATIONS
TAIJI SABER CLASSICAL YANG STYLE
TAIJI WRESTLING
TRAINING FOR SUDDEN VIOLENCE
UNDERSTANDING QIGONG SERIES
WATER STYLE FOR BEGINNERS
WHITE CRANE HARD & SOFT QIGONG
YANG TAI CHI FOR BEGINNERS
YOQI: MICROCOSMIC ORBIT QIGONG
YOQI QIGONG FOR A HAPPY HEART
YOQI:QIGONG FLOW FOR HAPPY MIND
YOQI:QIGONG FLOW FOR INTERNAL ALCHEMY
YOQI QIGONG FOR HAPPY SPLEEN & STOMACH
YOQI QIGONG FOR HAPPY KIDNEYS
YOQI QIGONG FLOW FOR HAPPY LUNGS
YOQI QIGONG FLOW FOR STRESS RELIEF
YOQI: QIGONG FLOW TO BOOST IMMUNE SYSTEM
YOQI SIX HEALING SOUNDS
YOQI: YIN YOGA 1
WU TAI CHI FOR BEGINNERS
WUDANG KUNG FU: FUNDAMENTAL TRAINING
WUDANG SWORD
WUDANG TAIJIQUAN
XINGYIQUAN
YANG TAI CHI FOR BEGINNERS

AND MANY MORE . . .

more products available from . . .
YMAA Publication Center, Inc. 楊氏東方文化出版中心
1-800-669-8892 • info@ymaa.com • www.ymaa.com